Positive Art Therapy Theory and Practice

Positive Art Therapy Theory and Practice outlines a clear, systematic approach for combining positive psychology with art therapy's capacity to mobilize client strengths; induce engagement, flow and positive emotions; transform perceptions; build healing relationships and empowering narratives; and illuminate life purpose and meaning. Woven throughout are clinical illustrations, state-of-the-art research, discussion questions, and reflections on how therapists can apply this approach to their work with clients and in their personal and professional development. The book also includes a comprehensive list of more than 80 positive art therapy directives, a robust glossary, and lists of strengths and values. Written in an inviting and amusing style, this manual is both entertaining and practical—an invaluable tool for any practitioner looking to apply the most current theory and research on positive psychology and art therapy to their clinical practice.

Rebecca Ann Wilkinson, MA, ATR-BC, LCPAT, is co-founder of Creative Wellbeing Workshops, which uses art and the creative process to help individuals and organizations manage stress, cope with adversity, and increase wellbeing. She serves as adjunct faculty at George Washington University's Graduate Art Therapy Program. Rebecca is also a practicing artist and author/illustrator of *Miraval Mandalas Coloring Book*.

Gioia Chilton, PhD, ATR-BC, LCPAT, also co-founder of Creative Wellbeing Workshops and adjunct faculty at George Washington University, has written extensively on the intersection of art therapy and positive psychology, collaborative art processes, and altered books. Her doctoral thesis, an award-winning inquiry into the expression of positive emotions in art therapy, was acclaimed for its innovative arts-based research methods.

Positive Art Therapy Theory and Practice

Integrating Positive Psychology with Art Therapy

Rebecca Ann Wilkinson
and Gioia Chilton

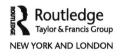

Routledge
Taylor & Francis Group

NEW YORK AND LONDON

First edition published 2018
by Routledge
711 Third Avenue, New York, NY 10017

and by Routledge
2 Park Square, Milton Park, Abingdon, Oxon, OX14 4RN

Routledge is an imprint of the Taylor & Francis Group, an informa business

© 2018 Taylor & Francis

The right of Rebecca Ann Wilkinson and Gioia Chilton to be identified as the authors of this work has been asserted by them in accordance with sections 77 and 78 of the Copyright, Designs and Patents Act 1988.

All rights reserved. No part of this book may be reprinted or reproduced or utilised in any form or by any electronic, mechanical, or other means, now known or hereafter invented, including photocopying and recording, or in any information storage or retrieval system, without permission in writing from the publishers.

Trademark notice: Product or corporate names may be trademarks or registered trademarks, and are used only for identification and explanation without intent to infringe.

Library of Congress Cataloging-in-Publication Data
Names: Wilkinson, Rebecca Ann, author. | Chilton, Gioia, author.
Title: Positive art therapy theory and practice: integrating positive psychology with art therapy / Rebecca Ann Wilkinson and Gioia Chilton.
Description: First edition. | New York : Routledge, 2018. | Includes bibliographical references and index.
Identifiers: LCCN 2017016054| ISBN 9781138908895 (hardcover: alk. paper) | ISBN 9781138908918 (pbk.: alk. paper) | ISBN 9781315694245 (e-book)
Subjects: | MESH: Art Therapy—methods | Happiness | Psychology, Social—methods
Classification: LCC RC489.A7 | NLM WM 450.5.A8 | DDC 616.89/1656—dc23
LC record available at https://lccn.loc.gov/2017016054

ISBN: 978-1-138-90889-5 (hbk)
ISBN: 978-1-138-90891-8 (pbk)
ISBN: 978-1-315-69424-5 (ebk)

Typeset in Minion Pro
by Swales & Willis Ltd, Exeter, Devon, UK

Dedication

This book is dedicated to our families who patiently humor and tolerate two wild and willful renegades. It is also dedicated to our clients, whose artwork has painted the landscape of our adult lives and who have taught us what it means to love humanity.

Contents

Figures

The figures can be found in the color plate section at the end of Chapter 8.

Foreword: A New Era in Art Therapy

Shaun McNiff

There is no question that the worldwide art therapy community shares a commitment to the life-enhancing powers of artistic expression, but there are differences in how we think about the work and the people we serve. I came to art therapy with a vision of bringing what I called the "positive" features of artistic expression (McNiff, 1974) to people living in the back wards of a state psychiatric hospital. There was a common-sense understanding of how art heals by immersing people in creative expression and by furthering human dignity in otherwise degrading conditions. The work gained public attention and we showed the patients' art in museums and university galleries throughout the Northeast as a manifestation of health rather than illness. The problems we faced were severe and obvious. It made no sense to focus on the negative, so we asked, how can we further a person's "strengths through art"?

But this approach did not carry as much weight within the larger mental health context. The distinctly negative view on the psychopathology of artistic expression prevailed and it was embedded in art therapy, where artistic expressions were approached as indicators of what was wrong. There was also an exclusive focus on "unconscious" expression, as distinguished from acts of spontaneous and unplanned creation, which effectively dismissed a person's deliberate efforts to create and reinforced the power of diagnosticians, since it was assumed that the artists did not know what they were "really" communicating.

We have made progress over the past five decades in offering alternatives to this way of operating as described by the authors in this book, but the dominant culture and its accompanying language and labels persist. Within the mental health field, both personal and collective human experience are too often reduced to something harmful occurring in the past, and within art therapy, less attention is given to how art heals (McNiff, 2004).

Rebecca Wilkinson and Gioia Chilton attribute art therapy's condition to a "negativity bias" in the mental health professions, and call for a more positive focus on abilities and wellbeing. Their book not only offers methods of practice but grounds them in a paradigm shift that I strongly support and whose time has come. Yet it is perhaps natural that the current emphasis on positive attitudes, resilience, and strengths is met with suspicion by some who see it as encouraging denial and avoidance, and possibly generating feelings of guilt and failure for people who struggle with daily life. Tendencies to look at experience with either doubt or optimism are ingrained in human nature and not going away. In this respect, I see "positive psychology" as an effort to correct the longstanding one-sidedness of mental health thinking.

In China, Taoist thought posits an indivisible life force, what I view as a palpable creative energy (McNiff, 2016), composed of interdependent elements and a creative tension between polar realities like positive and negative ideas. Ill health is caused by the absence of reciprocity, change, and fluid circulation. Rather than denying the negative, *positive art therapy* asks us to make a place for its complementary partner.

Advocacy for art's life-enhancing purpose does not in any way challenge the existence of dark and difficult conditions, nor propose an exclusive focus on positive ones. The differences in art therapy tend to involve how we envision the use of art to further the shared commitment to wellbeing. My position is that the artistic process is essentially transformative and a source of creative energy that circulates within persons and environments, as contrasted to apathy and despair. Artistic expression is an intelligence, a force of nature (McNiff, 2015), that is uniquely capable of finding its way through the most complex difficulties that are inaccessible to linear analysis. Art heals by engaging difficulties and wounds as a source of expression and hopefully changing our relationships with them. Sometimes it breaks and makes chaos and frustration, but in the service of life. Admittedly, this perspective opts for positive motivations and outcomes but it embraces the negative as reality and fuel for creative action. We might ask, can we better understand the affliction and its place in our lives, respond more compassionately and imaginatively to its presence, put it to use, and change our relationship to it?

Rebecca Ann Wilkinson and Gioia Chilton's comprehensive call for the positive features of artistic expression invites us all to begin a new era in art therapy, one dedicated to a better use of the whole creative process.

Foreword: Art Therapy, Inherently Positive

Robert Biswas-Diener

Years ago when I was a student working on an advanced degree in clinical psychology, I was taught the standard content: therapeutic orientations, diagnosis and treatment planning, biological approaches to psychopathology. On reflection, it is interesting to consider what I learned about conducting therapy without it ever being made explicit. Therapy happens in an office. The therapist and client sit while therapy occurs. The therapist—but probably not the client—might take notes. We face one another. It is remarkable how much of this process is simply assumed. It wasn't until years later, after I had shifted from clinical work to research, that it occurred to me that therapy might work just as well while standing, walking, or working together at a whiteboard.

These ideas are probably not revolutionary to you. Chances are, if you are reading this book you have an interest in expressive therapies in general and in art therapy specifically. If so, then "therapy as usual" means something different to you than it did to me. You are likely well acquainted with the idea that therapeutic intervention can occur in the absence of discussion or while using some medium such as paint, or while moving around the consulting room.

In fact, if you are working as an art therapist, you probably see yourself as a bold pioneer willing to venture into the less explored areas of clinical treatment. You have undoubtedly endured the rolled eyes of more conventional colleagues who see your approach as, well, pretty "woo-woo." You have had— somewhere along the way—to defend the legitimacy of art therapy against the presumptive superiority of cognitive and pharmacological interventions. It is precisely this experience with being on the vanguard of alternative treatments that makes you a good candidate for truly appreciating this book.

Make no mistake—just as expressive therapies offer both a compliment and challenge to therapy as usual—positive psychology offers a paradigm shift for the field of psychology as a whole. Sure, there are historical precedents in our field. The classical Greek scientist-philosophers, for instance, attended to positive topics such as courage and ethics. Similarly, humanistic psychologists such as Maslow, Rogers, and May were intrigued by potential, motivation, creativity, and self-improvement. It is only in very recent times, however, that the modern movement of positive psychology has offered something more.

Modern proponents of positive psychology bring sophisticated modern research to bear on life's best experiences. We can use hierarchical modeling, item response theory, meta-analyses, and other techniques to explore positive topics in a way that was—quite frankly—unavailable to the ancient Greeks and the humanists alike. We can use larger samples, multiple data collection methods, replication, and more rigorous peer review to continually raise the quality of positive psychological science.

These advances fly in the face of the concerns of the skeptics and critics of positive psychology. Some charge that it is a science focusing on Western and middle-class concerns. But I myself have spent my career researching happiness among the homeless and in non-Western cultures such as those of tribal Kenyans or Inuit villagers. Other critics worry that positive psychology is a form of naiveté; a whitewashing of the world's legitimate ills. There is, however, an increasing chorus of voices from within positive psychology who argue for an increased synthesis of the so-called negative and positive aspects of psychology. In the end, part of me just thinks that skeptics are shaken by the tectonic movement that positive psychology represents. At its core, this science offers a string of bold assertions: positive topics such as happiness are possible to study, are worth studying, and represent promising avenues for improving quality of life.

Nowhere is the core message of positive psychology more threatening than in the world of clinical psychology. For conventionally minded therapists, positive psychology intervention appears to ignore pain and to require a baseline level of resourcefulness that some clients might not have. It is appears to sidestep attention to the etiology of psychopathology and to replace a focus on symptoms with a focus on strengths. Just how challenging is this? I once spoke with a therapist in Europe who informed me that she was seeing a client who had no strengths whatsoever. A view, in my opinion, that speaks directly to the need for positive psychological approaches in clinical work.

It is with this—the marriage of positive and clinical psychology—that the authors of this book, Rebecca Ann Wilkinson and Gioia Chilton, are concerned. I first met them many years ago as they were just beginning the upward arc of expertise in applying positive psychology to art therapy. I have delighted in watching as they have pioneered this corner of psychology. Like the science they represent, these two trailblazers offer some challenging assertions. They say, unapologetically, that positive psychology is just too good to be confined to the healthy. They argue that positive psychology is not an adjunct to be offered after clients complete a course of therapy. Instead, it is appropriate from the very first session.

Wilkinson and Chilton dare to grab us by the shoulders and shake. Hard. They rightly argue for viewing art therapy as an inherently positive treatment modality. The more examples they point out in this book, the more obvious the truth of their thesis becomes. Art therapy enjoys a natural intersection with flow, creativity, positive emotion, and the list goes on and on. It is a refreshing reminder that therapy need not be somber, or even problem-focused, to be effective. It is hard to turn a page of this book without wishing that all people wrestling with anxiety, depression, and other ills had the opportunity to spend as much time on strengths and enjoyments as they do on symptoms and distress tolerance. It is my hope that you will find between the covers of this book a call to arms. I hope you are willing to take a look at your own practice and see how it might be improved.

In the pages that follow, Wilkinson and Chilton invite you to join them in a world where clinical intervention can be upbeat, inspiring, and flat-out positive. I hope you accept.

Acknowledgments

We start off with thanking you, dear reader, for taking time out of your life to honor our book with your attention.

We thank our families, who tolerated two years of countless Skype sessions, piles of books left randomly around the house, heated debates, and disappearances while we wrestled over this creative endeavor. We celebrate their perseverance, patience, and optimism while ours were flagging. It takes a village. We also thank each other for holding the light and appreciating the good in each other (and tolerating the bad) so that, even though it was often challenging, we had fun and we are not only proud of the book but also the process of writing it.

We thank Shaun McNiff for his inspiration and guidance, and Robert Biswas-Diener, who taught us so much about positive psychology and helped lift Creative Wellbeing Workshops off the ground. We are deeply grateful for the mentorship of Audrey DiMaria, Katherine Williams, Carol Cox, and Nancy Gerber. We thank the institutions that have supported us—George Washington University, Drexel University, and the American Art Therapy Association. In addition, we celebrate the many researchers and scholars whose work is the very foundation of this book. We are truly standing on the shoulders of giants.

We also thank Lee Wilkinson for her tireless editing, Tiffanie Brumfield for her insight and humorous feedback, and Paige Scheinberg for her contributions to the book and to scholarship in positive art therapy. We'd like to thank

Nina Guttapalle of Routledge and copy-editor Jeanne Brady for providing us with their thoroughness and persistence.

Last but in no way least, we thank the clients we have been blessed to know throughout the years. We are grateful to those who generously gave us permission to use their artwork in the book—although their names have been changed, their images serve as their unique signature in the world and in our hearts.

CHAPTER 1

Introduction

When we teach art therapy graduate students about positive psychology, we often start by having them make artwork about "what a happy and fulfilled life includes for you." We suggest that before you proceed any further, you might do the same—consider what a happy life means to you? What would you be doing and where would you be? Who would be there with you? How would you be feeling? You might refer back to this image occasionally as we examine the world of happiness, wellbeing, and art therapy.

And now we welcome you to the community of folks who, like us, are excited by the possibilities of combining art therapy with the science of positive psychology. Positive psychology, most broadly defined, is the study of the conditions and processes that contribute to the optimal functioning of people, groups, and institutions. Built upon existing foundations of mental health theory and practice devoted to relieving suffering and overcoming hardship, positive psychology expands our capacity to thrive in the face of adversity and fulfill our highest potential. *Positive art therapy* unites the unique benefits of art therapy with positive psychology's mission: to promote individual and global wellbeing by nurturing what is good and functioning in our lives.

We, the authors of this book, are two art therapists who found that this approach has had an invigorating and renewing effect not only in our clinical work but also in all aspects of our personal and professional lives. It has underscored our profound appreciation and love for art therapy while simultaneously opening our eyes to new ways that our field can be conceived of and practiced.

We think art therapy and positive psychology have a lot to offer each other. In the past, we have thought of the connection between art therapy and positive psychology as the intersection of two worlds. We also like the metaphor of a blossoming friendship. So, in the following pages, we are going to introduce you to our pal positive psychology and explain how it has infused and brightened everything we do as art therapists. We will acquaint you with different facets of this multi-dimensional friend and explore the unique ways that art therapy can contribute to the relationship.

We coined this dynamic synergy, at its simplest, "positive art therapy" (Chilton & Wilkinson, 2009). We believe that not only will art therapists benefit from delving into this exciting new approach, but that positive psychologists, when they learn about how art therapy so naturally and effectively promotes wellbeing, will also be inspired to do the same. We also hope that, by articulating more precisely how art therapy affects wellbeing, the book will serve as a celebration of the exceptional power of this work. And finally, we are excited to share this approach with you because we hope that, as it did for us, learning about the complementary nature of positive psychology and art therapy will also invigorate your practice and make *you* happier!

First, though, let us introduce ourselves. We first met as graduate students in 1991 at the George Washington University Graduate Art Therapy Program after finding a passion in the crossover between art and psychology. After two years of stellar training and mentorship by art therapists such as Edith Kramer, Audrey DiMaria, Carol Cox, and Katherine Williams, we began our careers at St. Elizabeth's psychiatric hospital in Washington, DC, for people with mental illness. There we became and have remained close friends, even though our work and our lives have taken us on very different paths.

Gioia worked for five years in St. Elizabeth's long-term wards and forensic units with people struggling with chronic mental illness, poverty, and racism. She thrived at "St. E's" in the Creative Arts Therapies Department—a community of art therapists, dance movement therapists, music therapists, bibliotherapists, and psychodramatists—gaining a deep appreciation for the breadth of the creative process to bring dignity, hope, and healing to those on the edge of society.

Gioia went on to work with children and adolescents with emotional disabilities in the juvenile justice and foster care systems. She also collaborated with the Potomac Art Therapy Association, the local chapter of art therapists, holding educational workshops and community events across the city. While taking time off in the early 2000s to raise her children, she discovered that she still wanted to stay connected to the art therapy world. She became active with the American Art Therapy Association (AATA) helping to organize their annual conferences, tapping into the realization that for her, art therapy was more than a job, it was a life calling.

Rebecca's love of wide-open spaces took her to the Arizona desert where she continued to work with adults in inpatient and outpatient psychiatric care. On many of the psychiatric units in which she worked, she was asked to develop art therapy programs which included generating all of the documentation for monitoring patient progress and contributing to treatment planning. Participating so fully in all aspects of patient care—not just the delivery of art therapy (which was almost always gratifying), but also in the evaluation and diagnosis of psychiatric illness was often disturbing for her. Not because of the patients, whom she loved, but because of the pervasively pathology-based lens through which they were seen. Even back then, long before she was introduced to the field of positive psychology, she could see that something was amiss both with the way patients were viewed—and how they viewed themselves—and with the assumptions that governed the delivery of their care.

In 2005, Rebecca moved to Costa Rica for a couple of years with her husband. During that time, Gioia, at home nursing her second child, discovered the *Artist's Happiness Challenge*, an online course being offered by art therapist Lani Gerity (2009). The class was designed to explore ideas about happiness and wellbeing, chock-full of exercises derived from the field of positive psychology and modified with an art therapy twist. Lani's course seemed like a great way that we could "play" together even though we were in two different countries! At the time, we had no idea how much that whimsical interlude would reveal to us about ourselves and how it would change the course of lives.

For example, Gioia, who had resumed working part-time at what she thought of as the perfect job—getting well-paid for doing art therapy with children with emotional disabilities in a public school—was bored and restless. And Rebecca—who was by most measures living in paradise—was miserable. As we started to look at our beliefs about happiness, we realized that our assumptions were often superficial and ineffective. And as we experienced positive changes from the exercises we were doing, it became clear to us that this was something we wanted to bring not only to our clients but to other art therapists as well.

In 2007, after having made changes in our lives as a result of what we were learning—Gioia finding work that invigorated and challenged her more, and Rebecca and her husband returning to the DC area to be near family—we proposed a class, "The Art of Happiness," to our alma mater, GW's graduate art therapy program. At that time, we did not realize that positive psychology was at such a tipping point.

In 2009, we joined the International Positive Psychology Association (IPPA) (www.ippanetwork.org), which facilitates collaboration among psychology researchers, economists, social policy makers, educators, students, and practitioners of positive psychology across academic disciplines and around the world. While attending the First IPPA Congress in Philadelphia, we ran into Tarquam McKenna, an art therapy colleague from St. Elizabeth's, who had returned to his home in Sydney and was now editor of the Australian and New Zealand Arts Therapies Association (ANZATA) journal. He invited us to write an article describing the impact that positive psychology might have on the field of art therapy.

That summer we outlined a model for positive art therapy that integrated positive psychology principles with art therapy practice, *positive art therapy* research, and training (Chilton & Wilkinson, 2009). We also began conducting workshops showing art therapists how to incorporate these concepts into their work. In addition, it became clear that this material also had significance in their personal lives—blending positive psychology principles with art interventions increased *their* wellbeing, vitality, and engagement.

At around the same time, we were also invited by hospital administrators and mental health agencies to bring our trainings to other "frontline providers"— professionals in high-stress roles such as caregivers, medical staff, and other mental health providers—to help them manage stress, prevent burnout, and stay connected with the values and passion that initially moved them to join their field.

We also began to receive referrals from other organizations, e.g., the Government Accountability Office (not surprising—we were in DC) and the Office of the Capitol, and private corporations such as Genentech, Microsoft, and Full Picture (an international marketing company). In 2010, we advanced our mission to help reduce stress and burnout and increase wellbeing by forming Creative Wellbeing Workshops (CWW). CWW provides guidance, training, continuing education, and consultation on how to create sustainable happiness and wellbeing.

Shortly thereafter Gioia, who has the strengths of curiosity and love of learning, recognized that in order for her life to be most fulfilling, she needed to pursue endeavors which would challenge her in new and different ways. She decided to explore the intersection of positive psychology and art therapy through formal academic research. Serendipitously, a doctoral program in Creative Arts Therapies at Drexel University was launched, where she was able to explore positive art therapy through artistic inquiry and arts-based research—both of which fit her creativity and passion for artmaking with others. Gioia's research focused on positive emotions and art therapy (which we will explore in more detail in Chapter 5, "Positive Emotions and Emotion Regulation"). After graduating, she felt drawn to resume clinical work and found what was for her the perfect art therapy position—working at a drug and alcohol addiction center with a strength-based treatment philosophy and a deep appreciation for the value of the creative arts therapies.

In the meantime, Rebecca balanced what felt like competing values—her love of her family, most of whom were living on the East Coast, and her love of the Arizona desert where her husband's family lives. In order to sustain these geographical challenges while fulfilling her mission to help herself and others experience more happiness and wellbeing, she continues to provide workshops and teach on positive art therapy with Gioia on the East Coast for half of the month and serves as a visiting art therapy specialist and wellness counselor the other two weeks at Miraval Resort in Arizona, a mindfulness-based retreat center and wellness spa.

Regardless of other pursuits and commitments, our dedication to articulating and sharing with others the crossover between positive psychology and art therapy has persisted. We would not have guessed that interest in it would also resonate as much and for as long as it has in the art therapy world. Presentations on positive art therapy (led by us and others who are expanding this realm of inquiry) are heavily attended at national art therapy conferences and we are consistently asked to provide trainings on this topic for local and regional art therapy associations. Chapters on art therapy and positive psychology were included in Rubin's *Approaches to Art Therapy* (Chilton & Wilkinson, 2016) and *The Wiley Handbook of Art* (Isis, 2015).

As the relevance and value of combining positive psychology and art therapy continues to be recognized, the academic discourse is growing rapidly. Gioia published her research on art therapy and positive emotions (Chilton et al., 2015; Chilton, Gerber, Councill, & Dreyer, 2015). Art therapy and hope theory has been explored by Scheinberg (2012) and Johnson and Sullivan-Marx (2006). Art therapists are also adding to the research literature in the area of flow (Burkewitz, 2014; Chilton, 2013; Hovick, 2014; Lee, 2009; Voytilla, 2006), character strengths (Riddle & riddle [*sic*], 2007), meaning (Darewych, 2014), positive assessment (Betts, 2012) and positive ethics (Hinz, 2011). Research into art therapy's overall impact on wellbeing is also growing (Puig, Lee, Goodwin, & Sherrard, 2006; Stuckey & Nobel, 2010; Donald, 2008; Radel, 2015).

Just as the research into topics relevant to positive psychology is exponentially growing, so too will exploration and discourse related to positive art therapy continue to emerge. In addition, credit belongs to many others whose work is not only related but extremely relevant. This includes but is not limited to Laurie Rappaport's work on focusing, Mimi Farrelly-Hansen's and Patricia Isis's work on mindfulness, Michael Franklin's work on empathy and the transpersonal approach, Noah Hass-Cohen and Johanna Czamanski-Cohen's work on the body-mind connection, Pat Allen and Shaun McNiff's work on spirituality and arts-based research, not to mention the many contributions of others inside and out of the field who have added to the literature on the contribution of the arts in fostering resilience and contributing to individual, communal, and global welfare.

In the decade since we playfully experimented with Lani's *Happiness Challenge*, we have painstakingly challenged ourselves and each other to apply a positive psychology perspective to our work and to practice with the tools we have learned. As a result, it has completely altered our approach not just to engaging with clients and the people we encounter in our professional roles—workshop participants, clients, co-workers, students, colleagues, corporate sponsors, etc.—but to working with each other as co-facilitators, business partners, and friends. It has also greatly enhanced our relationships with our family members and loved ones, and helped us to better manage challenges and capitalize on opportunities that come our way.

To be sure, this isn't always easy; however, through doing so we have reaped many of the benefits that this approach promises. This includes feeling more enthusiastic and hopeful about our work; finding sustainability in it even when it is frustrating and stressful; having a clearer sense of our strengths and weaknesses and recognizing the strengths of others more; being more mindful and appreciative of our experiences, ourselves and others; acknowledging and being more accepting of our own and others' vulnerabilities; developing more resilience in the face of hardships and losses; getting and staying more connected to our vision, mission, and values; feeling better in general, and having more fun! Last but not least, we also feel much better equipped to help our clients. This book grew out of our desire to make those benefits available to other art therapists so that they, too, can experience and share them with others. Bottom line, *we* needed this work and think *you* might too.

We discovered the world of positive psychology by immersing ourselves in the positive psychology community, by extensively examining research and literature available on the topic, by experimenting with the material we were learning with our clients, our workshops participants, and our students, and by actively applying these tools in our own lives. What follows is our attempt to interweave the broad array of theory, application, and resources related to positive psychology that we have encountered over the last ten years with the research, training, and practice of art therapy.

This book is designed primarily for the art therapy world; however, because we believe that it has universal applications, we think that positive psychology practitioners, as well as those from other mental health and arts-related fields, will also appreciate its value. We suggest that much of the content could be useful to therapists at all stages of professional development, from students and entry-level therapists to seasoned clinicians, educators, and researchers.

Those of you who want to jump right into Positive Art Therapy can go straight to Chapter 4. However, we suggest that the preceding chapters may serve as useful refreshers and provide context for this approach within the broader scope of mental health. In the first section, Chapter 2 reviews historical factors that contributed to emergence of positive psychology. Chapter 3 provides an overview of "the science of wellbeing" and examines myths and facts about happiness. Chapter 4 introduces Positive Art Therapy, an approach to applying positive psychology to art therapy structured primarily around Martin Seligman's model of wellbeing, PERMA, an acronym for Positive emotions, Engagement, Relationships, Meaning, and Achievement. We also look at parallels in the development of psychology and art therapy and ways that applying a "positive" lens may benefit both. We then present a Positive Art Therapy Manifesto which outlines the mission and goals of positive art therapy.

In the second section, we delve more deeply into each of the domains of PERMA. We define their relevance to art therapy and then explore art therapy's contributions to each. Chapter 5 outlines the benefits of positive and negative emotions, as well as strategies for regulating affect. Chapters 6, 7, and 8 examines engagement as it manifests in three areas: creativity, flow, and strengths. Chapter 9 addresses relationships. Chapters 10 and 11 explore meaning through two lenses—Chapter 10 meaning in life and sense of purpose and Chapter 11 meaning-making and perception. Chapter 12 examines achievement, mastery, and goals.

In the final chapter, we explore ways to use this model with professionals in danger of burnout and compassion fatigue and in need of greater *compassion satisfaction*, with employees and management in corporate environments, in continuing education with mental health practitioners, and in the training and supervision of therapists. We close with a discussion of some of the limitations of this book and suggest future directions for research and practice in a positive art therapy approach.

We include several useful appendices: Appendix A, Positive Art Therapy Directives; Appendix B, Glossary; Appendix C, List of Strengths and Appendix D, List of Values.

Each chapter features relevant vignettes and discussion questions that we hope will evoke further contemplation of the content. Woven throughout the book are reflections on how this applies not only to our work with clients, but also to our practice and development as therapists, to the field of art therapy in general, and to our personal lives.

We highly recommend that you experiment with the techniques and directives that we have presented here before applying them in your clinical work. As Chris Peterson (2006), one of the eminent figures in positive psychology, put it "positive psychology is not a spectator sport" (p. 25). We believe you will most be able to appreciate a positive art therapy perspective if you are first able to experience more of its benefits *yourself*.

The immense challenges in the world today call for all of us to be functioning at our highest capacities—using all the creativity, love, inspiration, resilience, hope, and appreciation of beauty and excellence that we can generate! We suggest that positive art therapy, because it so powerfully combines the unique benefits of art therapy with positive psychology's charge to promote optimal functioning and wellbeing, provides us with an empowering approach and effective strategies to do so. So let's get going!

Discussion Questions

1   When you look back over your professional career, what were pivotal moments that shaped your choices and how has that affected your happiness?
2   What are some of the myths and stereotypes around happiness and wellbeing that you personally recognize? That you see in your clients and others?

CHAPTER 2

A History of Positive Psychology

How We Found Positive Psychology

In early 2000, while working as a counselor on an acute psychiatric unit in Tucson, Rebecca was asked to develop an art therapy program for a newly launched inpatient psychiatric unit. Along with all of the other requirements for creating such a program, she needed to include some way of documenting client progress. Initially, this seemed like a straightforward task—take the existing clinical progress note that was being used by the social workers and counselors and modify it to art therapy. However, in doing so, something which before had only hovered below her consciousness now seemed glaringly obvious. This document, and for that matter most of the forms that she had filled out in her years of assessing patients and recording their progress in treatment, consisted almost entirely of observations about either the presence or absence of symptoms! For example, the inpatient note that she was trying to revise was limited to the following options for affect: labile, restricted, apathetic, blunted, flat, euphoric, and appropriate. Only "appropriate" offered an option that indicated anything other than troubled or exaggerated affect.

The same seemed to be true of other domains. The descriptors for mood included words like manic, depressed, angry, sad, fearful, anxious, and happy. Although happy was at least positive, it didn't describe someone whose mood was neutral. Rebecca, herself, had difficulty defining such a state. She later discovered that it was "euthymic."

In an effort to create progress notes that were more inclusive, Rebecca searched online for other language for describing the ways that patients might present; however, she found the same limitations. For example, options for thought processing included long lists of aberrations which, however useful, failed to provide a selection of healthier possibilities: illogical, tangential or loose associations, poverty of content, flight of ideas, broadcasting, word salad, obsessions, ruminations, or delusions. Positive alternatives like logical, congruent, or decisive were limited or non-existent. Options for behavior and attitude included combative, agitated, defiant, hyperactive, passive, aggressive, passive-aggressive, bizarre, rigid, restless, or manipulative. Occasionally a couple of words like cooperative or, again, "appropriate" might appear.

Gioia, having worked in a variety of clinical settings, commiserated with this frustration. Even recently, while reviewing a patient's medical record, she was struck by the limited choices given on one of the "self-report" forms. Asking clients to describe their childhood, they were given the option to circle one or more of the following: traumatic, painful, uneventful, or other. Apparently, if your childhood was helpful, or constructive, let alone happy, your only option was to describe it as "uneventful" or "other."

When we first recognized this kind of oversight, we decided to make it our mission each time we went to another institution to modify the clinical documentation so that it presented a wider range of human functioning. This included bringing in language like hopeful, calm, engaged, self-initiating, motivated, comprehending, future-oriented, able to focus, tracking, organized, relevant, relational, responds well to support, independent, positive self-image, self-control, able to regulate affect, animated, insight-oriented, or psychologically minded.

Years later, when we encountered positive psychology, the broader context of our efforts began to make sense. Positive psychology was devoted to shifting the lens of psychology from focusing predominantly on pathology and disease to presenting a more balanced view of human behavior and motivation. It defined wellbeing and optimal functioning using concrete descriptions of associated thoughts, feelings, and behavior. Like a counterpoint to the American Psychiatric Association's (2013) *Diagnostic and Statistical Manual of Mental Disorders (DSM)*, it essentially outlined the "symptoms" of *mental health.*

Positive psychology also provided theoretical grounding for other aspects of our work. For example, in workshops we provided with clients affected by cancer, we were struck that often, despite dire prognoses, many of the participants talked about a fundamental shift in their priorities and a heightened sense of spirituality as a result of their diagnosis. The positive psychology paradigm shed light on our growing realization that, although some problems may be *unresolvable,* people might achieve a high quality of life despite these challenges and sometimes *as a result of them.* In fact, one could paradoxically be quite ill and impaired in some ways and yet thriving in others.

Disconcerted but also intrigued by the disruption of some of our fundamental assumptions about therapy, change, and human nature, we set about exploring positive psychology more deeply. This included looking at current literature in positive psychology, but also relevant material emerging in art therapy, education, and other related fields. It also involved looking back over the historical context surrounding the formation of this "new" field and the theoretical foundations upon which it is grounded.

In the next few chapters, we share some of what we discovered. We have tried to distill what, for us, has taken over ten years to learn. For some of you, this material may be redundant. On the other hand, perhaps it can serve as a useful refresher and set the stage for exploring art therapy from a positive psychology perspective. We felt that that could best be done by first describing the circumstances around which positive psychology emerged. Especially because, despite being seasoned clinicians as well as art therapy educators ourselves, we were often surprised by gaps in our knowledge or misconceptions that we had about the historical, social, economic, cultural, and political factors that led to development of different psychological schools of thought and that shaped mental health practices today, in general, let alone in the field of positive psychology.

Positive Psychology Defined

Positive psychology, also known as the *science of wellbeing*, is the study of human potential and optimal functioning. It is an in-depth exploration of the conditions and processes that allow individuals and communities to flourish and thrive (Seligman & Csíkszentmihályi, 2000). The field was christened in 1998 when Martin Seligman (1999), in his role as the president of the APA, identified that although we had made tremendous advances in understanding mental illness and reducing suffering, we had not devoted equal resources to exploring what is positive and functional in our lives. Positive psychologists have set about correcting this imbalance—not to diminish or replace the importance of addressing and attending to pathology and pain—but to complement this with an exploration of healthy, adaptive functioning. They wanted to establish for *mental health* the same depth and breadth of research, theory, and practical application as has been done for *mental illness*. Not only because mental health and wellbeing are worthy of exploration in their own right, but because doing so builds resilience, helps buffer against hardship, and prevents illness.

Seligman (1998), who up until the late 1990s had been most known for his research into *learned helplessness*, observed that psychology as a field was predominantly preoccupied with identifying and treating pathology rather than with understanding and building the characteristics that make life worth living. A task force of seasoned psychologists and promising new researchers joined together to create the *Positive Psychology Manifesto* which called for "a new commitment on the part of research psychologists to focus attention upon the sources of psychological health, thereby going beyond prior emphases upon disease and disorder" (Sheldon, Frederickson, Rathunde, Csíkszentmihályi, & Haidt, 2000, paragraph 1).

The Evolution of Positive Psychology

To provide context for exploring the field of positive psychology, we have pooled together historical factors which have been identified as having shaped its emergence and subsequent development. To be sure, it is not the only version of this history that one could write. For example, we skim over some of the economic forces at play, such as how capitalism has affected the persistence of the medical model and the role of pharmaceutical companies in "promoting" specific diagnoses for which their medications were prescribed. In addition, we do not delve as much into the role of gender and culture as we might have liked. Instead, we have tried to introduce the conceptual factors that appear to have contributed most significantly to the rise of a positive psychology perspective in the broader context of psychology as a whole.

Early Psychology in the 1800s

The field of psychology began crystallizing into its own discrete profession in the late 1800s as a synthesis of philosophy, neurobiology, and anthropology. Before then, mental aberrations were "treated" in asylums—if people showed signs of mental illness, they were essentially removed from society. At the turn of the century, efforts to understand and address human suffering and abnormal behaviors surfaced. Debates about the dichotomy between subjective experiences of the mind and observable phenomena in the physical world emerged. Early psychologists like William James (1890), one of the forerunners of modern American psychology, attempted to study and define consciousness. James emphasized the intimate relationship between the physical and mental life. He believed that what sets us apart from other living beings was free will—the power to determine how we respond to our environment.

Psychodynamic Theory: The First Force

Speculations about the role of self-determination and consciousness were eclipsed by *psychodynamic theory*, often called *the first force* in psychology. Psychodynamic theory originated with Freud, a European neurologist who discovered that many of his patients were relieved of medical symptoms when they were able to talk about their concerns. Freud noticed that many of their verbalizations related to early childhood experiences, particularly to traumatic memories, which at first he determined were real but which he later speculated might be imagined. He concluded that mental disorders originated during critical stages in childhood in which developmental challenges and needs were impeded or unmet.

Freud (1957b) proposed that human behavior was motivated by two essential impulses—seeking pleasure and avoiding death. However, because these drives were primitive and unacceptable to the part of ourselves that knows it must engage cooperatively with others, we develop elaborate strategies to mask them from our conscious awareness. Freud suggested that consciousness, which he called the *psyche*, was comprised of three levels, much like an iceberg. In this topographical metaphor, the conscious mind is the top point visible above the water, the pre-conscious domain is the portion just below the surface of the water, and the unconscious realm is the bulk of the structure underneath.

Psychoanalysis, the term for Freud's *talking cure*, involved unveiling unconscious material and integrating it with the conscious mind. This included identifying defense mechanisms—e.g., denial, repression, displacement, projection, reaction formation, and sublimation—which, although helpful in protecting the psyche from what it perceives as internal and external threats, also perpetuated maladaptive coping. According to Freudian theory, awareness of these defenses leads to catharsis—the release of repressed material—and improved insight and, as a result, to the resolution of mental and emotional disturbances.

Initially, psychoanalysis was also conducted exclusively by physicians and psychiatrists. This changed in the US in the late 1940s after a high incidence of psychiatric symptoms in returning veterans (what we now identify as *post-traumatic stress disorder* but what was then termed *shell-shock* or *combat stress reaction*) led the Veteran's Administration to channel federal resources toward addressing this epidemic. The VA funded the inception of programs designed to train psychologists, who previously had only worked in laboratories, in the practice of clinical psychotherapy. Similar to the training of doctors and psychiatrists, these programs combined medical research with supervised field experience, most of which happened on psychiatric wards (Frank, 1984).

Shortly thereafter, President Truman signed the National Mental Health Act which led to the inception of the National Institute of Mental Health (NIMH), designed to research and treat mental disorders. The growing national recognition that mental suffering required focused attention was profound—it established a universal mandate to attend to people struggling with psychological and emotional challenges. However, these federally funded developments created decisive shifts in the field of psychology. Psychology moved from a more expansive blend of philosophy and science devoted to exploring *all* aspects of mental functioning to a more restricted science of researching and treating *mental disorder*. In addition, the practice of psychology became firmly rooted in institutional settings which operated within a medical model. It was now focused predominantly on identifying pathology and treating symptoms and much less on *preventing* mental illness and exploring mental health and wellbeing (Gable & Haidt, 2005).

Behavioral Psychology: The Second Force

Concurrently, the *behavioral* movement—also known as *the second force*—was gaining prominence in the psychology world. Behaviorists rejected the psychoanalytic approach, criticizing it for relying too heavily on speculations about subjective and intangible internal states—e.g., thoughts, beliefs, and desires. Behaviorists such as Pavlov, Watson, and Skinner advocated the study of *observable* phenomena. They maintained that behavior is shaped by the interplay between environmental stimuli and the responses those generate.

The first edition of the *Diagnostic Statistical Manual* (*DSM*) was released during this era. Published in 1952 by the American Psychiatric Association, the *DSM*, much like a *Physicians' Desk Reference* (2013), was an effort to provide psychiatrists and psychologists with a standardized system for diagnosing symptoms associated with mental illness. It fit well with the behavioral mission to provide systematic ways of treating discrete conditions and observing measurable responses to those interventions.

Humanist Psychology: The Third Force

In the late 1950s, in reaction to the deterministic and mechanistic perspectives that characterized psychodynamic and behavioral theories, humanist aspirations began to resurface in the psychology world. Inspired by early philosophers such as Aristotle and Plato and nineteenth-century thinkers such as James, Kierkegaard, and Kant, humanists rejected the notion that we are only driven by base unconscious instincts or that we are passively manipulated by external influences. *Humanism*, coined *the third force*, proposed that we are propelled by *actualizing tendencies* and that mental and social problems arise from disruptions in these efforts. Humanists believed that human nature is inherently good and motivated by fundamentally noble intentions. They advocated taking a *phenomenological* approach which presumed that consciousness can only be understood through the lens of the individual subjectively experiencing it.

Neo-Freudian Contributions to Humanism

Several neo-Freudians—psychologists who were heavily influenced by Freud but who departed from strict psychoanalytic theory—contributed significantly to the evolution of the humanist psychology. Jung (1959), Freud's closest disciple, agreed with his mentor's theory that behavior was driven by unconscious forces within the individual, but he believed that all humans shared a *collective unconscious* which taps into more universal aspects of humanity. He was particularly moved by Eastern religions which led him to conclude that human beings naturally strive to find metaphysical and spiritual purpose.

Adler (1979), another disciple of Freud, defied the latter by insisting that we are driven not just by sexual and aggressive urges, but also by social interests both to receive affection and to further the welfare of others. Adler also believed that although we are all born with an *inferiority complex* which we are trying to overcome, we are also endowed with a *creative self* that can consciously shape our personality and destiny.

Otto Rank broke from Freud by designating *creativity* and *will* as core elements in the development of personality (Lieberman, 1985). Rank is also credited with proposing that therapists explore the *here and now* rather than the transference dynamic in the therapeutic relationship. Karen Horney (1951) argued against Freud's drive theory, suggesting instead that cultural and environmental influences shape personality. Horney also balked at male bias in Freudian theory, suggesting that *penis envy* for women was less powerful than *womb envy*—the ability to biologically grow and sustain life—for men. Horney focused treatment on current stressors in a patient's life, rather than on early childhood development. Henry Stack Sullivan (1953) maintained that personality and mental disorders develop only through interpersonal relationships and that individuals cannot be understood outside of the context of their connection to others.

Humanism Proper

Abraham Maslow (1971) and Carl Rogers (1951) are perhaps the names most associated with humanism in psychology. Others also contributed significantly: Victor Frankl's (1985) work on meaning in the face of adversity; Rollo May's (1975) work on creativity and love; and Fritz and Laura Perls's (1947) work on awareness and perception.

Maslow (1971) maintained that humans have a fundamental desire for self-fulfillment, growth, discovery, and change and that pathology resulted from frustration of our intrinsic needs, emotions, and capacities. Maslow outlined the *hierarchy of needs*, with levels representing basic needs for shelter, safety, love, sense of belonging, and self-esteem which must be fulfilled in order to achieve the upper tier of growth and self-actualization. Interestingly, Maslow is credited with first proposing a *positive psychology* (Peterson, 2006) which would focus on promoting human excellence.

Rogers (1951), Maslow's contemporary, coined the phrase *client-centered therapy*, suggesting that the dynamic between therapists and patients be more egalitarian—that therapists think of the latter more as *clients* than as patients. Rogers believed that pathology occurred when our self-image is not congruent with our ideal self. Full potential is achieved when we are able to be authentic and genuine.

Frankl (1985), an Austrian psychiatrist held prisoner in concentration camps during the Holocaust, proposed that even in the face of profoundly painful and dehumanizing experiences we search for meaning and a reason to live. Having survived years in captivity, he believed that true freedom lay in the attitude we take toward, and the meaning we derive from, the circumstances we encounter. Depression and illness arise when we experience a sense of *meaninglessness*.

May (1975) agreed with Freud's supposition that we are driven by primitive instincts, but he believed that love and genuine caring for others were equally powerful motivators. May suggested that loneliness, loss, despair, and death give rise to *existential anxiety*. These acute encounters with uncertainty and suffering provide the opportunity to forge meaning out of our lives. He also believed that creativity emerged not as a compensatory response to weakness, as was the prevailing assumption in the Freudian approach, but rather from attempts to overcome limitations and discover new ways of seeing the world.

Fritz and Laura Perls (1947), credited with formulating American *gestalt therapy*, applied the concept of *holism* to understanding human behavior. They maintained that people cannot be fully understood without understanding the context within which they are operating. Pathology arose from broken-off and polarized aspects of the self and from *unfinished business*, aspects of experience that had not been integrated. Gestalt therapy employed dynamic verbal and non-verbal techniques to promote self-awareness, self-responsibility, and awareness of the present moment.

Contributions and Critiques of Humanism

As humanist psychology gained popularity in the second half of the twentieth century, there is little doubt that it revolutionized not only fundamental assumptions about human nature and the relationship between therapist and client, but also public perception of therapy and its role in helping us enjoy more fulfilling lives. Perhaps the greatest legacy of the humanist movement was the recognition that clients are active agents in their treatment and their lives. Humanist psychology was also instrumental in the evolution of the *self-help movement* which promoted personal development, self-actualization, personality responsibility, and reaching our fullest potential.

Nevertheless, despite the tremendous influence humanist psychology had on popular culture and on psychological theories of human motivation, it was heavily critiqued for lacking systematic application and empirical validation. In addition, and perhaps as a consequence, it had much less impact on formally endorsed treatments for mental disorders, especially in institutional settings. Instead, the behavioral model persisted, although it evolved to include more nuanced understanding of the role of cognition in shaping responses to environmental stimuli.

Cognitive Behavioral Therapy

Strictly behavioral approaches fell out of favor in the later part of the twentieth century. For example, linguist Noam Chomsky (1965) famously challenged behavioral models of learning when he pointed out that children have an innate understanding of grammar that precedes instruction. Albert Bandura's (1977) model of social learning also transformed behavioral approaches. Bandura proposed that, rather than learning through direct interaction with our environment, we often model our choices and actions based upon observing others—both their behaviors and the results of those behaviors.

Cognitive approaches opened the *black box of cognition*—a term borrowed from engineering to describe the unseen processes that occur between the initiation of a stimulus and the subsequent response that is observed. Cognitive Behavioral Therapy (CBT) emerged during this time, which outlined strategies for addressing the mediating role of mental processes in shaping behavior

(Ellis, 1977; Beck, 1993). Practitioners of CBT proposed that behavior resulted from a complex interaction between beliefs and actions and that challenging dysfunctional assumptions could lead to change. Although different from traditional behavioral approaches, CBT fit well with the medical model because it followed a logical sequence of steps designed to correct faulty cognitions. They maintained that resulting behavioral changes could be measurably observed and replicated.

Dominance of the Medical Model

The medical model, which revolves around identifying symptoms and tailoring treatment toward their resolution, continues to be the operating paradigm guiding most approaches to treatment. The medical model has had an undeniably positive impact—we have substantially increased our understanding of many mental illnesses, the effects of trauma on the brain, and we can now effectively treat and even cure some psychological conditions (Seligman & Csíkszentmihályi, 2000). However, even in the face of these advances, the medical model is ultimately reductionist and limiting (Maddux, 2002). In the end, it leaves us not much better equipped to prevent mental illness and it does little to account for what has become increasingly evident: the relief of suffering does not always lead to wellbeing. Wellbeing is a process over and above the absence of anger, depression, illness, and mental and emotional pain (Duckworth, Steen, & Seligman, 2005).

The Medical Model and the DSM

The dominance of the medical model has also led to a myopic, socially constructed view of human experience whereby clients' thoughts, feelings, behaviors, life histories, and reasons for seeking help are matched to symptoms and diagnoses. Medical professionals and clinicians operating in this model are often unwittingly forced to justify treatment based upon criteria from the *Diagnostic Statistical Manual* (APA, 2013; Frances, 2012). The *DSM* and its various revisions have been useful in providing a language for conceptualizing categories of emotional and behavioral problems. However, it operates within an *illness* analogy in which psychological concerns are likened to physical diseases with discrete and measurable symptoms (Maddux, 2008). It tends to overlook the relevance of context and culture in symptom presentation and it does not adequately incorporate character strengths, social resources, and functional capabilities in its assessment process.

The *DSM* has also been criticized for being heavily biased toward Western conceptions of psychological phenomena, not the least of which assumes that emotional or behavioral dynamics lie exclusively within the person rather than resulting from complex environmental and socio-cultural interactions. It does not acknowledge that models of psychological health and pathology are also social constructs grounded in cultural values. In addition, the *DSM* has been accused of *medicalizing* normal aspects of human experience into psychiatric symptoms, e.g., labeling grief and worry as depression and anxiety (Horwitz & Wakefield, 2007).

Even more troubling, there has been insinuation that the some of the authors of more recent editions of the *DSM* have had potential conflicts of interest with pharmaceutical companies (Cosgrove, Krimsky, Vijayaraghavan, & Schneider, 2006). The pharmaceutical industry "through its pursuit of profits and skillful use of marketing, its control of science, and its disease mongering, has been a major driving force in . . . extending the boundaries of illness and encouraging use beyond the meeting of health needs" (Busfield, 2010, p. 940).

Despite these critiques, the influence of the *DSM* in the mental health world continues to be so pervasive that almost all textbooks on abnormal psychology and all guides to assessing and treating psychological disorders are organized around it (Maddux, 2008). The illness analogy now permeates most conceptions of normal and abnormal psychological functioning. It has led to implicit assumptions about the practice of psychology and by extension, other mental health professions such as counseling, social work, and, yes, art therapy, which train their practitioners using similar paradigms. For example, most of art therapy graduate schools tailor their assessment classes to *DSM* categories and, as Betts (2012) noted, most of our art therapy assessments correspond to diagnostic criteria.

One of the consequences of the *DSM*'s dominance in the mental health world is that instead of being seen as exaggerated variations of common life stressors, psychological problems are believed to be discrete illnesses that require separate theories to be understood and addressed. This has led to a tendency to *pathologize*—to diagnose as symptoms of a disease—normal responses to everyday challenges (Horwitz & Wakefield, 2007). Therapy, itself, is considered to be fundamentally different from other helpful relationships in the patient's life (Maddux, 2008). The therapist's role, like other medical practitioners, is to assess symptoms, diagnosis disorder, recommend interventions, and provide evidence-based treatment. This may exacerbate power differentials in the relationship and not allow for other dynamics that might be more egalitarian, such as mentor, guide, collaborator, participant-observer, co-researcher, etc.

In the late 1970s, psychotherapists, like psychiatrists, were awarded the opportunity to receive reimbursement from insurance companies for psychological services (Elkins, 2009). This was certainly a benefit for them and for their clients. However, clinicians were now faced with a quandary—in order to have psychotherapy covered, clients had to be assigned a qualifying diagnosis from the *DSM* and their symptoms had to meet a certain threshold of severity. Even therapists who ally themselves closely with client-centered models have been inadvertently drawn into applying the medical model in their practice. David Elkins, who writes about the hazards of the medical model, provocatively speculates about the ethical implications of "pushing the diagnostic envelope" if/when clinicians are pressured into labeling clients with diagnoses for which therapy is reimbursed by insurance (2009, p. 78).

Now, what might before have been described as "support and guidance" for someone trying to address personal challenges, or seeking personal growth, has to be couched in clinical terminology, with corresponding diagnoses and recommendations for "evidence-based" treatment. Ironically, we can see this dilemma in our own backyard. Art therapy students are often expected to receive therapy themselves in order to have that experience first-hand. Even though, in this case, therapy is for professional development, if the trainee needs to have her health insurance cover the cost of this service, she would need to be given a *DSM* diagnosis. Gioia, who had five years of individual psychotherapy through her insurance benefits, wonders what diagnosis she could possibly have been given to warrant coverage for that long.

Labeling clients with diagnoses has benefits and hazards. On the one hand, clients often find their diagnosis provides a helpful framework for understanding their difficulties. For example, Rebecca worked with a very high-functioning client who was feeling overwhelmed and extremely anxious. When Rebecca reviewed with her the criteria for generalized anxiety disorder, her client realized that her responses were more than just "stress" from the high demands in her job—that she had actually been experiencing anxiety *all of her life*. She recognized that her anxiety was significant enough that it deserved focused attention and that managing it was more important than getting rid of the stressors that she had thought were causing it.

On the other hand, in diagnosing clients with specific disorders, there is a danger they will internalize their diagnosis and symptoms to the exclusion of their strengths, their capacity for coping, and their own unique experience. For example, a patient diagnosed with borderline personality disorder may believe that she is doomed to emotional extremes. This may keep her from discovering that although self-destructive behaviors might initially have served as coping strategies to manage intense feelings, they may have more damaging effects in the long run and they may keep her from developing other, more productive, ways of coping.

Other potential pitfalls emerge in the business of compressing clients and their presenting issues into diagnostic categories. Most insurance companies not only require a qualifying diagnosis from the *DSM* to justify reimbursement for services, but they also require that clients continue to exhibit impairment in order for coverage to continue. This might skew a clinician's perception toward the persistence of symptoms. In addition, clients themselves may feel pressure to highlight their ongoing struggles rather than their progress. As a result, both therapist and client may overlook positive changes.

Finally, the vast majority of clients in psychotherapy are actually there for reasons other than severe mental disorders and rather are seeking support for challenges in their daily lives (Seligman, 2011). Many clients may not even perceive that have "problems" per se—instead they are looking for opportunities to improve the quality of their lives and, like therapists-in-training, for personal growth. Whereas the medical model might provide us with highly articulated approaches for viewing and treating mental disorders, there is far less vision of what it means to be well and far fewer systematic approaches for helping clients who want to increase their happiness and general wellbeing.

The Negativity Bias

It should be noted that the medical model, with its emphasis on identifying and addressing illness and disease, understandably derives from compassion and noble intentions. When we see others suffering and in pain, we want to help. We are also hard-wired to notice disturbances in ourselves and our environment. Because our conscious mind cannot devote all of its resources to sorting through the overwhelming amount of data inundating our perceptions, it selectively attends to negative cues that may be more salient to our survival. This evolutionary mechanism, known as the *negativity bias*, alerts us to threats and disruptions in our environment and expectations. It then propels us to channel resources toward fixing these disturbances.

The negativity bias can be likened to a figure/ground metaphor, such as in a photograph, in which the generally positive field of everyday human experience forms a diffuse background against which negative experiences *pop out* (Vaish, Grossmann, & Woodward, 2008). The negativity bias helps to explain why the medical model has dominated the field of psychology (Maddux, 2002). "We study the negative conditions of our lives primarily to become free of them" (Young-Eisendrath, 2003, p. 171). However, as a result of the negativity bias, the medical model, and the disproportionate focus of research on mental illness, we have a clear idea of what is *wrong* but much less of what is *right* (Baumeister, Bratslavsky, Finkenauer, & Vohs, 2001).

Positive Psychology Emerges as Part of the Fourth Force

Positive psychology is an attempt to correct for this imbalance. Positive psychology parallels other approaches emerging as part of *the fourth force* in psychology. Although this movement seems to be evolving as we speak and thus may be difficult to define, it appears to include practices which refute reductionist models of illness. It is characterized by trans-disciplinary, transpersonal approaches which include holistic mind-body integration, spirituality, and ecological sustainability.

The fourth force originated from the work of humanists such as Maslow, who believed that spirituality and higher states of consciousness were critical elements of human experience that had been overlooked in the scientific study of human behavior. They advocated practices such as extrasensory perception, altered states of consciousness, yoga, body-centered therapies, and creative arts such as dance, music, art, and poetry to access other realms of transpersonal experience.

The larger social change movement, with its increasing emphasis on diversity and multicultural awareness, has also highlighted the strength and resilience of oppressed peoples worldwide. This has led to growing attention to social justice and human rights in the mental health system, including the growth of disability rights and consumer/survivor/ex-patient empowerment (Morrison, 2013).

As this fourth force is underway, we also find new therapeutic approaches which combine cognitive strategies with interventions that build upon clients' strengths. For example, *solution-focused therapy* served to balance the dominance of "problem-focused" work. This approach identifies *exceptions* (times when things are going well) and areas of our lives with which we are already happy and uses these as guides for moving forward (De Shazer & Dolan, 2012). Narrative therapy examines the social values and assumptions that underlie the *stories* we tell about our lives. It helps people *re-author* their personal histories by creating narratives that are most congruent with their strengths and what gives their lives meaning (White & Epston, 1990).

Other emerging cognitive approaches include Mindfulness-Based Stress Reduction (MBSR) (Kabat-Zinn, 2003), Acceptance and Commitment Therapy (ACT) (Hayes, Strosahl, & Wilson, 1999), Dialectical Behavioral Therapy (DBT) (Lineham, 1987), and Eye-Movement Desensitization and Reprocessing (EMDR) (Shapiro & Laliotis, 2010). These methods differ from traditional cognitive therapy which revolves around disputation of dysfunctional beliefs. Instead, they focus on developing more psychological flexibility by concentrating less on attempts to reduce and control the quantity of negative cognitions and emotions and more on shifting our relationship with those internal experiences. MBSR, ACT, and DBT blend Western cognitive-behavioral strategies with Eastern concepts such as developing an observing self that witnesses other parts of the self that are having thoughts and feelings, refraining from judgment, and accepting rather than avoiding unpleasant experiences. EMDR utilizes bilateral stimulation (e.g., tapping on the left and right knee) to desensitize patients to traumatic memories and introduce positive cognitions.

Positive psychology emerges alongside these *fourth force* approaches. In fact, many positive psychologists may even identify as practitioners of these other therapies. What unifies positive psychology is a call for the mobilization of resources toward establishing what constitutes and promotes healthy functioning in *everyone*, from those who are gifted and high functioning to those who are challenged and "mentally ill". Positive psychology suggests that we devote more focus, effort, funding, research, and scholarship toward exploring wellbeing and related topics which in the past have received much less attention and institutional support (Seligman & Csíkszentmihályi, 2000, Snyder & Lopez, 2002). We need a psychology devoted to "repairing weakness as well as nurturing strengths . . . remedying deficits as well as promoting excellence, and . . . reducing that which diminishes life as well as building that which makes life worth living" (Seligman, Parks, & Steen, 2004, p. 1381).

Positive psychologists believe that the factors that make up wellbeing—such as positive experience, strengths, meaning, and purpose—do not automatically emerge when the causes of suffering are removed (Duckworth, Steen, & Seligman, 2005). If we want to improve wellbeing, we need explore these factors more fully. In addition, because improving wellbeing naturally builds resilience and buffers against future stressors, it may actually, as a byproduct, reduce suffering (Fredrickson, Tugade, Waugh, & Larkin, 2003).

Some positive psychologists even provocatively suggest that pathology may arise as much from thwarted attempts to realize our inherent capacities for wellbeing and fulfillment as from dysfunctional childhoods and trauma (Seligman, Rashid, & Parks, 2006). In fact, optimal functioning occurs when people experience high levels of wellbeing *despite* or even *as a result of* the challenges they have faced or are facing in their lives. In positive psychology, the components of mental health—i.e., feeling better, feeling more love and connection, identifying and developing interests and strengths, increasing autonomy and mastery, broadening our perceptions, finding meaning and purpose, and developing resilience—come to the center and fore. Because these are the elements that create a life worth living, we are best served by giving them more focused attention.

Positive psychologists agree that some clients may have indeed struggled with significant physical and/or mental challenges; however, despite and sometimes even as a consequence of these limitations, they may be coping well and experiencing high levels of fulfillment in their lives:

> Viewing even the most distressed persons as more than the sum of damaged habits, drives, childhood conflicts, and malfunctioning brains, positive psychology asks for more serious consideration of those persons' intact faculties, ambitions, positive life experiences, and strengths of character, and how those buffer against disorder. (Duckworth, Steen, & Seligman, 2005, p. 631)

We think often of the resilience and empowerment our clients have modeled, such as people whose cancer diagnoses propelled them to embrace what was left of their lives, or people whose lives were ravaged by substance abuse but who later found direction, purpose, and meaning in helping others in recovery.

Inversely, some people may be free of significant problems and yet experience their lives as bereft of pleasure, engagement, and meaning (Seligman, Rashid, & Parks, 2006). In this case, we are reminded of some of the participants in our organizational workshops or resort guests with whom Rebecca works who are at the pinnacle of their careers but are disenchanted with their lives and who, despite their wealth and influence, are searching for something more. What would it look like if we could consistently help all our clients not just return to, but to go above and beyond their baseline of functioning? Or, as Seligman put it, get them not just from −8 to 0 but from 0 to 8+ (Gable & Haidt, 2005).

How is Positive Psychology Different from Humanism?

Although positive psychology's focus on optimal functioning has obvious roots in humanist principles, several elements set it apart from those predecessors. Because it is trying to correct for what is perceived as an imbalance that has led to a predominantly pathology-driven view of human behavior, it is essentially *more positive* than humanism. Unlike humanism which might be identified as more neutral, the primary aim of positive psychology is to study the positive side of human experience—positive emotions, positive meaning, strengths, positive relationships, optimal functioning, and even the positives in negative experiences! Positive psychologists have attempted to create an overarching framework and to advocate for funding and rigorous inquiry into the many diverse areas that contribute to happiness, mental health, and wellbeing (Seligman & Csíkszentmihályi, 2000; Seligman, Rashid, & Parks, 2006).

Critiques of Positive Psychology

Ironically, positive psychology seems to generate quite a bit of negativity! Positive psychology has met with substantial criticisms, some warranted and others misinformed, e.g., that focusing on the positive is, in and of itself, pathological—delusional even. To this, we are stumped to respond. If living a higher-quality life does not hold some promise, we are not sure what makes life worth living. Positive psychologists have also been accused of naiveté, of adopting a Pollyanna view that denies negative or unpleasant aspects of life (Diener, 2003). Positive psychologists have also been criticized for minimizing suffering, for jumping too quickly to the positive and trying to make people mindlessly "happy" (Lazarus, 2003; Peterson, 2006).

We get this a lot. Dubious colleagues disapprovingly remind us that advocating positivity for our clients might lead students/clinicians to prematurely glide past suffering and trauma. There is also the suggestion that therapists who adopt a positive psychology approach do so as a form of denial and reaction formation, as a way to avoid addressing their own pain and loss. Leading positive psychotherapists addressed these concerns:

> We do not in any way suggest that positive characteristics are emphasized over negative ones, or that a focus on the negative is removed. Quite the converse, we suggest that the field fully integrates the study and fostering of positive and negative characteristics equally; the positivity comes from developing a better and more integrated field rather than narrowly focusing on only one domain of life (Wood & Tarrier, 2010, p. 820).

Some have cautioned that this approach may be too sophisticated for novice therapists who might overemphasize the positive because they don't have the skills to address deeper pain and suffering. However, most students and early professionals we've worked with are thirsty for this kind of a life-affirming approach in the face of what they perceive to be the unrelenting focus on pathology still so common in clinical practice. They also grasp the delicate balance inherent in simultaneously attending to suffering and promoting wellbeing.

Positive Psychology versus Psychology-as-Usual

The word "positive" in positive psychology has also been a bone of contention—both for critics and proponents of the field. It has led to the unfortunate but unfounded implication that positive psychologists believe that the rest of psychology is "negative." In fact, most positive psychologists see the field of psychology as neutral or, as some have coined it, *psychology-as-usual* (Gable & Haidt, 2005). The excitement that positive psychologists experience about exploring wellbeing does not mean that they reject traditional psychological theories and practices. Nor do they seek to take credit for groundbreaking research into creativity, wellbeing, and strengths that were developed before the term "positive psychology" emerged. Positive psychologists do not wish to disparage those who have furthered our understanding of human nature, but instead to honor them. Positive psychology is built upon their foundational work!

Is Positive Psychology Only for the Working Well?

Another critique is that a positive psychology approach is a luxury that applies only to the working well—wealthy and/or "high functioning" individuals—rather than people with emotional and psychological problems or who struggle with socio-economic challenges. Along the same lines are misconceptions that it is only useful when clients are stable, receptive, and self-initiating rather than when they are in crisis and impaired (Diener & Ryan, 2009). This is not true.

Although income and life satisfaction are correlated, happiness, purpose and meaning, engagement and flow, accomplishment and connection are universal needs, and valued worldwide at all levels of functional ability and income (Diener & Biswas-Diener, 2008). Robert Biswas-Diener (2010) in his book, *Positive Psychology as Social Change*, outlined ways that positive psychological science can address pressing social ills. Anecdotally, we have invariably found that this approach works just as well with people who are struggling with the very worst of financial, social, and psychological challenges as those with the highest levels of income and functioning.

On the other hand, the critique that positive psychology is only about and for the high-functioning, exceptional, and gifted is not necessarily unfounded. Positive psychology emerged at the turn of twenty-first century, before 9/11 and the global economic collapse of 2006/2007 (King, 2011). At that time, it seemed right to shift the focus to optimism, wellbeing, and prosperity. *Finally* we could be less preoccupied with pathology and devote ourselves more to the exceptional and gifted, the good life, and optimal functioning! However, this focus seemed suddenly ill-placed with the violence, terror, war, economic hardship, wealth disparities, and political strife that has characterized the start of the twenty-first century.

Ironically, positive psychology, with its focus on character strengths, resilience, and posttraumatic growth, may be even more relevant during hard times. It calls us to revisit part of positive psychology's original mission—to build upon the "ordinary strengths and virtues" that help us survive and thrive (Sheldon & King, 2001, p. 216). We want to explore what makes *everyday* humans feel better, be happier, live more rewarding lives and experience overall physical, psychological, spiritual, and emotional wellbeing.

Do You Have to Be Happy Yourself to Adopt a Positive Psychology Approach?

Finally, we have also been told that only "happy" therapists can be positive psychologists; that it is not for therapists who are realists or curmudgeons, like Rebecca, who describes herself as dark, fussy, and cynical. On the contrary, these are the folks who gain the most from improving their wellbeing, as Rebecca and other naturally pessimistic folks like Marty Seligman can attest. And because wellbeing is associated with health, improved relationships, and success, it is well worth learning (Forgeard & Seligman, 2012).

Positive psychology can also be useful for people who, like Gioia, are naturally joyful and optimistic. Even the most hardy and buoyant can benefit from learning ways to enjoy a higher quality of life. In addition, none of us are immune to difficulty and hardship, whether we are generally happy-go-lucky or we struggle with anxiety, depression, trauma, pain, confusion, or other challenges. Positive psychology is about helping us all experience the highest quality of life possible with whatever assets, resources, limitations, and challenges we have.

Positive Psychology Is Still Going Strong

Interestingly, when positive psychology was first conceptualized, many positive psychologists speculated it would be assimilated into psychology-as-usual (Gable & Haidt, 2005). They believed that by bringing attention to the need for more robust exploration of mental health and wellbeing, the broader field of psychology would gradually become more balanced and that imperative would subside—that it would be considered just a passing fad. However, 17 years after its formal inauguration, it is still relevant and timely. This is perhaps because its mission—"to discover and promote the factors that allow individuals and communities to thrive" (Sheldon et al., 2000, paragraph 1) and to focus upon "sources of psychological health"—continues to be as relevant, and perhaps even more so, today as it was in 2000.

In the last few years, positive psychology has gained further legitimacy in the psychology world. It is now included in most psychology textbooks. Courses on the topic are now regularly being offered at universities in the US, the UK, Denmark, Spain, South Africa, and Australia. Several comprehensive hand-books have been published on positive psychology with contributions from a broad range of scholars on an array of subjects related to the field. Publications such as the *Journal of Positive Psychology*, the *Journal of Happiness Studies*, the *International Journal of Applied Positive Psychology*, and *Applied Research in Quality of Life* have been launched over the last few years. Robust online forums have also emerged, such as the APA's *Friends of Positive Psychology* listserv and several LinkedIn and Facebook groups, including ones devoted to positive psychology and art therapy.

In addition, there is increased funding for research in the areas of wellbeing, character strengths, positive emotions, positive health, positive education, and other relevant topics from sources such as the John Templeton Foundation, the Robert Woods Johnson Foundation, National Institute of Mental Health, and the US Army. Overall, positive psychology has become an established part of the broader field.

Despite projections that positive psychology would render itself obsolete, it appears that it is still going strong. With that in mind, we will now dive deeper into the realm of happiness and wellbeing and share with you what we have learned about combining the science of positive psychology with the magic of art therapy.

Discussion Questions

1 Have you felt pressure to diagnose clients with psychiatric conditions?
2 How has the medical model influenced your practice?
3 Have you ever been in therapy and received a *DSM* diagnosis? What was that like?
4 How do you see the negativity bias emerging in your personal and profes-sional life?
5 What role might positive psychology play in your line of work?

CHAPTER 3

Happiness and Wellbeing

When we enrolled in Lani Gerrity's *Happiness Challenge*—the online course that introduced us to positive psychology—one of our first assignments was to explore the self-assessment section on University of Pennsylvania's Authentic Happiness Website. Among the many questionnaires looking at qualities such as gratitude, grit, resilience, optimism, and strengths, Lani recommended we take the *Approaches to Happiness* and the *Authentic Happiness Inventory* (Peterson, Park, Steen, & Seligman, 2006).

The *Approaches to Happiness* questionnaire involved rating how much given ideas resonated for us, e.g., "My life serves a higher purpose," "I love doing things that excite my senses," and "I seek out situations that challenge my skills and abilities." The results measure happiness in three different areas: the pleasant life, the engaged life, and the meaningful life. The *pleasant life* includes our capacity to experience and savor pleasure and the mindfulness skills to amplify those sensations. The *engaged life* involves using our signature strengths to experience more flow. The *meaningful life* includes using our signature strengths in the service of something greater than ourselves. Seligman suggests that we experience a *full life* when we find fulfillment in all of those domains.

The next questionnaire, the *Authentic Happiness Inventory*, provided a measure of our happiness on a scale of 1–5. Each question provided a range of responses from "I have sorrow in my life" to "I have much more joy than sorrow," "Most of the time I feel bored" to "Most of the time I feel quite interested in what I am doing," and "I do not know the purpose of my life" to "I have a very clear idea about the meaning of my life."

Our results were quite illuminating. They explained why Gioia could be bored with what seemed like a dream job and why Rebecca could be living in paradise and yet still be miserable. Gioia's general happiness score was fairly high. This made sense with her naturally buoyant disposition. Not surprisingly, she scored high in the pleasant life. In addition, because she derives a great deal of meaning from being an art therapist and from spending time with her family, she also scored high on the meaningful life. However, she was low on the engaged life because she was in a job that neither challenged nor inspired her.

Rebecca, like Gioia, also scored high on the meaningful life—she has a strong sense of mission, particularly related to using art to help others; however, she was lower on the engaged life and quite a bit lower on the pleasant life. It occurred to her that, although she was supposedly "living the good life," she felt restless because she wasn't working regularly and, even though she identifies herself as an artist, she didn't really enjoy painting alone in her studio. In addition, it was no surprise that she scored low on the general happiness scale and on the pleasant life because not only was she far away from family, but she is by nature anxious, she has a history of depression, and she has a chronic pain condition.

Even though we are both therapists in the business of helping others feel better, we were struck by these insights into *our own* happiness. Equally important, we had been introduced to a model for looking at happiness that we had never been exposed to before. Shortly thereafter, Gioia quit her job to go back to school and get her PhD, which she found much more challenging and engaging. Rebecca channeled her efforts toward yoga, meditation, and other techniques to help increase her level of emotional and physical wellbeing. She and her husband also moved back to the States to be closer to family. And she and Gioia decided to look more deeply into this happiness business.

Happiness

Happiness matters. It does for us and we can probably guess with some certainty it does for you too. It is what most people want in their lives. Aristotle said that happiness transcends all other considerations—that it is the ultimate goal in life "because we choose it for itself and never for any other reason" (Thomson, 1953, p. 73). We are reminded of the many times that our clients, our friends, our family members, and even we, ourselves, have said, "I just want to be happy."

However, when we ask people to describe what happiness means to them, they are often at a loss. Although we seem to implicitly know that it essential to what makes life worth living, many of us have not examined what that actually means. Is it peace of mind, having our burdens lifted, having more energy and vitality, feeling, getting along better with our loved ones, finding adventure, having more fun, more structure, more freedom, being successful and recognized for our talents, or feeling like we've accomplished something with our lives?

Wellbeing

In many ways, our ideas about happiness are often more poetic and ephemeral than objective and quantifiable. Rather than trying to establish scientific definitions of happiness, positive psychologists instead opted for the broader concept of *wellbeing*, which they believed could be more precisely defined and measured. As we proceed, we will outline discourse on wellbeing, which has essentially been shaped by two theories: 1) Subjective Wellbeing (SWB) and 2)

Psychological Wellbeing (PWB). We also examine Keyes' model of *flourishing* and Seligman's model of wellbeing, PERMA.

> Health is a state of complete physical, mental and social well-being and not merely the absence of disease or infirmity. Mental health is defined as "a state of well-being in which every individual realizes his or her own potential, can cope with the normal stresses of life, can work productively and fruitfully, and is able to make a contribution to her or his community." (World Health Organization, 2014)

Subjective Wellbeing

Subjective wellbeing (SWB) was initially conceived by Ed Diener, also known as "Dr. Happiness," one of the senior researchers at the Gallup Institute. SWB grows out of the field of hedonic psychology (Kahneman, Diener, & Schwartz, 1999), the study of what makes life more pleasant and unpleasant. It should not be confused with *hedonism*, the single-minded pursuit of pleasure. It suggests that the more positive emotions (e.g., joy, hope, curiosity, love) and the fewer negative emotions (anger, fear, sadness) we have, the happier we feel. SWB is most closely associated with "felt" happiness; however it also includes cognitive evaluations of important areas in our lives (such as health, work, and relationships) and how satisfied we think we are in meeting our desires and goals in those domains (Diener, 2012).

Psychological Wellbeing

Psychological wellbeing, also known as *eudemonic wellbeing*, refers to meeting and overcoming challenges in life and reaching our fullest potential (Ryff, 1989)—being resilient, knowing ourselves, and becoming the best that we can be. Carol Ryff, a psychologist whose work has focused on *optimal aging*, based this approach to wellbeing upon the notion that pursuing happiness for its own sake appears to produce fleeting pleasure but rarely more enduring happiness. In fact, it often seems to make people to feel *less* happy (Oishi, Diener, & Lucas, 2007). Instead, engaging in activities that give us purpose and meaning seem to be the most fulfilling.

Ryff maintained that the hedonic model—feeling better more and worse less—does not account for the importance of strengths, meaning, and virtue in happiness. Feelings of accomplishment and elevation can be more rewarding than momentary pleasure. In addition, people often do things that are unpleasant and involve tremendous sacrifice for a higher good (most parents, who know the joys and tribulations of raising children, would likely confirm this). In contrast, some things, such as indulging in foods high in sugar and fat, which are seemingly pleasant may be detrimental to our overall wellbeing.

Ryff's (1989) credits her approach to wellbeing on the seminal work of Marie Jahoda (1958), a social psychologist who was commissioned in the late 1950s by the National Institute of Mental Health to study mental health needs in the United States. Recall that the National Mental Health Act of 1947 had been ratified after World War II to address the growing awareness of psychological problems in veterans and in the general public. Jahoda was one of the first to recommend that there was as much of a need to attend to wellbeing as there was to address psychological illness. With this in mind, she set about articulating the variables that contribute to what she called *positive mental health*.

Ryff used Jahoda's framework to operationalize *psychological wellbeing* (PWB). It includes: 1) finding meaning, purpose, and direction in our lives; 2) having a sense of autonomy and personal standards to guide us; 3) experiencing personal growth and employing our strengths and talents; 4) connecting meaningfully with others; 5) mastering the complexities of life; and 6) knowing and accepting ourselves.

There is some debate about which approach to wellbeing most accurately captures what it means to be happy and well—SWB or PWB. Advocates of SWB agree that components of PWB which are not outlined in the SWB model— autonomy, positive relationships, environmental mastery, etc.—are important; however, they suggest this is because they *lead* to a sense of satisfaction with life and to positive feelings of contentment and wellbeing. They are the *means* to the end—happiness. Because our subjective sense of wellbeing is so closely tied to the emotional quality of our lives, people naturally use it to evaluate their *overall* sense of happiness. From that perspective, psychological wellbeing might then be seen as happiness *plus* meaningfulness (McGregor & Little, 1998; Ryan & Deci, 2001), a concept we will explore in much more detail in Chapters 10 and 11 on meaning.

There are compelling arguments for both approaches and they are not mutually exclusive. Both offer ways to objectively measure wellbeing, which has become increasingly important as research reveals the significance of wellbeing in helping people move from beyond just surviving to thriving and *flourishing*.

Flourishing and Languishing

Corey Keyes (2007), a psychologist who collaborated with Ryff, was one of the first to fully articulate *flourishing*—a state of optimal functioning that combines the elements of SWB and PWB as well as detailed criteria for *social functioning*. Keyes was also influenced by Jahoda's work, particularly her conclusion that neither mental health nor mental illness could be defined by the absence or presence of the other. He pointed out that, for example, the absence of delusional ideation does not necessarily lead to healthy perceptions of reality; the absence of depression and apathy does not mean the presence of joy and sense of purpose.

Keyes (2007) challenged the notion that mental health and mental illness even belong on the same continuum—that as one moves down in mental illness, one would correspondingly move up in mental health and vice versa. He also proposed that mental health, just like mental disorder, can be "diagnosed" by measuring "symptoms" of mental health. In other words, just as we use the *DSM* to look at the presence of a certain number of symptoms in several dimensions and level of impairment in social, occupational and educational functioning, we can also determine whether someone is mentally well, or *flourishing*, by measuring the presence of hedonic "symptoms" and *positive* functioning.

For example, with depression, one would show depressed mood or loss of pleasure/interest in daily activities for more than two weeks, along with five out of nine symptoms; e.g., disturbed sleep, changes in weight, fatigue or loss of energy, difficulty concentrating, and thoughts of death or suicide. In order to be flourishing, one would consistently show high levels of SWB (more positive affect, less negative affect, and a sense of satisfaction in life) and high levels of at least six out of eleven measures of psychological wellbeing; e.g., self-acceptance, acceptance of others, sense of autonomy, purpose in life, and positive social relations. People who exhibit *low* levels of positive affect or satisfaction in life and *low* scores in least six of the measures of positive functioning are considered to be *languishing*—they may not be not mentally ill but they are also not flourishing.

Keyes (2007) maintained that languishing can be as harmful as mental illness. Although people who are languishing may not be experiencing any *overt* signs of mental disorder, they often describe their lives as "hollow" or "empty." They might not meet criteria for a psychiatric diagnosis, but they still show impaired functioning. For example, they are more prone to chronic physical disease, poor work performance, and strained interpersonal relationships.

Not surprisingly, Keyes (2007) identified that people who are *both* flourishing and have *no* mental illness show the highest levels of wellbeing. However, he also discovered that people *with* mental disorders, despite the challenges that they face, often show indicators of flourishing—of experiencing significant emotional, psychological, and social wellbeing. It is interesting to note that, although people with a diagnosis who are *flourishing* and people who have no diagnosis but are *languishing* both exhibit health limitations and work impairment, they differ in that people with a diagnosis who are flourishing show *higher* levels of psychosocial functioning than the latter. In other words, although people with a diagnosis who are flourishing still have challenges, the quality of their relationships is better. This is particularly significant when we consider the importance of social connection and support in wellbeing.

Seligman's PERMA Model of Flourishing and Wellbeing

Growing recognition for the critical role relationships play in flourishing also influenced Seligman's approach to happiness. As mentioned earlier, Seligman initially conceptualized happiness as the convergence of three main avenues: the pleasant life, the engaged life, and the meaningful life. However, he recognized that the three paths failed to adequately account for the significance of relationships to happiness. In other words, when people describe what they enjoy and makes them feel good, what engages them, and what is meaningful to them, it almost always includes people—family members, friends, lovers, patients, colleagues, etc.

Seligman also realized that "happiness," itself, was an untenable construct—it focused too much on "feeling good" rather than on resiliency, tenacity, and the pursuit of activities which might not be pleasant but which provide an overarching sense of accomplishment and connection. He shifted his focus from *happiness* to *wellbeing*—outlining PERMA, a model which served as an acronym for the five elements that he believed contributed most to wellbeing: Positive emotions, Engagement, Relationships, Meaning, and Achievement (Seligman, 2011).

Seligman (2011) suggested that PERMA incorporated the affective components of SWB, as well as critical elements of PWB; e.g., the need to be engaged, to optimize our highest strengths and live up to our highest potential, to find meaning and purpose, and to experience autonomy and a sense of accomplishment. Seligman maintains that the PERMA model has applications beyond the scope of positive psychology. For example, he advocates for Positive Education and Positive Health which he believes will generate not only personal but also global wellbeing.

There is clearly value in all of the models of wellbeing—Subjective Wellbeing, Psychological Wellbeing, Flourishing, and PERMA—and throughout the book we will refer back to each. However, in general we found that Seligman's PERMA model was, for our purposes, the most effective framework for illustrating the ways that positive psychology and art therapy combine to improve wellbeing. As a result, we have used PERMA—Positive emotions, Engagement, Relationships, Meaning, and Achievement—as the structure of the book. Before diving into these domains more fully, we will first outline some of the variables that deserve consideration when exploring wellbeing.

Factors that Influence and Are Influenced by Wellbeing

Culture

In examining different models of wellbeing, we must not fail to acknowledge the role that culture plays in our assumptions about happiness. Christopher (1999) has identified that because it has not been conceptualized with the same specificity as psychopathology, we often rely uncritically upon "common-sense" assumptions about wellbeing which, in fact, are much more culturally bound than we realize. For example, high self-esteem, autonomy, independence, and individual achievement matter much more in Western cultures;

whereas social acceptance, harmony, and communal identity matter more in Eastern cultures (Diener, Oishi, & Lucas, 2003; Fulmer et al., 2010).

Christopher (1999) suggests that the prevailing models of wellbeing derive most from Western humanism. In these paradigms, the individual is seen as a self-contained entity and society as a collection of other similarly autonomous and self-defining beings who possess their own needs, interests, and desires. Although these perspectives may be relevant in Western cultures, they might conflict with more collectivist viewpoints.

For example, signs of mental health identified in psychological wellbeing such as autonomy, self-expression, high self-esteem, and personal growth, may reflect a bias towards individualism. In addition, when measuring subjective wellbeing, someone in a collectivist society may be less concerned with evaluating their personal satisfaction in life and more concerned with whether or not he/she is contributing to an organized social order (Diener, 2012). Not only that, measures of positive and negative affect operate on the assumption that emotions are experienced within the individual which does not properly account for their interpersonal nature.

In approaching wellbeing, we need to exercise the same degree of sensitivity that we have been called to apply in *psychology-as-usual* when addressing assumptions about pathology, suffering, and mental illness. Christopher (1999) recommends that we develop awareness of the *cultural embeddedness* which naturally prevents us from being neutral on matters that are so fundamental to our identity. This bias is not intrinsically unhealthy; however, it needs to be explored so that we can identify blind spots that might be inherent to the models of wellbeing we adopt. In addition, as a result of examining our own assumptions about happiness, we are better able to help our clients do the same.

Socioeconomic Impact

Socioeconomic influences on wellbeing and conversely, the impact of wellbeing on socioeconomic status, are also relevant. Keyes (2007) has identified that because languishing is highly correlated to increased healthcare utilization, it is as much of a strain on the healthcare system as mental illness. In the US, although only about 50 percent of the population will experience symptoms of a mental disorder and only 23 percent will exhibit a full-blown mental illness, less than 20 percent of the US adult population is flourishing—therefore, conversely, more than 80 percent are languishing.

Keyes lamented that, given Jahoda's suggestion more than fifty years ago that we focus as much on positive mental health as on mental illness, very little effort has been put into channeling resources towards building the factors that improve wellbeing—mental health remains "a catchword of inept good intentions" (Keyes, 2002, p. 208). Public policy and funding continue to be funneled predominantly toward researching and treating mental illness, not toward studying and promoting the factors that promote mental health and wellbeing.

Along these lines, Seligman (2011) and Diener (2012) have identified that even though the Gross Domestic Product has tripled over the last fifty years in the US, life satisfaction has not. In fact, statistics on depression, anxiety, and suicidal behaviors have actually *increased*. They suggest that, because of the *downstream* benefits of flourishing—improved health, increased productivity, greater civil peace—we need to measure and then make policy around wellbeing and quality of life, not just around economic growth. Seligman pointed out that, especially in the US, focusing on measuring financial wealth has shaped our policies to ensure we are securing wealth. It follows, therefore, that if we focus more on measuring life satisfaction and psychological health, then policy will also change to capture those aspects of wellbeing.

Global Wellbeing

It should be noted that there is promise in this area. For example, data is being collected measuring happiness and subjective wellbeing both in the US and around the world by organizations such as the Gallup Institute, the World Happiness Report, and the Happy Planet Index. The World Happiness Report identified six factors that appear to contribute most to happiness levels in different countries. These include GDP per capita, social support, healthy life expectancy, freedom to make life choices, generosity, and perception of corruption. Their research revealed that, for 2015, Switzerland had the highest level of happiness, followed by Iceland, Denmark, and Norway. The US, just behind Mexico, ranked only 15th. The lowest levels were found in Afghanistan, Rwanda, Benin, Syria, Burundi, and Togo (Diener, 2012), places where there is not only significant poverty, but also war and political unrest.

This type of data is gaining more visibility on the global stage. For example, the United Nations is adopting Sustainable Development Goals which move from focusing exclusively on economic objectives to including social and environmental goals as measures of growth. It is being recommended that happiness indicators, such as SWB, be included in the tools used to measure progress towards these goals. This may bode well for the bold vision Seligman put forth at the First World Congress of Positive Psychology held in Philadelphia in 2012— that by the year 2051, 51 percent of the people in the world will be flourishing.

Benefits of Happiness and Wellbeing

Beyond being rewarding in and of itself, wellbeing is also correlated to and/ or causal in all areas of our mental and physical health. Improved wellbeing leads to better physical health, improved immune functioning, greater longevity, improved relationships, higher income, and superior work performance. People who are happier appear to be more cooperative, charitable, and self-confident. They experience more creativity, energy, and flow. They have greater capacity to self-regulate. They are more likely to get married (Diener, 2012), less likely to divorce (Harker & Keltner, 2001) and they are also more satisfied with their marriages (Ruvolo, 1998). Wellbeing is also highly correlated with *resiliency*: the capacity to bounce back from adversity, and to preventively buffer against future stress (Fredrickson et al., 2003).

There is some debate about the causal arrows for happiness (Myers & Diener, 1996). A classic example is that people who are happier tend to donate more money to charities and, conversely, donating to charities makes people happier (Diener, 2012). Generally speaking, people who are constitutionally happier naturally exhibit the markers of wellbeing—they are healthier, more satisfied with their lives, more optimistic, have higher self-esteem, are more decisive and cooperative, and they perform better at work. On the other hand, feeling better and engaging in activities that improve wellbeing makes people happier (Myers & Diener, 1996).

Set Point or Set Range

There is evidence that we are genetically disposed to a *set point* of happiness (Lykken & Tellegen, 1996)—a general level of happiness toward which we are naturally inclined. Diener, Lucas, and Scollon (2006) suggested that, because our set point may fluctuate a little bit and even improve over the years, it might be more useful to call it a *set range*. Not surprisingly, we return to this baseline more slowly with negative events. What may be unexpected is that we return to it much more quickly with positive ones.

The Hedonic Treadmill

The *hedonic treadmill* (Lykken & Tellegen, 1996) refers to our tendency to adapt to changes in our environment. Related is our tendency to overestimate what we think will make us happy—we often believe, whether consciously or unconsciously, that if we win the lottery, get a promotion, find the perfect job, the perfect home, the perfect mate, etc., *then* we will be happy (Wilson & Gilbert, 2003). Although initially we usually do feel happier when those things happen, we also "adjust" fairly quickly and return to our previous level of happiness.

We may also exhibit the *adaptation-level phenomena*, whereby we judge our current circumstances based upon past experiences (Myers & Diener, 1996). Positive events, particularly ones that create feelings of euphoria and elation, may create a new "normal" against which subsequent experiences are compared. And then, because our neutral level has been raised, we may require more to feel better and feel deprived by what used to be satisfying.

What We Think Will Make Us Unhappy

As mentioned earlier, we tend to be genetically predisposed towards a set range of positivity to which we return after adjusting to external events. Although our baseline might be permanently affected by trauma and loss, our inherent disposition and coping style appears to determine our responses more than the event itself. For example, although people who become blind or paralyzed do not fully return to their baseline, they do adapt, even though that process may take a while (Diener, Lucas, & Scollon, 2006). Positive events have much less impact on our lives. People who win the lottery report an initial increase in wellbeing within the first year, but then they usually return to their initial set point.

We also to tend to misjudge what will make us *unhappy*. Although, understandably, we imagine that we will be devastated by loss and trauma and *we do suffer* when bad things happen, most of us actually recover and manage much better than we would have expected (Gilbert, 2009; Lyubomirsky, Sheldon, & Schkade, 2005). In fact, although most people would certainly not say that they were "happier" because of hardships they encountered, they often report a higher quality of life as a result of these challenges. They experience a shift in their priorities and a greater appreciation of life, an increased sense of personal strength, a richer spiritual life and more meaningful relationships—a phenomenon coined *posttraumatic growth* (Tedeschi & Calhoun, 1996). What seems to help people bounce back most from negative experiences is their capacity to cope (Diener, Lucas, & Scollon, 2006) and their ability to derive some kind of meaning from what they went through, also known as *benefit-finding* (Tedeschi & Calhoun, 1996). We will explore these concepts in greater detail in Chapters 10 and 11 on meaning and perception.

What Actually Makes Us Happier

Finally, we tend to underestimate what actually *does* make us happy. As mentioned before, we often focus more on what we *think* will make us happy (wealth, romance, success, material possessions) without recognizing that peripherals—our health, our daily experiences, and the quality of our personal connections—have much more impact on our wellbeing (Gilbert, 2009): "Happiness is produced not so much by great pieces of good fortune that seldom happen as by little advantages that occur every day" (Benjamin Franklin, in Myers & Diener, 1996, p. 17).

Emotions

People who experience more positive emotions and fewer negative emotions tend to have high subjective wellbeing (Diener, 2012). It also appears that higher frequency of positive emotions is better than more intensity. Although feeling more positive emotions is generally good, there is a tipping point. Having *too many positive emotions* is associated with risk-taking and reduced effort to meet objectives—in other words, people who are *too* happy may be manic or overly optimistic; they may show less judgment and lower motivation to make changes in their lives (Diener, Oishi, & Lucas, 2003; Gruber, Mauss, & Tamier, 2011).

It is also important to note that the total absence of negative emotions does not lead to improved wellbeing—negative feelings are critical to our survival because they provide us with important feedback about the quality of our relationships, what matters to us, our values, and our safety and security. And, as we know as therapists, suppressing negative emotions is detrimental to wellbeing. It appears that the ability to effectively *regulate* emotions is most conducive to wellbeing. We'll come back to this important point throughout the book.

Personality and Disposition

Personality appears to play a significant role in the experience of wellbeing, particularly the traits identified by the Five Factor Model of Personality which lists five essential characteristics that form the core of all personality profiles: openness to experience, conscientiousness, extroversion, agreeableness, and neuroticism. Neuroticism, the tendency to be anxious, self-conscious, tense, and self-defeating, is a strong predictor of negative affect, pessimistic thinking, and lower psychological wellbeing (Sharpe, Martin, & Roth, 2011). Of the other personality traits, extroversion, conscientiousness, and agreeableness appears to be the strongest predictors of positive effect, but only the first two are strongly related to psychological wellbeing. Openness to experience appears to be highly correlated with sense of fulfillment but less with positive affect and subjective wellbeing.

People who are more dispositionally optimistic and hopeful also appear to be happier. They are also more likely to be healthier and to recover more quickly from medical interventions. In addition, when they get sick, they tend to return to their previous level of activity more rapidly and they also appear to cope with stress better (Scheier & Carver, 1993). Similar benefits appear to emerge for those who exhibit a *growth mindset* rather than a *fixed mindset* (Dweck, 2006). Growth mindset assumes that intelligence and learning result from trial and error, rather than that intelligence is a fixed quality with which one is either born or not. Decades of research show people with a growth mindset tend to be more resilient, to overcome barriers more readily, and to experience greater self-esteem (Dweck, 2006).

Relationships

As mentioned earlier, supportive relationships are fundamental to wellbeing. Not surprisingly, people who also experience secure attachments are happier. In addition, the *quality* is more important than the *quantity* of relationships. People who are married appear to be happier, partly because of the support and companionship that it provides and also because it often adds socioeconomic security. On the other hand, single women appear to have higher levels of autonomy and personal growth. Divorce appears to be negatively correlated to wellbeing. Single and widowed women appear to be happier than single and widowed men (Ryff, 2014).

Family connection and family rituals have a positive impact on wellbeing. Although parenting is often considered challenging, in general it enhances wellbeing. However, it suffers if parents feel their children are struggling. Certain losses have significant impact on wellbeing—losing a child affects wellbeing for years, even decades, and losing a parent in childhood also predicts lower wellbeing. In addition, caring for a family member with high needs negatively impacts wellbeing (Ryff, 2014).

Money and Success

The effects of money on wellbeing are intriguing—some predictable but others surprising. Not surprisingly, being wealthier has important benefits—access to more medical and educational resources, safer living conditions, better health and nutrition, greater sense of security, autonomy, and control. These advantages help buffer against adversity, a benefit in and of itself. In addition, people who are wealthier report more overall satisfaction with their lives. However, being wealthier has much less effect on day-to-day experience. Once we get beyond sustenance levels, wealth has very little impact on happiness (Myers & Diener, 1996).

An important caveat about money—although increases in happiness relative to income level off after a point (about $75,000/year), *poverty* appears to adversely influence happiness. This is likely because of its negative impact on health, stress, autonomy, and ability to contribute meaningfully to one's community. In addition, economic inequality has increased over the last half-century in much of the world. Places with greater disparities of wealth have lower life expectancies and higher rates of crime, obesity, drug and alcohol abuse, and anxiety, all of which reduce wellbeing (Diener & Ryan, 2009).

It appears that when we are *preoccupied* with financial wealth and status, we are *less happy*, especially when we use money to prove ourselves or to gain power. This may be because it leads to focusing more on material goals than on personal growth or psychological wellbeing. It may also be a result of engaging in *upward social comparison* whereby we compare ourselves unfavorably with others (they have bigger houses, nicer cars, etc.), and we feel inadequate or powerless in the face of these inequities (Ryff, 2014). We also tend to feel worse if we believe that we are not as successful as whomever we think of as our peers. For example, we feel better about making $50,000 if our peers are making $40,000 than if we are making $100,000 when our peers are making $150,000 (Myers & Diener, 1996).

If we spend our money on experiences rather than possessions, we seem to be happier (Dunn, Gilbert, & Wilson, 2011). Also, although paradoxically counter-intuitive to the more selfish parts of our nature and yet fundamentally valued in most spiritual paradigms, we seem to derive more pleasure by spending money on other people rather than ourselves. In other words, if we channel money toward basic psychological needs for meaningful connection, autonomy, mastery, and personal growth, we are more likely to be happier. In addition, when we engage in *downward social comparison*, whereby our attention is focused on someone worse off than we are, we may experience an appreciative shift in our perceptions of our own assets: "I thought I was struggling, but at least I have a job, my health, etc. . . . and that person just got laid off, lost a family member, got diagnosed with a terrible illness, etc. . . ."

Social Comparison

As alluded to earlier, social comparison has an impact on our wellbeing (Suls, Martin, & Wheeler, 2002). Social comparison serves as a way to set expectations for ourselves of how we should be in comparison to people whom we perceive as peers—people in our age group, our neighborhood, our social networks, or in the same occupation (Festinger, 1954). Upward social comparison can increase feelings of inferiority, particularly if we have low self-esteem or we have recently suffered a setback that challenged our self-concept. On the other hand, upward social comparisons can also serve as motivation to improve ourselves. Downward social comparison can enhance our esteem by making us feel better about our circumstances. For example, people who are struggling with hardship, such as cancer patients, evaluate their situation more favorably when they perceive that others are suffering even more than they are (Wood, Taylor, & Lichtman, 1985). It should be noted, though, that cancer patients show a preference for upward comparisons to people who have been *more fortunate* because it gives them hope.

Diener (2012), who has ambitiously attempted to explore wellbeing throughout the world, warns that because of the pervasiveness of television and social media across the planet , social comparison is no longer exclusively within peer groups. As a result, *world standards* of success and happiness, which emerge from some of the wealthiest of countries, may lead to unrealistic and unfavorable comparisons and negatively impact wellbeing.

Work

Although we may at times pine for a life of leisure, people actually feel better if they work. Work provides focus, purpose, personal identity, a network of support, and a sense of pride and belonging. In addition, people who are happier enjoy work more. They also seem to secure more job interviews, are valuated more positively by their employers, earn more, work harder, are more productive, and experience less burnout (Diener & Ryan, 2009). Unemployment, even for short periods, has been shown to have a significant and lasting negative impact on wellbeing. However, that effect is lessened when unemployment levels are high for everyone, presumably because it normalizes the experience (Diener, 2012; Ryan & Deci, 2001).

Religion and Spirituality

Religiously active people are happier, healthier, and less vulnerable to depression, drug and alcohol abuse, delinquency, divorce, and suicide (Myers & Diener, 1996). They also seem to cope better with adversity. Religious practice is positively associated with interpersonal wellbeing, purpose in life, and personal growth, but less with autonomy. On the other hand, *general* spirituality is associated with all aspects of wellbeing (Ryff, 2014).

Helping Others

Volunteering seems to make people happier, especially later in life, and inversely, people who are happier tend to volunteer more. Volunteering seems to serve multiple functions—it is prosocial, it can involve downward social comparison, and it is engaging. In addition, it can provide healthy distraction for people who are struggling with challenges such as illness or depression (Miller, 2012).

Age

Generally speaking, as people age, they experience more emotional wellbeing, mediated by lower affective arousal and more emotional maturity—they experience fewer and less intense positive *and* negative emotions. If people *feel* younger than they *actually* are, they have higher wellbeing. But if they *wish* they were younger than they actually are, they feel *less* happy (Diener & Ryan, 2009). In other words, people who have fewer illusions and who are more realistic about their age tend to fare better (Ryff, 2014).

Health, Exercise, and Sleep

People with higher wellbeing have fewer chronic health problems, better biological regulation (such as lower stress hormones and lower inflammation), less physiological reactivity, and lower healthcare utilization (Ryff, 2014). Ryan and Frederick (1997) have identified that people who are happier feel like they have more energy, suggesting that physical vitality is correlated with wellbeing. Not surprisingly, exercise and physical health appears to have multiple positive effects on wellbeing, such as the release of endorphins, improved immune functioning, elimination of toxins, improved sleep, enhanced self-esteem and a sense of accomplishment. In addition, people who have high-quality sleep also experience wellbeing in all areas. Conversely, people who have insomnia have reduced enjoyment in their lives, although no less meaning (Ryff, 2014). Our physical health also impacts our emotional wellbeing and our perceptions, a topic we will discuss in greater detail in Chapter 11 on meaning and perception.

Trying to be Happy

One of the paradoxical findings that has emerged in researching happiness is that people who focus too much on *trying to be happy* are *less happy* (Gruber, Mauss, & Tamir, 2011). When we are told we *should* be happy, it makes us *unhappy*. *Trying* to be happy appears to make us lonelier and more self-absorbed. It also seems to lead to unfavorable comparisons—we may believe that we should be happier than we are and experience a sense of disappointment that we are not. This is particularly problematic if our set range is generally lower or we are naturally more anxious in temperament, since our expectations may be out of alignment with what we might reasonably be able to achieve. The same is true if our efforts to be happier include *avoiding* being unhappy or feeling bad. What seems to be most helpful is if we focus less on trying to be happy and more on building wellbeing.

Chronic Happiness Level and Intentional Activities

Lyubomirsky, Sheldon, and Schkade (2005) maintained that the following factors contribute to happiness in these ratios: set point 50 percent, circumstances 10 percent, and intentional activities 40 percent. The latter two numbers are most significant. They suggest that, although we tend to attribute much of our happiness to our histories and to variables outside of ourselves, in fact they only account for 60 percent of actual happiness. Although this is significant, it leaves 40 percent which we can cotrol by utilizing strategies that help us cope with set point, environmental factors, and exposure to adversity. We will explore this further when we look at ways we can intentionally boost our happiness and wellbeing despite challenges that we are either prone to inherently or that we have encountered along the way.

Practical Applications for Increasing Happiness and Wellbeing

As we can see from operating theories of wellbeing, many factors contribute to and are affected by wellbeing. At times, it has seemed daunting to find ways to systematically conceptualize the breadth of this material and initiate utilizing it in therapy. Before attempting to do so, we begin with the caveat that, as decades of research has firmly established, therapy in and of itself, because it is founded upon an empathic and supportive interpersonal relationship, is effective regardless of approach (Lambert & Barley, 2001).

In addition, just as we, the authors, were initially trained in a particular clinical paradigm, most practitioners reading this book, whether they are art therapists or other mental health professionals, are also undoubtedly guided by their own orientation—be it psychodynamic, gestalt, family systems, solution-focused, client-centered, or an eclectic blend of those approaches. They may also have further training in specific interventions—Eye Movement Desensitization Reprocessing Therapy, Cognitive Behavioral Therapy, Dialectical Behavioral Therapy, Mindfulness-Based Stress Reduction, etc. Rather than refuting or contradicting any of this training and background, we suggest that a positive psychology approach may be seen more as a means of building upon existing theoretical foundations with complementary strategies for *exploring and increasing happiness and wellbeing*. With this in mind, positive psychology may be distinguished as much by a focus as by a method (Biswas-Diener, 2013).

As positive psychologist James Pawelski has suggested, positive psychology *actively aims* at optimal functioning whereas *psychology-as-usual* focuses *more* on identifying and solving problems, reducing suffering, and returning people to normal functioning (in Biswas-Diener, 2013). It is important to note that alleviating suffering and helping our clients cope with challenges is critical to the therapeutic process. In actual practice, positive psychology and a *psychology-as-usual* approach are not mutually exclusive and perhaps should never be. We can alternately address problems and increase wellbeing at any given moment, and doing one will naturally affect the other.

On the other hand, it has been provocatively suggested that positive psychology interventions, when appropriately implemented and properly timed, might be as successful, if not more so, at reducing suffering and helping people cope as traditional "problem-focused" strategies (Seligman, Rashid, & Parks, 2006). For example, Seligman observed that although the curative nature of the therapeutic relationship is now implicitly understood, too little attention is paid in the training of clinicians to systematically cultivating the skills that promote this critical alliance. These include warming up clients to and engaging them in the therapeutic process, instilling hope, universality, and altruism (Yalom, 1995), and identifying the strengths and resources that have helped clients survive (De Shazer, 1985). They also include harnessing the *undoing effect* of positive emotions—the capacity of feelings such as love, compassion, gratitude, curiosity, and even amusement to help people cope in the midst of difficulties and to recover more quickly from stress and negative events (Fredrickson et al., 2003).

Positive interventions also capitalize on the ability of positive emotions to help people experience a shift in their perceptions and find positive meaning in the difficulties they have encountered. This promotes resilience which, in turn, buffers against future stress (Fredrickson et al., 2003). In addition, shifting from a problem-focused paradigm to one that attends more to positive experience, positive meaning, and positive relationships often by default lessens the stranglehold that stress, trauma, and pain have over our lives. It is not that difficulties and problems disappear, or that disease and mental disorder are cured, but that their prominence recedes so that other possibilities can become visible: "The aim of positive psychology is to begin to catalyze a change in the focus of psychology from preoccupation only with repairing the worst things in life to also building positive qualities" (Seligman & Csíkszentmihályi, 2000, p. 5).

We will now transition from a broader survey of positive psychology, happiness, and wellbeing, to journey into the specific interplay between those concepts and art therapy. As we mentioned earlier, we will predominantly be using Seligman's (2011) model of PERMA as a framework for approaching this endeavor. This is partly because, in our estimation, the PERMA domains—positive emotions, engagement, relationships, meaning, and accomplishment—effectively account for the components of both subjective wellbeing (SWB) and psychological wellbeing (PWB). In addition, the PERMA model seems to provide the best platform not only to demonstrate the relevance of positive psychology to art therapy, but, even more exciting for us as art therapists, to showcase the unique benefits that art therapy brings to positive psychology.

Discussion Questions

1   After visiting the University of Pennsylvania Authentic Happiness website (https://www.authentichappiness.sas.upenn.edu/testcenter) and taking the *Approaches to Happiness* questionnaire and the *Authentic Happiness Inventory*, what did you learn about your own happiness and wellbeing?
2   What factors contribute most to your happiness and wellbeing?
3   What cultural factors have influenced your beliefs about happiness and wellbeing?
4   As you think about the clients with whom you work, what factors contribute most to *their* happiness and wellbeing?

CHAPTER 4

Positive Art Therapy Emerges

From the moment we first learned about positive psychology, it forever changed not only our personal lives but also how we saw ourselves as art therapists, how we worked with our clients, and how we perceived our field relative to other professions. We were so inspired by this transforming work that we made it our mission to bring what we are learning about positive psychology to the art therapy community and, in turn, to bring the magic of art therapy to the world of positive psychology.

Positive Art Therapy and PERMA

When we initially conceptualized "positive art therapy" (Chilton & Wilkinson, 2009), we adopted Seligman's (2002) model of *Authentic Happiness* without much critical thought. The three paths to happiness—positive emotions (the pleasant life), engagement (the engaged life), and meaning (the meaningful life)—seemed to fit well with our efforts to apply positive psychology principles to the theory, research, and practice of art therapy (Chilton & Wilkinson, 2009).

When Seligman (2012) replaced Authentic Happiness with PERMA, we realized that we needed to go back to the drawing board and determine which approach to wellbeing would serve as the best framework for conceptualizing an updated version of positive art therapy. Subject wellbeing? Psychological wellbeing? Flourishing? This was especially relevant after we'd immersed ourselves in studying positive psychology and recognized the breadth of concepts wellbeing touches on: positive emotions, gratitude, mindfulness, stress management, hope theory, creativity, strengths, flow, positive relationships, purpose and meaning, perception, the negativity bias, the hedonic treadmill, set point, posttraumatic growth, benefit-finding, positive assessment, optimism/pessimism, motivation, self-determination theory, achievement, positive organizational development, appreciative inquiry, compassion satisfaction, and positive ethics. Whew!

Figuring out how to present all of these concepts relative to the field of art therapy seemed overwhelming. Over many Starbucks planning sessions, we argued about how to structure the wide range of material that we knew should be included. We needed a new framework—and more coffee! Thankfully the Starbucks baristas knew our orders by then and were happy to serve up as many grande vanilla lattes (Gioia's—sweet) and short triple decaf espresso macchiatos (Rebecca's—intense) as needed. Finally, almost knocking over her cup, Rebecca exclaimed, "PERMA!—it all fits in PERMA!"

Just as at the beginning of this journey we had naturally gravitated toward Seligman's Three Paths, we realized that his more recent model of wellbeing— PERMA—provided the most useful framework for updating our approach to the interplay between the world of positive psychology and art therapy. PERMA, which included five pathways—Positive emotions, Engagement, Relationships, Meaning, and Achievement—seemed to account for both the emotional components of *subjective wellbeing* and the optimal functioning characteristic of *psychological wellbeing*. It seemed to provide a structure upon which the field of art therapy could coherently be superimposed to illustrate how the latter can boost wellbeing.

Throughout this book, we'll explore the relevance of PERMA to the field of art therapy and how art therapy contributes uniquely to increasing wellbeing. Although we examine the PERMA categories as if they were discrete domains, in reality, they each have an impact on and are often integral to one another, especially when we combine artmaking and the art therapy process to the mix. For example, simply making art often leads to *positive emotions* and *engagement* as well as satisfaction, pride and a sense of *achievement.* Creating art with others and having it appreciatively received also fosters connection and positive *relationships*. These encounters help shift perceptions and lead to more expansive *meaning* and sense of possibility.

Parallels in the Evolution of Art Therapy and Positive Psychology

As we studied the emergence of positive psychology in the broader context of psychology in general, we were struck by parallels in the evolution of the field of art therapy. Because art therapy has profound roots in psychology, it has mirrored many of the latter's theoretical developments along with many of the same limitations and challenges. In the following brief survey, we compare some of these historical developments. There are many sources for more in-depth reviews of art therapy (Vick, 2003; Rubin, 1999). We draw from those here.

Foundations of Art Therapy

Art therapy was born from many traditions. It integrates diverse sources beyond the realm of psychology such as art education, art history, outsider art, art brut, and folk art (Lowenfeld, 1957; Malchiodi, 2006; Rubin, 1999).

Dissanayake (2003), an anthropologist, was instrumental in identifying that our impulse to create evolved from core human motivations, such as the need to communicate, to form social cohesion, and to "make special" (p. 95). She points to 40,000+-year-old cave paintings found around the globe which, through imagery, illustrate our first recorded history and, through action, one of the characteristics that defines humans—the desire to make art to honor and celebrate our experience. Evidence exists in all cultures of creative and artistic practices that contribute both to helping societies flourish and to archiving that experience.

Psychoanalytic Traditions in Art Therapy

Certainly the psychological relevance of art and the creative process was explored by early psychologists well before the field of art therapy emerged as its own profession in the 1940s and 1950s. For example, Freud (1930) viewed artistic expression as a manifestation of sublimation, one of the few defense mechanisms which—as opposed to others such as repression and displacement that reflected neurosis—led to better psychological adjustment. He suggested that creative expression was among the most valuable forms of sublimation because it allowed the artist to channel unconscious libidinal impulses into productive activities that were not only socially acceptable but highly valued. He also believed that art derived from the unconscious realm of the psyche and that, just as one could interpret dreams through the process of free association, so too could they determine the artist's mental state from their artwork. More specifically, that artwork could shed light on the artist's inner conflicts and repressed anxieties (Kofman, 1988).

Neo-Freudian and Humanist Influences on Art Therapy

Freud often dialogued with an Italian contemporary, Roberto Assagioli (1959) about the role of the arts and creativity in human development. Assagioli took a much more celebratory view of artistic endeavors, best articulated in his theory of *Psychosynthesis*, a holistic approach which championed positive aspects of humanity such as spirituality, wisdom, and creativity. Assagioli (1942) was influenced by Eastern practices which led him to conclude that if we undertook to live a spiritual life, we could overcome "the dark night of the soul" and arrive at *nirvana*, a state of transcendent joy (p. 168). Assagioli used artmaking, movement, visualization, active imagination, role-playing, and creative writing for dialoguing with and integrating conflicted parts of the self.

Jung also believed that art served as a means of bringing unconscious material to conscious awareness. Like Freud, Jung frequently encouraged his patients to draw and paint their dreams—to use the meaning derived from the imagery to cope with trauma and emotional distress. However, Jung saw art as a gateway to *all* aspects of consciousness—that it represented a synthesis between outside reality and the subjective inner world of the artist. Jung wrote, "in order to do justice to a work of art, analytical psychology must rid itself entirely of medical prejudice, for a work of art is not a disease, and consequently requires a different approach from a medical one" (Jung, 1966/2014, p. 71).

Jung was convinced that creative energy was driven by a "supra-personal force" that soared "beyond the personal concerns of its creator" (Jung, 1966/2014, p. 71). He believed that artistic imagery revealed archetypal symbols which transcended the individual and originated from the *collective unconscious*, a universal realm of human experience (Guttman & Dafna, 2004). Jung himself used the art process throughout his life as a means to explore his inner world and overcome moments of personal crisis, examples of which we now have the pleasure of viewing in *The Red Book* (Jung, 2009).

Winnicott (1971) was also influenced by Freud but believed that the latter placed too much emphasis on psychoanalyzing unconscious processes and not enough on the significance of relational phenomena. Winnicott observed that play behaviors which manifest in early infancy serve to create the *transitional space* that allows the developing child to connect their interior world with exterior "reality." Artmaking provided a creative and yet safe way to "play" in this transitional realm and the resulting artwork could serve as a *transitional object*, a comforting bridge between the self and others. Like Jung, Winnicott believed that symbols in artwork were culturally bound and could therefore communicate in ways that could intuitively be understood by others. He developed the "Scribble Drawing" technique—finding and developing an image from scribbles—as a means of warming children up to the drawing process and pulling for unconscious material.

Art Therapy in the United States

Art therapy crystallized as its own profession in the United States around the mid-twentieth century, articulated in the writings of Margaret Naumburg and Edith Kramer. These pioneers were part of the *first force* of psychology. Both were heavily influenced by Freudian psychoanalytic theory and both believed that unconscious forces were operating in the art process. However, they applied Freudian principles in different ways. Naumburg (1966) proposed that art allows for the uncovering and externalizing unconscious material. In her approach, *dynamically oriented art therapy*, the artwork and the art process serve primarily as a form of *symbolic speech* whose content could enhance the psychoanalytic process. In Kramer's (1958) approach, *art as therapy*, artmaking facilitates sublimation of unacceptable unconscious material. She maintained that it allowed for chaotic, primary process material to be channeled into constructive and ordered experience.

Behaviorism, the *second force*, which emerged in the early and mid-twentieth century, had less influence on the development of art therapy. Behaviorists used the scientific method to study observable phenomena—they were not interested in mental events which could not be seen and measured, such as imagination, memories, and consciousness (Roediger, 2004). These processes, as well as other elements inherent to art, such as creativity, visual symbolism, and the healing nature of engaging in artmaking, would have been outside the purview of behavioral science at that time. Those features were, on the other hand, of much interest to grassroots art therapists—then more often art educators or artists than therapists—who were not working in labs, but in schools, hospitals, and institutions.

For instance, in the US, Mary Huntoon, a Kansas art teacher and art therapist, worked from the 1930s through the 1950s with people with psychiatric diagnoses and World War II veterans in studio settings, focusing on art expression as a healing process (Wix, 2000). On the East Coast, Cliff Joseph, Myra Levick, and Edith Kramer, helped establish the American Art Therapy in 1967 (Joseph, 2006). Joseph taught at the Pratt Institute, in the first humanist art therapy program, established in 1970. Joseph, a civil rights activist, was influential in promoting multiculturally informed art therapy practices (Riley-Hiscox, 1997).

Art Therapy in the UK

Art therapy in the United Kingdom was also emerging in the grassroots, seen mid-century in the collaborative work of artists Adrian Hill and Edward Adamson. Although neither identified as art therapists, they both championed the healing benefits of doing artwork and Hill (1945) is actually credited with coining the term "art therapy." Hill, having used art to help recover from a medical illness, taught art classes and organized art shows in hospitals and institutions to help others do the same. Adamson saw Hill's work and was inspired to create studio spaces in psychiatric settings to give patients opportunities to express themselves artistically (Guttman & Regev, 2004). Adamson rejected the notion that patients' art should be used to psychoanalyze the artists—instead he adopted more humanist beliefs, e.g., that having the opportunity to create art in a safe and inspiring environment was healing.

Humanism and Art Therapy

Humanism also surfaced in the evolution of art therapy practices in the United States. For example, Mala Betensky (1977) combined art therapy with *phenomenology*—the study of the individual's subjective experience of consciousness. Betensky believed that psychodynamic art therapy and art-as-therapy did not adequately explain the creative process. Looking at the building blocks of line, form, color, shapes, and symbols, Betensky described artistic expressions as arising from our fundamental need not only to make things with our hands, but to find patterns and deeper meaning in this work and to convey that to others. Through visual perception, art therapy could induce the kind of self-discovery that brings about a "synthesis between the inside and the outside reality" (Betensky, 1977, p. 179).

Janie Rhyne (1973), another influential humanist art therapist, focused on what she called the *Gestalt Art Experience*. She applied Rudolf Arnheim's (1974) principle of *isomorphism*—the suggestion that the visual elements in artwork can be directly linked to the artist's internal experience—to art therapy. She used *visual thinking* to help clients perceive the *gestalt* of their images— beholding the unified whole of the artwork rather than focusing on specific elements. Rhyne foreshadowed the current focus on mindfulness through simple drawing activities designed to increase self-awareness, such as "begin where you are" to "bring yourself into direct contact with what you are feeling and thinking now" (Rhyne, 1973, p. 102).

Art therapy educator Bruce Moon (2009) articulated an *existential* approach to art therapy that addresses "the ultimate concerns of human existence"— meaning, aloneness, suffering, freedom, purpose in life, and death. He believes that art allows expression of that existential *angst* and helps bridge the separation between ourselves and others. Moon encourages art therapists to do art with and alongside clients as a way not only to witness and honor their pain, but to participate in a shared artistic journey.

Silverstone (1997) developed *person-centered art therapy* which applied Rogers' principles—authentic connection and unconditional positive regard— to art therapy. Many art therapists naturally gravitate toward this approach, intuitively grasping that artmaking inherently shows us the virtue of creativity and self-actualization, and adopting client-centered methods in their manner of engaging with their clients. Other art therapists have incorporated a humanist approach in their work. For example, Roger's daughter, Natalie Rogers (1993), combined her father's client-centered approach with dance, music, art, and poetry. Shaun McNiff (1992), another pioneer in the *expressive arts therapies*, adopts a multimodal approach to "creating a therapy of the imagination."

Developmental Models of Art Therapy

In the late 1950s, art educator Viktor Lowenfeld's (1957) work built on Jean Piaget's theories of childhood development which suggested that children perform certain tasks only when they progress through discrete stages of cognitive development. Lowenfeld identified that children do the same in their artistic development. For example, children first scribble, then, as fine and gross motor skills develop, scribbling becomes more controlled and refined until recognizable representational imagery emerges. Over time, the child's aesthetic, social, physical, intellectual, and emotional growth leads to progressively more complex imagery.

Rhoda Kellogg (1967/2007) conducted research related to children's artistic development, collecting almost a million children's drawings. Like Lowenfeld,

Kellogg identified stages of graphic development in which specific visual elements such as scribbles, diagrams, radials, mandala patterns, humans, and animals emerge (see the Child Art Collection, available at www.early-pictures. ch/kellogg).

Rawley Silver (2001) observed that language deficiencies can often mask intelligence and that imagery can help assess and develop cognitive skills. Silver used a series of *stimulus drawings* to determine a child's level of intellectual development. This included a series of exercises which measured the capacity to imaginatively form relationships between unrelated objects, to recreate visual arrangements (drawing shapes in particular sequence) and to project changes in a sequence (how sipping from a straw would reduce the liquid in a glass).

The *Expressive Therapies Continuum* (ETC) developed by Kagin and Lusebrink (1978), incorporated graphic and cognitive development into advances in our understanding of brain function and information processing. This foundational construct describes different levels of visual expression which range from spontaneous free-form activity to the representation of thoughts and feelings. The ETC serves as a guidepost for understanding how media choices both reflect levels of brain processing and influence how we, as art therapists, either consciously or intuitively choose media and directives for our clients (Hinz, 2009).

Cognitive Behavioral Approaches to Art Therapy

Art therapy educator Marcia Rosal is perhaps most associated with cognitive behavioral applications to art therapy (CBAT). Rosal (2016) observed that although most art therapists don't identify with cognitive behavioral approaches, they may intuitively be using them if they are teaching strategies for stress reduction, problem solving, emotional regulation, shifting perceptions, and increasing self-efficacy. Rosal suggests that CBAT is, at its core, about visualizing and reframing stressful and traumatic thoughts, actions, and events.

Rosal (2016) identified that cognitive strategies have been used in art therapy in a variety of ways: developing organized schemas from confused and dysfunctional thoughts and feelings, regulating emotional responses by exploring and analyzing personal constructs that create feelings, anger management by addressing stereotyped responses deriving from rigid cognitive constructs, problem solving and coping by creating shifts in dysfunctional thinking, modeling of pro-social behaviors, perspective taking, relaxation, visualization, stress management, and systematic desensitization to traumatic memories.

Malchiodi and Loth Rozum (2011) have also explored the use of cognitive behavioral strategies in art therapy. They suggest that art can help to identify schemas that underlie negative thoughts, to reframe negative experiences, and to experiment with more positive assumptions. Czamanski-Cohen and colleagues (Czamanski-Cohen, Sarid, Huss, Ifergane, Niego, & Cwikel, 2014) conducted research on CBAT with women struggling with pain, anxiety, and depression, having them first make art that focused on their symptoms, then combining psycho-educational strategies for accessing coping resources with modifying their artwork so that the images became more adaptive and the symptoms more manageable.

Other Developments in Art Therapy

Art therapy has followed other developments in the broader scope of mental health. Kwiatkowska (1967) articulated a system's approach to Family Art Therapy. Landgarten (1981) combined psychodynamic and systems theories in her work with families. Many art therapists have written on applications of art therapy with specific populations and in various settings—people with developmental delays, psychiatric patients, people with eating disorders, children with behavioral problems and learning disabilities, medical patients, substance abusers, clients with degenerative cognitive and physical conditions, dying patients, prison inmates, the list goes on.

Art Therapy and the Medical Model

Despite our diverse trans-disciplinary roots, art therapy as a profession has progressively gravitated toward a medical model. Art therapist Randy Vick observed that medical facilities "have long served as important incubators for the field of art therapy" (2003, p. 6). He added that, "for better or worse, medical model concepts such as diagnosis, disease, and treatment have had a strong influence on the development of most schools of thought within Western psychotherapy, including art therapy" (2003, p. 6).

Just as most training in counseling, social work, psychology and other mental health fields gravitates around a medical model, so now do most of the art therapy graduate programs. For example, as our field has attempted to stay relevant in the culture of managed care and mental health licensing, most of our graduate programs now include assessment and diagnosis. In addition, training related to treatment planning is usually based upon identification of clients' presenting problems, impairment in functioning, and interpersonal conflict.

Art therapy assessments such as the *Diagnostic Drawing Series* (Cohen, Mills, & Kijak, 1994), and the Formal Elements Art Therapy Scale (FEATS) (Gantt, 2009) are most often presented vis-à-vis their capacity to contribute to, or to correlate with, *DSM* diagnosis. Even drawing tasks whose titles sound less clinical and more metaphoric, such as the "Bird's Nest Drawing" (Kaiser, 1996), the "Person Picking an Apple from a Tree" (Gantt, 1990), the "Bridge Drawing" (Hays & Lyons, 1981) or the "Road Drawing" (Hanes, 1995) have been primarily used to evaluate dysfunction and pathology.

In addition, art therapy educator Sarah Deaver observed, "most research in this area focuses upon deviations from the norm—aspects of drawings assumed to represent maladjustment, impairment, or disturbance rather than upon what 'the norm' actually is" (2009, pp. 4–5). Recently, art therapy researchers have begun trying to establish baselines for what might be "normal" in children's artwork (Bucciarelli, 2011).

Congdon suggested that we shift from centering our focus on mental illness to developing art therapy theory which recognizes "normalized problem-solving" (1990, p. 19). We might suggest that *art therapy-as-usual*, like *psychology-as-usual*, might be critiqued for focusing so much on mental illness and symptomatology that it has overlooked what it means to be "normal" and yet struggle with the challenges of daily living. In addition, because "normal" and "healthy" are not always the same, art therapy might also go *beyond* establishing norms to developing clear and systematic indicators of mental health and wellbeing (Chilton & Wilkinson, 2009; Betts, 2012).

Art therapy has struggled to maintain its unique identity while trying to carve out its place as a viable field within the medical model and in the professional marketplace. Although art therapists are employed in a wide array of settings—psychiatric units, schools, clinics, homeless shelters, community health, and the fine arts world—they sometimes find that they do not quite fit in any of these venues. Art therapy is often an outlier, awkward for institutions to manage—it is not strictly verbal psychotherapy, art instruction, or recreation. Art therapists negotiating for positions in these settings have often been misidentified as counselors, activity therapists, occupational therapists, and art teachers. Their unique combination of skills—part expert in art, part expert in therapy—frequently presents a conundrum which is not easily resolved.

Who Are We?

The inherent interdisciplinary nature of art therapy has created an interesting dynamic in the evolution of our profession since its earliest formation. Art therapy pioneer Elinor Ulman (2001) suggested that art therapists, by balancing artmaking and psychotherapy, create a synthesis which streamlines the psychotherapeutic process. She explained that, although art therapists might at any given moment sacrifice artistic achievement for insight and vice versa, their skill lay in not straying so far from either that it lost its efficacy.

Judith Rubin, whose early work in the 1960s as the "art lady" on the television show *Mister Rogers' Neighborhood* gained her an enduring spot in pop culture, spent much of her career explaining the process of art therapy in accessible manner. In a short but seminal article published in 1982, titled "Art Therapy: What It Is and What It Is Not," Rubin masterfully presented art therapy's challenge—because so often art therapy, on the surface, looks like art for educational or recreational purposes, it can be easily confused as such. However, it is the therapeutic *intent* of the session which makes the difference between art for therapy and art for any other purpose, a nuance lost on many.

Rubin (2011) suggests that the *synergy* of the *art part* and the *therapy part* makes art therapy much more complex than either of those parts alone. The extensive training necessary to navigate the interface between these two processes is rarely understood and appreciated by practitioners outside of the field. Although they often "get" that art therapy is very helpful, they do not comprehend the delicate balance required in what art therapists do.

Art therapists such as Pat Allen (1992) have pointed out that social and economic pressures have led to the *clinification* of the field at the expense of what makes it unique. In addition, because of licensure issues, many art therapists have had to cross-train in counseling or other fields, such as marriage and family therapy; often having to take additional coursework to fulfill state licensure requirements. That might entail repeating content which was covered in graduate art therapy training—i.e., diagnosis, assessment, ethics, and even basic counseling— but was taught under the umbrella of art therapy.

For example, Virginia does not license art therapists. As a result, Gioia, in order to work as an art therapist in a drug and alcohol treatment center in Virginia, had to become a certified substance abuse counselor. Despite the fact that she has a doctorate in creative art therapy, is a nationally registered and board certified art therapist, and is licensed as an art therapist in the state of Maryland, she still had to take additional coursework and another comprehensive exam, not to mention the time and expense of fulfilling the continuing education requirements, acquiring additional supervision, and the annual fees for maintaining these other credentials.

On the other hand, one of the benefits of the push toward licensure and evidence-based practices is that students being trained in art therapy today have a much more research-informed comprehension of the field than those of us who were trained in the 1990s or before. In addition, they do not experience conflict between *art psychotherapy* and *art-as-therapy*—that is, art's capacity to communicate symbolically versus the inherently healing nature of engaging in the art process—with which many of us from an earlier era struggled. Thankfully, research is now confirming the validity of both (Hartz & Thick, 2005; Wadeson, 2002).

We also have a better understanding of the neuroscience and body-mind interface that occurs during the art therapy process. (Chapman et al., 2001; Chilton, 2013; Belkofer & Konopka, 2008; McNamee, 2005; Hass-Cohen, Kaplan, & Carr, 2008; Lusebrink, 2004). For example, Perry (2009) identified that the creative arts positively regulate core functions of the brain which effect heart rate, blood pressure, and body temperature. We also have an enriched view of the therapeutic nature of the art process itself—that artistic creation is more than just channeling aggressive impulses or, at best, sublimation. Instead, it is now understood to have multiple measurable healing effects, such as reducing anxiety, inducing the relaxation response, facilitating expression, fostering creativity, inducing flow, increasing the capacity to focus and reflect, promoting perspective taking and meaning making, and producing feelings of mastery (Czamanski-Cohen, 2016).

Positive Art Therapy Emerges as Part of Art Therapy's Fourth Force

Recall that we seem to be in the midst of a *fourth force*, a time of trans-disciplinary, transpersonal approaches which challenge the reductionism of the medical model with more expansive mind-body integration. We see this trend in the art therapy world as well. For example, Michael Franklin and his colleagues have incorporated transpersonal psychology and traditional wisdom into art therapy practice and training (Franklin, 2016, 2010; Franklin, Farrelly-Hansen, Marek, Swan-Foster, & Wallingford, 2000). Farrelly-Hansen (2001) edited a book titled *Spirituality and Art Therapy: Living the Connection*, featuring contributions from many of the art therapists we know and love.

In addition, as Eastern spiritual practices were finding their way into the broader spectrum of psychology, so too have similar practices emerged in art therapy. For example, art therapists have combined mindfulness techniques with art therapy to increase tolerance for negative affect, emotional regulation, and impulse control (Monti et al., 2006; Peterson, 2013; Heckwolf, Bergland, & Mouratidis, 2014; Huckvale & Learmonth, 2009). Laury Rappaport (2013) edited *Mindfulness and the Arts Therapies* which outlines current work in this area. Rappaport (2008) also developed *Focus-Oriented Art Therapy* (FOAT), which involves attending to the *felt sense*—i.e., bypassing limitations of the cognitive mind by tapping into what we feel and know through body sensations.

Art therapy has been combined with other emerging approaches. For example, Shirley Riley (2013) applied social constructivist theories to *narrative art therapy*, observing that art was particularly useful in creating "new resolutions to old scripts" (p. 284). Mooney (2000) did so as well, incorporating solution-focused interventions into art therapy. McNamee (2005), Talwar (2007), and Tripp (2007) have combined art therapy with EMDR, integrating traumatic memories through combining bilateral stimulation with negative and positive cognitions and artmaking.

We also include the efforts of art therapists to improve social justice in art therapy and increase awareness of the *intersectionality* of cultural influences in shaping us (Gipson, 2015; Hocoy, 2005; Junge, Alvarez, Kellogg, & Volker, 1993; Potash, 2011, 2005; Talwar, 2010; Talwar, Moon, Timm-Bottos, & Kapitan, 2015). We observe that social justice is a character strength that is naturally congruent with the sensibilities of art therapists—many of whom quietly (or audibly!) and persistently advocate for the needs of people who are often unseen, overlooked, and underrepresented. In addition, art therapists know that even though their beloved clients' voices may not always be heard, their artwork gives them a chance to be seen.

In some ways, art therapy in the fourth force reflects a diverse profession still finding ways to work within, but also to subvert and coopt, the medical model. *Positive art therapy* emerges in this current environment. We are noticing that students, practitioners, and researchers alike are keenly interested in how the science of wellbeing and positive psychology can intersect, partner with, and support art therapy research and practice. For example, both Rubin's most recent edition of *Approaches to Art Therapy: Theory and Technique*, one of the seminal textbooks in the field, and *The Wiley Handbook of Art Therapy*, edited by Gussak and Rosal, include chapters on positive art therapy (Chilton & Wilkinson, 2016; Isis, 2015).

Scholarship in Positive Art Therapy

In addition, the body of art therapy scholarship which addresses many of the elements of PERMA and wellbeing is growing. For example, the use of positive psychology tools such as quality of life measures demonstrate art therapy's overall impact on health for people with cancer (Nainis et al., 2006; Öster et al., 2006; Puig, Lee, Goodwin, & Sherrard, 2006; Svensk et al., 2009). DeLue (1999) conducted research with school-aged children and determined that drawing mandalas induced the relaxation response. Research has also shown that artmaking repairs mood and increases positive emotions (Babouchkina & Robbins, 2015; Bell & Robbins, 2007; Kimport & Robbins, 2012; Smolarski, Leone, & Robbins, 2015). Artmaking with a positive focus appears to produce even more increases in positive emotions (Dalebroux, Goldstein, & Winner, 2008; De Petrillo & Winner, 2005; Henderson, Rosen, Sotirova-Kohli, & Stephenson, 2009; Manheim, 1998).

Art therapy and artmaking have also been linked to other aspects of wellbeing. For example, Visser and Op'T Hoog (2008) in their research with cancer patients, established that the creative art therapies promoted positive social interaction and coping skills. Trauger-Querry and Haghighi (1999) determined that art therapy helped cancer patients experience a reduction in their pain and helped them feel more peaceful in the face of challenges that cancer posed to their mortality. Reynolds and Prior (2003) also found that art therapy was helpful in distracting cancer patients from their pain, as well as in restoring self-image and regaining an ability to project themselves into the future, filling an occupational void, and giving them a sense of choice and control.

Öster and colleagues (Öster et al., 2006; Öster, Magnusson, Thyme, Lindh, & Åström, 2007) established that art therapy improved self image, quality of life, and coping resources for women with cancer, particularly in the area of social support. Svensk and colleagues (2009) reported that art therapy interventions improved physical and psychological health, self-image, and future orientation with breast cancer patients undergoing treatment. Czamanski-Cohen (2012) and Czamanski-Cohen and colleagues (2014) determined that art therapy helped patients with chronic illness cope better with their symptoms, manage distress about and move forward with decisions in their treatment, and reconcile conflicted feelings they had about treatment choices they had made in the past.

Positive psychology co-founder Mihaly Csíkszentmihályi's (1991) research into *flow* has also been studied by art therapists (Kaplan, 2000; Malchiodi, 2006; Lee, 2009, 2013; Chilton, 2013; Burkewitz, 2014; Hovick, 2014). For example, Voytilla (2006) found that participants in an open-studio art therapy setting measurably experienced flow during the artmaking process. Hovick (2014) determined that using Cane's (1951) gestural movements—such as broad sweeping arm motions—to warm participants up to the art process enhanced the intrinsically rewarding aspects of the flow state. Flow leads to feelings of engagement, mastery and accomplishment, factors that we know are fundamentally important in art therapy (Kramer, 1971).

Other art therapy therapists are also addressing topics related to PERMA. For example, Darewych (2013, 2014) modified the bridge drawing to assess hope and life meaning in institutionalized orphans in the Ukraine and college students in Britain and Canada. She found that asking people to draw a bridge with a path and to relate a narrative about what they had made was an effective tool for exploring meaning and purpose in life. Participants who scored higher in "presence of meaning" drew more sources-of-life-meaning paths (such as to relationships, careers, or spirituality) in their images than participants with lower scores (Darewych, 2014).

Betts (2012) advocates for *positive art therapy assessment* which involves using strengths and the assessment process to build the therapeutic alliance. In the realm of professional development, Hinz (2011) has inspired art therapists to adopt a positive approach to ethical decision-making, moving from a fear-based risk-management perspective to more aspirational striving for ethical excellence. Riddle and riddle [*sic*] (2007), in their research with male art therapists using the *Values in Action Survey*, determined that, above and beyond other strengths, they shared "appreciation for beauty and excellence" and "curiosity and interest in the world." Riddle and riddle speculated that these strengths would generalize to all art therapists.

In the chapters ahead we will explore these lines of inquiry in more detail. We expect interest, scholarship, and research into the interplay between well-being, positive psychology, creativity, and art therapy to continue growing, even as we are writing this book.

Positive Psychologists Recognize the Value of the Creative Arts Therapies

As we proceed with conceptualizing positive art therapy, our intention is not only to illustrate how art therapists can benefit from learning more about the science of happiness, but also to articulate how art therapy uniquely contributes to improving mental health and wellbeing.

Because art therapy is such a small field and its base of research is still limited, it has yet to gain significant recognition in the world of positive psychology. However, unlike in the broader scope of mental health where art therapy is often viewed as peripheral or adjunctive to "real" therapy, in positive psychology there is broad-based assumption that creativity and art have a fundamental role in wellbeing and the life well-lived. For example, Peterson and Seligman observed that "creativity is often seen as a sign of mental health and emotional well-being. In fact, various art and music therapies emerged that promote psychological adjustment and growth through creative expression" (2004, p. 96).

Other positive psychologists have recognized the value of the expressive arts in wellbeing. For example, when we attended the 2009 IPPA Congress, we participated in an art therapy focus group led by art therapist/coach Poppy Spencer. At this same conference, Australian psychologist Dianne Vella-Broderick (2009) identified that most of the research on positive psychology interventions had focused on verbal and written activities and that non-verbal interventions might be more useful for some populations. More recently, art and music therapy were recognized in a chapter on rehabilitation psychology in the textbook *Positive Psychology in Practice* (Peter, Geyh, Ehde, Muller, & Jensen, 2015).

Positive psychologist Barbara Fredrickson (2009) recommends building *portfolios* or *scrapbooks* of photographs, images, poems, and inspirational messages to gain insight into and celebrate what uplifts and enlivens us. Michael Steger, who articulated the crossover between *Acceptance* and *Commitment Therapy* and positive psychology, suggests that, as a way of eliciting "growth narratives" from clients, that they become "photojournalists" and document "what makes their lives meaningful" (Steger, Sheline, Merriman, & Kashdan, 2013b, p. 235). Michael Frisch, who developed *Quality of Life Therapy*, identifies creative self-expression as "a major ingredient of a client's happiness stew" (2006, p. 281).

In addition, Diener and Ryan (2009) identified that many of the most effective positive psychology interventions are based upon a mix of cognitive-behavioral therapies and *activity theories*. They point to flow theory and propose that interventions designed to improve wellbeing are most effective when coupled with activities that are inherently engaging and rewarding. They note that many positive psychologists such as Lyubomirsky, Frisch, Seligman, Rashid, and Parks suggest combining strategies for promoting positive thinking and improved mood with relevant and enjoyable activities. Art naturally falls into such categories. In fact, engaging in art has been found to increase retention in therapy *just because it is enjoyable* (Pizarro, 2004).

Practicing Positive Art Therapy

In the last ten years, we have connected with many art therapists who are combining art therapy and positive psychology. For example, while we were developing our ideas about positive art therapy, across the world in Australia, art therapist Megan Booth and psychologist Jane Sleeman had been formulating their own thoughts on the topic. They developed "Strengths in a Box," a collection of 150 gorgeous flash cards which we often use with clients to help them identify their character strengths (Booth, 2007). We had the chance to meet Megan at the second IPPA Congress but, sadly, Jane had succumbed to cancer. Megan still carries forward their mission to bring creativity and art to the practice of positive psychology.

Two French-Canadian art therapists, Jacinthe Lambert and Diane Ranger (2009), also wrote about their approach to "*L'art therapie et la psychologie positive.*" Here in the US, Patricia Isis (2015) incorporates positive art therapy and mindfulness into her practice with adolescents, and Cathy Malchiodi teaches positive psychology and art therapy at Prescott College's graduate Creative Arts Therapies Program.

In Tennessee, art therapist Paige Scheinberg developed *Wellness Arts* which combines her "love for art therapy, positive psychology, happiness, art, design, discovery, and life!" Just as we had, Paige observed that in all of the institutions where she worked, there was a focus on "what is wrong with people, what labels they have, and how we can work with them to decrease their symptoms" (in personal communication). She has since made it her mission to advocate and educate about art therapy and the practice of positive psychology:

> For me, positive psychology and (positive) art therapy have become a way of life … I strive to live the science of happiness and well-being in my relationships, in my goals, and in my daily experiences. And, it seems the more I step into it and live it, the happier and more "successful" I become! (Personal communication, 2016)

Our students have also taught us how they are incorporating a positive psychology worldview into their work. For example, GW graduate art therapy student Amelia Zakour wrote to us that, for her:

> Positive Psychology marries beautifully with Art Therapy because both fields are inherently strength-focused and client-driven. In my work with medically ill children, the artmaking itself is a strength and an accomplishment. Often times, patients lie in their beds unengaged or passively watching television. So when a patient feels empowered enough to even just choose a material, I view this as a strength. Strength-spotting and validating have been important with my individual adult client as well. We live in a culture that often asks us to examine our flaws, but less frequently enables us to celebrate our strengths. When I asked my client about her strengths, she could not even think of one. So we have been exploring this through directives like strength stones and writing down positive affirmations. These affirmations have started out with simply trying to identify one small thing she did well or enjoyed that day. (Personal communication, March 5, 2016)

Although much of the book outlines how positive art therapy can be applied with clients, in the end it is perhaps most important to think about the ways that we can directly apply it to *ourselves*. Exploring the world of positive art therapy should be more than just an intellectual exercise—it should be a full immersion of mind, body, and spirit. That means that *we* experience more positive emotions, that *we* find the benefits that we have gotten from and ways that we have learned to regulate negative emotions or, as art therapist Tiffanie Brumfield says "feeling positive about being negative." It means that *we* experience more creativity and flow; that *we* recognize and engage more of our energizing strengths, that *we* become strengths spotters, and that *we* celebrate the unique strengths that we share with others in our field.

Applying a positive art therapy lens to our lives also means that we find what brings passion, purpose, and meaning to our lives. It means that we use the art process to look at our assumptions and beliefs about the world, to tell our stories, and if we need to, to shift those narratives to find more positive meaning, and to experience growth and resilience from the adversity we have encountered.

It means that we use the art process as a witness and testimony to our triumphs. It means that we find a sense of accomplishment and pride from the artwork that we make and the work that we do. Finally, because practicing a positive art therapy approach improves the quality of *our* lives, we experience more satisfaction and enjoyment of *our work*. This will make it more sustainable and makes us much better able to help our clients, our communities, and humanity as a whole.

In the following chapters, we will outline the theory and practice of positive art therapy. As we mentioned, we will be using the PERMA model to structure this content. Before we do so, we introduce you the *Positive Art Therapy Manifesto* which highlights how we imagine positive psychology can positively impact art therapy and, in turn, the unique strengths that art therapy brings to the world of positive psychology.

Discussion Questions

1   How do the people/institutions that you interact with perceive art therapy with respect to other professions in your workplace?
2   Have you seen evidence of the medical model affecting your art therapy practice?
3   How have economic pressures and licensure requirements influenced your ability to practice as an art therapist and your professional choices?
4   As you get a glimpse of positive psychology, what are ways that you or others might already be practicing a positive psychology approach?

Interlude: The Positive Art Therapy Manifesto

How to Transform Art Therapy with Positive Psychology

- Apply it:
    - With clients of all levels of abilities/disabilities and functioning
    - At all stages of therapy
    - In any setting.
- Validate but do not dwell on problems and history of trauma.
- Induce positive emotions such as hope and feelings of universality to:
    - Warm up clients to therapy process
    - Foster willingness to engage in behaviors which require effort and/or risk
    - Increase investment in treatment.
- Empower clients by:
    - Finding exceptions when they have felt better
    - Visualizing what it would be like to experience more wellbeing
    - Exploring what happiness and wellbeing means to them
    - Recognizing the strengths and resources that have helped them persevere
    - Identifying positive motivations behind behaviors that may have become dysfunctional.
- Educate clients around factors that contribute to and interfere with happiness and wellbeing.
- Educate clients about the benefits of positive and negative emotions.
- Provide strategies to regulate positive and negative emotions, by:
    - Becoming more mindful of all emotions
    - Harnessing negative emotions—reducing but not eliminating them
    - Increasing the ratio of positive to negative emotions.
- Improve mood by using directives with a positive focus.
- Promote creativity by inducing positive emotions.

- Foster the healing benefit of flow by promoting creativity.
- Educate clients about strengths:
  - Identifying and developing strengths
  - Differentiating between those that are energizing and those that are depleting
  - Partnering with others to manage weaknesses and accomplish activities that are draining
  - Developing strengths-spotting skills—noticing strengths in others.

- Explore meaning, purpose, values, vision, mission, interests, and passions.
- Recognize that clients are more likely to experience posttraumatic growth than posttraumatic stress as a result of the challenges they have faced.
- Shift perceptions by increasing positive emotions, expanding creativity, experiencing flow, and focusing on strengths, beliefs, worldviews, and meaning and purpose.
- Find positive meaning, promote posttraumatic growth, and increase resilience through shifting perceptions and experiencing feelings of gratitude, appreciation, insight, improved relationships, empowerment, sense of possibility, and positive change.
- Increase our own wellbeing by:
  - Exploring our own ideas about happiness
  - Identifying the unique strengths, values, and beliefs that bring us to art therapy
  - Creating sustainability in our work by developing the strengths that energize, revitalize, and put us into flow
  - Minimizing learned strengths that deplete us
  - Discovering what gives our lives passion, purpose, and meaning
  - Finding positive meaning in the hardships we face
  - Increasing compassion satisfaction, feelings of accomplishment, and pride in our work.

- Engage in positive ethics by identifying the values and aspirations that ground our ethical standards rather than adopting only a risk management approach that seeks to avoid ethical violations.
- Use supervision to explore the ethical dimensions of our work, rather than waiting to address ethical dilemmas.
- Celebrate our pioneers, leaders, and organizations for the contributions they have made and are making toward advancing the field of art therapy.
- Collaborate with researchers from positive psychology and other fields to examine the interaction among artmaking, art therapy, and wellbeing.
- Celebrate the unique strengths that art therapy brings to the mental health professions.
- Use these strengths to solve pressing social needs and help the institutions we work with, the field of art therapy, the communities we live in, and the world as a whole to flourish and thrive.

How Art Therapy Can Transform Positive Psychology

Art Therapy

- Accelerates the therapeutic alliance by providing art materials and a place to create;
- Safely facilitates affective engagement and feelings of connection through visual stimulation and sensorimotor, kinesthetic manipulation of art supplies;
- Promotes future-orientation, hope, and optimistic thinking by visualizing and illustrating positive states;
- Encourages curiosity, creativity, play, and experimentation;
- Induces the positive emotions (enjoyment, interest, amusement) that come from engaging in play behaviors;
- Provides positive distraction from physical pain and emotional distress;
- Fosters group cohesion through parallel participation in enjoyable artistic endeavors or through collaborative artmaking (murals, mosaics, collective mandalas, etc.);
- Promotes flow through directives and art media designed to optimize skill/challenge balance;
- Initiates the relaxation response through focused engagement and the experience of flow;
- Providing pro-social avenues for flow in group settings;
- Provides a highly efficient form of information processing by retrieving parts of consciousness, implicit and explicit thoughts, feelings, and memories not accessible through other means;
- Creates shortcuts to communication by promoting uncensored externalization and expression of internal processes—a message from the self to the self and from the self to others;
- Simultaneously arouses and provides opportunities to regulate strong emotions;
- Encourages more nuanced expression of thoughts and emotions, both positive and negative;
- Promotes awareness of and distance from thoughts and feelings (mindfulness) and opportunities to reflect upon them more objectively;
- Provides a visual signature that, however simple and/or primitive, is unique and helps increases awareness of:
  - Identity
  - Personality
  - Tendencies toward positive/negative emotionality
  - Physical dispositions
  - Beliefs/worldviews
  - Memories
  - Values, passion, purpose, and meaning in life
  - Internal/external resources
  - Personal strengths

- Strengths in others (inside and outside of the therapeutic relationship)
- Interpersonal dynamics
- Resilience
- Motivations
- Goals
- Explanatory styles of attribution (optimistic/pessimistic)
- Growth/fixed mindset
- Sense of agency
- Beliefs about pathways to meet goals
- Patterns of perception, cognitive biases, and insights
- Beliefs that interfere with or contribute to happiness
- Accomplishments

- Organically shifts perceptions by seeing different aspects of the self simultaneously, as a gestalt—a unified whole;
- Facilitates sophisticated exploration of meaning and perception by comparing and contrasting metaphors that emerge in:
  - The process of making the artwork
  - The visual elements
  - The intention behind the artwork
  - The verbal associations to it

- Fosters positive meaning, benefit-finding, and posttraumatic growth by revealing parts of the self, memory, and consciousness through visual imagery;
- Changes "the story"; creates new narratives that include more empowered perceptions of experiences, especially those that were traumatic or involved loss;
- Cultivates optimism and "attending to the good" by revealing nuances of and challenging negative beliefs;
- Increases positivity (love, appreciation, gratitude, empathy, compassion, forgiveness) in relationships by illustrating interpersonal dynamics and strengths that had not been evident before;
- Visualizes aspirations and leads to more self-concordant goals by illustrating what is important and relevant in highly personalized visual language;
- Illustrates potential barriers;
- Provides opportunities to "virtually" explore and experiment with a range of possibilities and solutions;
- Illustrates where to most congruently channel resources;
- Literally accomplishes something—making art!
- Encourages impulse control, skill-building, experimenting with novel behaviors, autonomy;
- Enhances self-efficacy, pride, and mastery as a result;
- Provides a visible record of the therapeutic process;

- Reveals recurrent visual and metaphorical themes which reflect core aspects of the self;
- Identifies ongoing concerns and areas which need more attention and additional resources;
- Gives concrete evidence of the evolution of therapy; reveals consistencies and highlights change;
- Provides opportunities to "capitalize"—to celebrate progress;
- In groups, strengthens cohesion and fosters appreciation for others, strengths spotting, and empathy through seeing artwork of other members and witnessing them explore its visual content and metaphors;
- Helps therapists learn more about their clients and the intersubjective dynamics of the therapeutic alliance through making response art;
- Deepens the therapeutic alliance through sharing response art and engaging in collaborative artmaking with clients;
- Illustrates and encourages new perception of broader elements of experience such as aesthetic beauty, spirituality, and finding the sacred in the mundane;
- Moves beyond and challenges the medical model's reductionist focus on problems, symptoms, and diagnosis by providing complex and personalized information;
- Enriches supervision and consultation by revealing unique perspectives on our work:
  - Professional identity and career aspirations
  - Relationships with client(s), colleagues, supervisors, work setting, and other institutions
  - Ethical dimensions vs. ethical dilemmas

- Adds to the knowledge base of art, art therapy, and wellbeing;
- Engages research methods, such as arts-based research, congruent with our unique strengths that empowers participants to discover knowledge that is difficult to access through other means;
- Builds community and provides novel approaches to social activism;
- Makes the world more beautiful!

CHAPTER 5

Positive Emotions and Emotion Regulation

We open most of our workshops with a simple exercise, "Think of three things that went well this morning or three things for which you are grateful" (Seligman, Steen, Park, & Peterson, 2005). Small blessings often get mentioned: "I was able to find a parking space close by" or "I had a tasty cup of coffee." Weightier reflections also emerge: "I'm grateful for my husband and my kids"; "that I can walk and talk"; "I am able to work and provide for my family." Although most of us, when specifically asked, can readily identify what is functioning and good in our lives, because of the *negativity bias* we tend be more aware of and distracted by what is problematic and out of alignment with how things "should" be.

In other words, most of our experience is uneventfully positive—that is, we can walk, talk, eat, work, and play. When something disrupts this baseline, it naturally grabs our attention. This makes sense—it signifies that some concern may need to be managed. To go back to the metaphor of a photograph, you could say that the good forms the background, it frames the picture but it is less distinct and may even go unnoticed; whereas difficulties, like the main subject, appear in the foreground more sharply and distinctly. So, we use the "Three Good Things" exercise to bring this overall backdrop of positivity to the fore, to notice what is already working just fine.

But why bother, if we are more naturally inclined to notice what is problematic? Because focusing on what is good in our lives makes us feel more hopeful, it relaxes us, it makes us more receptive to others and to possibilities, it keeps us from taking things for granted, and it counteracts negative feelings. In other words, it makes us feel better, and when we feel better, we are more better able to cope with and feel empowered to handle the difficulties that confront us.

The "P" in PERMA

It is no accident that the "P" for positive emotions comes first. Seligman identified that it was "a cornerstone of well-being theory" (2011, p. 16).

As we know, happiness and wellbeing have strong emotional components that include experiencing more positive emotions—hope, love, amusement, contentment—and less negative emotions—guilt, anger, worry (Diener, Suh, Lucas, & Smith, 1999). For example, when we ask clients, "If your situation were to improve, what would be better?" their replies are most often couched in emotional language: "I wouldn't feel so sad, or lonely and anxious anymore," "I would be happier, feel more peace, more energy and joy."

The vital role that positive emotion plays in wellbeing makes intuitive sense. However, up until recently, the evolutionary function of positive emotions was not as clearly understood as that of negative emotions. Through the lens of evolutionary theory, it was assumed that expression and regulation of *all* emotions increased adaptive functioning (Turner, 2000). However, negative emotions were considered more critical to immediate survival. For example, emotions such as fear, anger, and anxiety not only alert us to problematic situations but they also mobilize urges that enable us to act quickly in response to perceived environmental threats. Fear mobilizes the fight/flight/freeze response, anger the urge to strike out; etc. Although we might not necessarily act upon these impulses, they have evolutionary value in that they prepare us to spring into action if needed and are, therefore, more likely to lead to our survival (Fredrickson, 1998).

Positive emotions were challenging to fit within this evolutionary framework. Positive emotions were thought to facilitate approach behaviors and elicit continued action ("Gee, this is pleasant, I'm going to keep doing it"). Approach behaviors encourage engagement and cooperation with others. Continued action promotes productivity and goal attainment. In other words, positive emotions motivate us to step outside of ourselves, to interact with others, and to make things happen in the world. Although these behaviors may serve evolutionary function, they do not appear to correlate to any *specific* tendencies. Instead, they appear to produce vague inclinations—general urges to do "anything or nothing at all." This initially led to the assumption that positive emotions had less evolutionary relevance; however, Barbara Fredrickson's research (1998) has given us a framework for understanding the critical role positive emotions play in our survival.

Benefits of Positive Emotions: The Broaden-and-Build Theory of Positive Emotions

Fredrickson (1998) proposed that positive emotions serve to *broaden* our thinking and to *build* enduring psychological, social, and physical resources. Whereas negative emotions were thought to narrow attention and initiate quick, decisive action, positive emotions widen perception and expand options. They increase our ability to take in new information, to engage in creative ways of thinking, to perceive multiple options, and to experiment with novel behaviors.

Positive emotions such as joy and interest promote play, an activity that has been well-documented to increase physiological and psychological flexibility and responsiveness (Burdette & Whitaker, 2005). Positive emotional states facilitate faster cognitive processing and increase intuition, creativity, and adaptive thinking. Emotions such as gratitude and love build social capital and cultivate community; when people are feeling better they are more likely to initiate contact with others, they are more curious and welcoming, and they tend to display more affection, all of which strengthen social bonds (Wood, Froh, & Geraghty, 2010). These connections tend to outlast the positive experiences that inspired their inception. Positive emotions such as hope and serenity boost the immune system and help us recover more quickly from illness (Davidson, Mostofsky, & Whang, 2010).

The Undoing *Effect of Positive Emotions*

The *broaden-and-build* nature of positive emotions can also "undo" the lingering effects of negative emotions (Fredrickson, 1998). The negativity bias leads us to notice and focus more on negative emotions because they are intense and indicate potential danger in one's immediate environment (Vaish, Grossmann, & Woodward, 2008). When appropriately induced, positive emotions can help release the grip of negative emotions. An example might be when we are grieving but we see a friend engaged in charming antics that, by making us chuckle, allow us to experience a temporary lift in our sadness.

When we experience positive emotions, our bodies also appear to recover more quickly from the damaging physiological effects of negative emotions. For example, people who have been exposed to a negative event (with the associated biochemical arousal that event produces) appear to return to their baseline heart rate and blood pressure more rapidly when they experience positive emotions. Positive emotions also appear to improve immune function, lower cortisol, and have favorable effects on the heart's vagal tone which serves to regulate the parasympathetic branch of the autonomic nervous system. The vagal tone both predicts and positively responds to positive emotions and affiliation (Kok et al., 2013). This mind-body connection explains why positive feelings are correlated with longevity—people who feel better more often live longer (Diener & Chan, 2011; Xu & Roberts, 2010).

The Upward Spiral of Positive Emotions

Positive emotions, the broadening of perception, and the building of physical, social, and psychological resources appear to be reflexive in nature and to aid with coping well in the face of adversity. In other words, an initial experience of positive emotions expands awareness, promotes novel thinking and inspires pro-social behaviors which in turn fosters increased knowledge, expanded possibilities, social connection, and improved physical health (Fredrickson, 1998).

This contributes to the capacity to cope with and bounce back from negative experience. Building and strengthening coping resources and the ability to manage stressors promotes greater resilience, which leads naturally to more positive experiences and emotions. This cycle generates the *upward spiral* of positive emotions, a reversal of the downward spiral that commonly manifests in depression, hopelessness, and pessimistic thinking (Garland et al., 2010).

The beneficial impact of positive emotions on resilience appears most pronounced when we are able to find positive meaning in the difficulties we encounter. This process of *positive reappraisal* does not mean that we minimize our losses but that we are able to extract something positive from what we have experienced (Sears, Stanton, & Danoff-Burg, 2003). The relationship between finding positive meaning in challenges, also called *benefit-finding* (Helgeson, Reynolds, & Tomich, 2006), and positive emotions appears to be reciprocal as well—finding positive meaning induces more positive emotions, which in turn broadens thinking and inspires more positive perception of events. We will explore this critical dynamic more fully in Chapter 11 on meaning making and perception.

What Are Emotions?

Before we continue discussing positive emotions, we might step back and take a moment to consider what emotions are in general. The etymology of the word "emotion" traces back to old French and Latin terms meaning "to move" and even "to dance"! This makes sense because most of us experience our emotions in the body—from the heart-pounding sensation of fear, to the bounce in our step from joy, the tear-jerking pull of grief and sadness, and the serene exhale of contentment and peace. This also makes sense because our emotions often *move* us into action, spurring us on to do things.

Emotions also *move on by*, like the weather, quickly changing. Whereas mood indicates longer-term experiences, emotions are thought to be temporary and fleeting (Scherer, 2005). In Western science, emotions were long thought to be the enemy of rational thought. Plato (1992) believed that we had to tame our emotions lest they carry us off like runaway horses. However, separating emotions from thoughts is misleading. Our thoughts and what we believe shape how we feel about what we are experiencing but, conversely, what we feel also shapes our perceptions and our thoughts.

Emotions appear to have multiple functions—they prepare us to respond to our environment, they facilitate thinking and decision-making, they provide us information about the congruence between our internal experience and the external environment, and they help us evaluate whether something is "good or bad." Emotions also serve social purposes—they influence and shape social interactions, give us information about others' intentions, and promote moral behavior through helping us make empathic connections to each other (Pham, 2007).

What Are Positive Emotions?

Positive emotions are feelings that are considered desirable, that subjectively make us *feel* good. These include but are not limited to feelings such as love, serenity, joy, interest, awe, excitement, pleasant surprise, contentment and hope. Positive emotions about the past include forgiveness and gratitude; positive emotions in the present include savoring the moment, humor, or being profoundly moved by awe when we witness something that is inspiring; positive emotions about the future involve feeling hope, optimism, and faith (Seligman, 2002a, 2011).

What Are Negative Emotions?

Negative emotions are ones that we find difficult and cause unpleasant sensations. As we know, they are critical to survival—they indicate a disturbance in our environment that requires attention and spur us into action. They also serve a critical developmental role. For example, Bowlby (1988) argued that secure attachment is formed *only* when a child experiences fear and anxiety that is then assuaged by the comfort of a primary caregiver. *Guilt* tell us that we may have compromised our values, *anger* that a boundary (ours or someone else's) has been encroached upon, *fear* that we may be in danger, and *grief* that we have lost something that was important to us.

Appropriate and Inappropriate Negativity

Let's be clear—negative emotions are essential. They should not be ignored or repressed. In addition, when we experience *appropriate negativity*, it actually promotes flourishing. For example, negative emotions such as guilt not only alert us that we have done something wrong, but they can also steer us from engaging in or repeating behaviors that might jeopardize trust. Anger can be a useful catalyst to energize us into action—e.g., getting pumped up with anger can help people perform better in competitive situations and it helps us confront someone we believe is in the wrong (Tamir, 2009).

Negative emotions serve to anchor us to reality—they keep us tethered to the world. Without them, we might float away. People with sociopathic tendencies show a *deficit* of negative emotions, particularly anxiety and fear. People with manic tendencies often experience excessive positive emotions without compensatory negative emotions that might inhibit risk-taking behaviors (Gruber, 2011).

Not only is it critical and useful to *feel* negative emotions, we also need to *express* them. There is substantial data that *suppressing* negative emotions is harmful to our health (Gross & Levenson, 1993). It lowers our immune functioning and activates the sympathetic nervous system. Expressing emotions appropriately is not only beneficial for the person experiencing the negative emotion, but it serves to communicate important information to others. For example, a frown indicates displeasure and discourages people from approaching and tears show sadness and perhaps a need for comfort. If appropriately communicated, the expression of emotions is socially productive, regardless of their positive or negative valence.

Persistent Negative Emotions

On the other hand, experiencing persistent negative emotions has detrimental consequences to our health (Salovey, Rothman, Detweiler, & Steward, 2000). When we chronically experience anxiety, anger, fear, and sadness, it takes its toll mentally, physically, and psychologically. Persistent negative emotions can lead to difficulties concentrating, racing thoughts, rumination, and poor judgment. We may also experience symptoms such as feeling overwhelmed, irritability, loneliness, and depression. Physical symptoms may also emerge such as headaches, nausea, rapid heartbeat, chronic pain, inflammation, and reduced immune function. We may also exhibit changes in behavior such as agitation, increased or reduced appetite, disturbed sleep, withdrawal and isolation, and/or addictive behaviors (Kiecolt-Glaser, McGuire, Robles, & Glaser, 2002; Smith, Glazer, Ruiz, & Gallo, 2004).

Corrosive Negative Emotions

In addition, corrosive negative emotions such as disgust, contempt, or shame appear to be damaging both intra- and interpersonally. Positive psychologists suggest that negative emotions are appropriate when they are time-limited and they provide useful feedback about a specific situation; whereas inappropriate negativity, so common with chronic depression and anxiety, is not helpful because it dominates one's life and impedes the capacity to usefully cope with internal and external stressors (Fredrickson & Kurtz, 2011). In other words, it isn't just whether and how often we experience positive or negative emotions, but how deeply we experience them, for how long, and how we manage them. And, as we will explore further when we discuss meaning and perception, our beliefs about the value of emotions in general are also critical in both the affective and the cognitive realms.

Emotional Sensitivity and Emotion Regulation

Emotional sensitivity and regulation are key to any discussion about positive and negative emotions (Gross & Thompson, 2007). Emotional sensitivity describes how easily and quickly we may enter an emotional state, as well as how deeply we experience it. Emotion regulation determines how we manage and/or leave that state. At times, this may occur naturally, such as when we instinctively tense up from something threatening in our environment, but then subconsciously instruct our body to relax when we realize that we are safe. Other times, regulation may result from conscious intention, such as reminding ourselves to breathe when we are anxious.

Our capacity to regulate our emotions is heavily influenced by core affect— basic states of feeling good or bad, energized or drained. It appears that people who naturally experience more positive affect not only experience less sensitivity to negative affect, but they are more effective at short-circuiting negative affect (Larsen, 2009). People who naturally experience more negative affect seem to be more responsive to negative states. This may be further heightened if they also seek to *avoid* those states.

Personality traits, especially those accounted for in the Five Factor Model (Digman, 1990), are considered to be particularly relevant in emotional sensitivity. OCEAN is an acronym for the Five Factor Traits which are considered to be most common: Openness to experience, Conscientiousness, Extroversion, Agreeableness, and Neuroticism. People who exhibit extroversion (energetic and outgoing), and agreeableness (friendly and cooperative) appear to experience more positive emotions such as hope and enjoyment. People who exhibit neuroticism (sensitive and nervous) are more vulnerable to feelings such as anxiety and fear. People who are high in extroversion tend to be more energetic and cheerful (McCrea & Costa, 2003).

Emotion regulation usually serves as an attempt to prevent pain and promote pleasure—i.e., to feel worse less often and feel better more often. However, we may employ some emotion-regulation strategies to do the opposite, e.g., generating anger in order to induce determined concentration. Emotion regulation involves a range of strategies that may be more or less functional. For example, some people high in extroversion are more likely to attend to and *seek out* positive experiences. People high in neuroticism are more likely to attend to and devote resources toward a*voiding* anxiety-provoking input (Derryberry, Reed & Pilkenton-Taylor, 2003). In other words, our temperament can impact whether we focus more on approaching positive experiences or avoiding negative ones.

The Positivity Ratio

Fredrickson (2009) and others suggest that we cannot and do not want to eliminate negative emotions. However, because of the negativity bias and the fact that negative experiences outweigh positive experiences, the weight of their impact should be countered with a *higher ratio* of positive emotions. Negative experiences register immediately in our emotional memory, whereas positive experiences have to be held in awareness for 5–20 seconds for the same to occur (Hanson, 2009). We adapt to negative events much less quickly than positive events. Our bodies recover more slowly from negative affect than positive affect. We also devote more attentional resources to negative events and negative internal data is more readily accessible than positive information.

The positivity ratio is especially relevant with people who are suffering because they tend to experience a significantly higher ratio of negative to positive emotions. We know this is true for our clients who are have experienced loss or trauma, or who are suffering from depression. It also includes people who are generally anxious, pessimistic, and emotionally sensitive. On the other hand, Fredrickson (2009) has pointed out that even people who are *functioning well* may not be experiencing adequate amounts of positive affect.

Fredrickson suggests that in order to move from languishing to flourishing, in which we experience more expansiveness, generativity, and growth, we need to have a minimum of 3:1 positive to negative affective experiences. Although there is some controversy about the exact number of positive emotions required to favorably tip the positivity ratio (Brown, Sokal, & Friedman, 2013), Fredrickson argues that even twice as many positive to negative emotions is not enough. A caveat to this formula—as we mentioned above, there appears to be an upper limit to this ratio. More than 12:1 may be associated with excessive and risky behaviors leading to negative consequences, as in manic phases of bipolar disorder (Gruber, 2011).

In short, we now view emotions as complex, transient, embodied states both linked to and influencing our thoughts. We know that negative emotions such as anger, sadness, and guilt are useful and necessary. There is also evidence that supports the *Broaden-and-Build Theory* (Fredrickson, 1998) regarding the evolutionary usefulness of positive emotions. Because of the many benefits of feeling better—experiencing relatively more positive emotions to negative emotions—our goal should be to reduce inappropriate negativity, to help value and regulate appropriate negativity, and to boost moments of positivity.

Positivity in Clinical Practice

The importance of positive emotions in clinical practice may be the most important take-away that we have gotten from positive psychology. Because of their capacity to induce hope and reduce feelings of isolation, to warm people up to the therapy process, to promote more effective coping, and to build relationships, we introduce them strategically at the very onset of therapy (Rashid, 2014). As we know, the therapeutic alliance consistently emerges as the most salient variable in effective therapy, regardless of the therapist's treatment approach (Lambert & Barley, 2001). Positive emotions may be the most effective tool for fostering that connection. Before we explore how we combine positive emotions and art therapy for that purpose, we will first describe the interface between art therapy and emotions in general.

Art Therapy and Emotions

We know that, in general, expression of positive, negative, or any kind of emotion is a crucial part of psychological growth and change. We also know that *suppressing* emotions, particularly negative ones, is harmful. Expressing negative emotions such as fear, shame, grief, and anger is key to learning to differentiate and process emotions (Pascual-Leone & Greenberg, 2007). Exploring emotional experience within the safety of the therapeutic alliance has been positively correlated with improved treatment outcomes (Coombs, Coleman, & Jones, 2002).

Art therapy is perhaps best known for its capacity to facilitate expression—through art we bring feelings into awareness and shape them into tangible form (Langer, 1957). Through art, we can express a wider and more colorful range of emotions than we can through words alone. Although artmaking may be frustrating at times, we also know the deep satisfaction that comes from giving form to tangled-up emotions. That process and the resulting product also helps us find emotional clarity and discover new insights. Art therapists support this effort, providing compassionate witnessing and artistic know-how to boost expression and contemplation.

In art therapy, as opposed to artmaking in other contexts, the unique support of the art therapist (and often other group members) powerfully increases the therapeutic value of artistic self-expression. As we will discuss more in Chapter 9 on relationships, the therapeutic alliance adds a depth to the experience that increases its relevance. Through exploring emotions in a supportive environment, individuals can "unfold" the essence of their experience which allows them to identify and organize it (Rimé, 2009, p. 81).

People also tend to find making art pleasurable. There is growing research showing the activity of making art can repair and improve mood and increase positive emotions in the short term (Babouchkina & Robbins, 2015; Bell & Robbins, 2007; Smolarski, Leone, & Robbins, 2015). For example, researchers found that artmaking positively affected mood whereas completing a simple but engaging task—doing a puzzle—did not (De Petrillo & Winner, 2005).

The growing body of research on positive emotions and art therapy just scratches the surface of what is happening in the art therapy process. For example, in a study with people with cancer, art therapy was associated with increased positive emotion—that is, improvement in self-reports of happiness, positive affect, hope, and benefit finding (Shapiro, McCue, Heyman, Dey, & Haller, 2010). Improved well-being, reduced anxiety, and less global distress were also seen in hospitalized cancer patients receiving art therapy (Thyme et al., 2009; Nainis et al., 2006). Reynolds and Prior (2006), in their study of women with medical conditions, determined that art served as a positive distraction and as a way of experiencing flow and spontaneity. Davis (2010), in a study with international students exploring how art therapy was used to express emotions and organize thoughts, found that art creation transformed their emotional chaos into more manageable emotional experiences, such as feelings of calm.

How Art Therapy Engages Emotions and Improves Mood

- Warms up clients to the therapeutic process;
- Provides healthy distraction;
- Induces positive emotions via enjoyment in making art;
- Relieves acute distress and induces the relaxation response;
- Facilitates externalization, expression, and regulation of emotions;
- Provides distance from and opportunities to mindfully observe overwhelming feelings;
- Transforms complex emotions into symbolic visual communication;
- Helps "undo" the effects of negative emotions;
- Aids in visualizing and experiencing more positive emotions;
- Fosters pride, self-esteem, and mastery;
- Boosts hope, connection, comradery and micro-moments of love;
- Promotes creative and expansive thinking.

How We Use Positive Emotions in Positive Art Therapy

Because of the broadening potential of positive emotions, we employ them strategically in all of our work. In many ways, it forms the foundation of a positive art therapy approach. Without fail, they serve as the principle agent in all of the therapeutic interactions in which we engage. To borrow language from the field of psychodrama, we think of positive emotions as the "warm-up" for all subsequent work that we do. It serves to reduce anxiety provoked by new or unpleasant situations and encourage new responses to familiar situations.

Positivity Early in Treatment

Therapeutic encounters are simply more effective if participants are physically, emotionally, and mentally prepared. Warm-up involves social and psychological *awakening* and focusing. Warm-up helps mark the formation of a psychological space that encourages trust and "spontaneity for response in the here and now—to enable participants to relate and act and become involved, so that the end results are moments of personal freedom, discovery, creative expression and a new awareness of reality" (Weiner & Sacks, 1969, p. 85).

Positive emotions are ideal for warming people up to therapy, in general, and art therapy in particular. They promote intrinsic motivation—people are more likely to participate when they are feeling better. There is also evidence positive mood promotes social-behavioral engagement and group cohesion—people are more likely to listen to, engage with, and support their fellow group members when they feel good. In addition, they are more receptive and better able to process negative information when they are experiencing positive emotions (Linnenbrink-Garcia, Rogat, & Koskey, 2011; Bramesfeld & Gasper, 2008).

In art therapy, the warm-up also takes place through visual stimulation when clients (and therapists) see art supplies. Often, regardless of whether they are excited or anxious about the prospect engaging in a therapeutic encounter (which may be heightened or lessened by the expectation of making art), they will often pick up and experiment with the art supplies. Even if they don't touch the art materials, just by seeing them participants' senses are engaged and they begin, either consciously or unconsciously, to contemplate making art. Art materials which are easy to use reduce anxiety and increase positive emotions of curiosity, interest, and inspiration.

We should be clear that the strategic use of positive emotions is in the service of creating a safe environment that promotes engagement and willingness to take risks. It is not for the purpose of avoiding unpleasant affect. In fact, negative emotions readily emerge when people feel safe and being able to express them freely is the hallmark of a good therapeutic relationship (Hill, Thompson, & Corbett, 1992). We are suggesting that the depth of content, including negative feelings and experiences, is likely to emerge more readily when people are properly warmed-up and engaged. Positive emotions facilitate this process.

As mentioned above, clients often seek help because of a presenting problem, something which is distressing them. It is obviously important to gather some information about how they perceive their situation and to acknowledge the challenges they have faced. For example, in psychiatric settings, we ask people to share briefly whatever they are comfortable revealing about what brought them to the hospital, whether they are there involuntarily or not. This applies even when the initial contact is not with the primary client, such as with a parent/spouse/teacher. It provides the client and/or relevant parties the opportunity to express the discomfort and pain they've been experiencing and to receive acknowledgment and support for the suffering it has caused them. This exchange is critical in establishing trust. However, gathering extensive bio-psychosocial histories and detailed information about the complaint is not necessary to begin addressing it (Molnar & de Shazer, 1987).

In fact, it may be more important to look for *exceptions*—times when they have experienced some relief from the problem, that they were feeling better, and/or they were coping well with the situation (Molnar & de Shazer, 1987). Exception finding, in and of itself, often produces positive feelings, leading to expanded thinking and upward spirals of positivity (Fredrickson, 1998). Similarly, Resnick, Warmoth, and Serlin (2001) suggest that it is not enough to be concerned only with our clients' pain, anxiety, guilt, and shame, we also need to be interested in moments when they have felt better and had more joy and peace in their lives.

So, although we are careful to validate the concerns that brought clients to us, we want to look for exceptions and ask "if our work together were to be most helpful, what would be different?" Many times clients have difficulty articulating what it would look like if things were better, but they are very clear about what looks like when they are not! We frequently have clients compare and contrast, "When it's bad," "When it's good," and "What makes it better." Usually, for "bad," they rattle off a slew of words—anxious, sad, lonely, depressed, worried, etc. Identifying "bad" paradoxically warms them up to the "good," i.e., articulating negative feelings they have struggled with provides the springboard from which to identify their opposites.

Visualizing Positive Emotions

Helping clients conceptualize what it might look like if the problem were resolved often creates an affective shift (Carter, 2006)—imagining positive feelings induces those feelings. We may also provide lists of positive emotions and ask them which ones they would like to feel more often. Conceptualizing treatment within the context of their affective aspirations—wanting to be "more relaxed," "less anxious," or "more joyful"—can inspire and sustain motivation.

In her work with clients with substance abuse and dependence issues, Gioia often uses the directive to depict a positive emotion they would like to feel more often. Lamont, one of her clients, was inspired by the feeling *serenity*. Through delicate marks and curvilinear lines on soft blue-colored paper, he depicted a soothing and inviting landscape (Figure 5.1). In visualizing and imagining himself watching the flowing ocean waves, he was, in essence, transported into that experience and, even if only for a few moments, into the sensation of *low-key joy*.

Another client, Kristin, decided to focus on love (Figure 5.2). She began by drawing a heart on a small 4.5-inch circular paper with oil pastels, encircling it with bright white paint. She then extended the image by attaching it to a larger piece of paper, adding dramatic strokes of paint radiating from the heart. The expansive nature of this emotion led her not only to more fluid and expressive media but also to literally expand the image—*broaden and build* made manifest.

Evoking positive emotions such as hope and feeling connected to others—both considered to be essential curative factors in treatment (Yalom, 1995)—is critical at the inception of therapy when feelings of isolation are often prominent and belief in the possibility of change may be tenuous. In groups, positive emotions such as compassion can also provide temporary relief for clients who are anxious and depressed. This often occurs with clients who are in crisis and receiving inpatient psychiatric care. They are frequently consumed by their distress but when they witness others who have equally difficult or worse situations, they often experience a spontaneous rush of compassion which temporarily overrides their own pain and gives them a sense of shared humanity (Rashid, 2014; Yalom, 1995).

Positive Emotions During Other Phases of Treatment

Hope

Hope is critical throughout all stages of therapy, especially during times when clients may be discouraged or experience setbacks in their progress. This is particularly relevant when we consider the pervasively debilitating impact of *hopelessness*. Farran and colleagues describe hope as "a delicate balance of experiencing the pain of difficult life experiences, sensing an interconnectedness with others, drawing upon one's spiritual or transcendent nature, and maintaining a rational or mindful approach in responding to painful life experiences" (Farran, Wilken, & Popovich, 1992, p. 7).

Farran and colleagues (1992) identified that hope engages four processes—experiential/feeling, spiritual, cognitive, and relational. In addition, hope not only serves as a coping strategy, but it also initiates and is an outcome of coping. Scheinberg (2012) developed an art therapy protocol for increasing hope in patients with lupus, modified from an eight-week Hope Intervention created by nursing educator Herth (2001) for cancer patients. Herth included art activities in her program—e.g., visually chronicling one's *hope journey* and drawing a *success map* of the steps to maintain hope—intuitively understanding that art provides unique ways for patients to express their feelings, tell their story, and visualize positive outcomes. Scheinberg's protocol includes other art therapy directives such as making *hope kits/boxes* to hold symbols for things that bring hope and joy into their lives and creating murals which represents messages of hope they would want to share with others who are struggling.

Gratitude

Gratitude helps clients notice positive elements in their lives which have endured despite their challenges. There are abundant directives which promote gratitude, e.g., *visual gratitude journaling*—cataloguing events and experiences that we feel good about or for which are grateful—thank-you cards, and gratitude for the sacred in one's life (Malchiodi, 2002). *Inspiration* may give them renewed motivation—thinking about someone they admire or something that they once witnessed (a place or an event) that moved them and inspired awe. *Forgiveness*, focusing on what it would look like if conflicted relationships were better resolved, may help clients feel some relief from trauma and resentments.

Humor

Humor can serve as a welcome relief at any stage of treatment (Pomeroy & Weatherall, 2014; Yalom, 1995) and amusement and delight can promote further connection, intimacy, and disclosure. The best humor makes uncomfortable truths and awkward or painful aspects of our experience more approachable.

Humor builds social bonds by reminding us of our common humanity. It's been well established that laughter fortifies our immune system, boosts emotional well-being, and increases life satisfaction (Hasan & Hasan, 2009). Humor in psychotherapy can reduce anxiety and fear as well as promote spontaneity, playfulness, intimacy, trust, and hope.

Art therapy can be the perfect place for a lighter look at life. Participants might find humor or irony in imagery that was at first meant to represent something very challenging. They might make funny cartoons or silly drawings and depict themselves or others in a humorous manner. Humor can gently nudge over-seriousness and defended beliefs about oneself (Franzini, 2001). It often emerges when clients are experiencing a shift in self-perception and when there is a working therapeutic alliance (Fitzpatrick & Stalikas, 2008).

Savoring

Using savoring or positive reminiscence to recall and take pleasure in the best moments in one's life is another means of inducing positive emotion. In savoring, a person places deliberate attention onto pleasant experiences. Art directives that promote savoring can include doing artwork about positive memories, celebrating beauty in nature and in others, and focusing on sensations that feel comforting.

Art with a Positive Focus

The benefits of using interventions with a positive focus such as those we listed above have been supported by research. For example, Henderson (2012) conducted a study with 359 undergraduate students in which they were randomly assigned to four experiential groups, including one where participants drew mandalas after they were instructed to "think of an experience where you felt love, complete acceptance, amazing grace, gratitude, abiding joy, humility, compassion, kindness, happiness, and hope" (p. 68). Participants whose drawings had focused on love and joy felt higher positive affect than those directed to simply draw their thoughts and emotions at that moment.

In research comparing the effects of assigning artmaking with a positive versus negative focus, Curl (2008) found that college students who were directed to create artwork in response to something positive that had happened to them experienced greater reduction in stress than those who were asked to focus on something that had been stressful. There is also research that shows that *venting* negative emotions through making art, although helpful, is less effective at improving mood than focusing instead on something more positive (Dalebroux, Goldstein, & Winner, 2008; Smolarski, Leone, & Robbins, 2015).

In Gioia's qualitative arts-based research, she looked at the process of doing artwork about emotions in general and then positive emotions in particular. She asked participants to make artwork about "how you are feeling at this time," and to discuss if their art helped them to express *any* emotions. She then had them make a follow-up art piece to further express any *positive* emotions that might have emerged in the first drawing. According to one participant, Gretchen K., making the first piece of artwork about how she felt overall was enjoyable, because it helped her to gain "a little more insight into the emotions that I do have . . . so now it's a little more organized as to what is what" (Chilton, 2014, p. 134). She stated that the subsequent piece boosted her positive emotions even further. "It felt good to make a piece focusing just on the positive emotion; it made that emotion larger and more real" (p. 155) (Figure 5.3).

We often use this kind of sequence—general expression and then shifting to a positive focus—in inpatient care. It allows clients in crisis to both express and experience some relief from their distress. For example, Laura, a young woman with a history of childhood sexual abuse, represented the depression and pain she experienced by surrounding a stick figure with red and black scribbled lines (Figure 5.4). She explained that the yellow arrows bouncing off of this "shell" meant that "no good can get in or out." When asked what it would look like "if the good got in," Laura recreated the image so that the black and red marks "let the good flow through." As she did this, she became more animated and group members observed that she looked brighter and sounded more hopeful.

Positive psychology interventions that have reliably been found to increase positive affect (Layous, Chancellor, Lyubomirsky, Wang, & Doraiswamy, 2011; Sin & Lyubomirsky, 2009) can also be adapted to art therapy. These include activities like the "Best Possible Life" exercise, using *Character Strengths*, and *Love-Kindness Meditation*. The "Best Possible Life" (King, 2001) involves imagining that we are advanced in years and reflecting back upon our lives—if things had gone as well as we would have wanted, what would it look like? What would have happened? Using Character Strengths, as we will explore more in Chapter 8, involves developing those that energize us most. In love-kindness meditation, we direct compassion and kindness toward ourselves and others. We will explore love in greater detail in Chapter 9, which focuses on relationships.

Psycho-education About Positive and Negative Emotions

Aside from increasing positive emotions, we also want to educate ourselves and our clients about the benefits of *all* emotions, positive and negative, and the role they serve in our lives. It can be helpful to differentiate our personal experience of certain emotions from how others might experience them. We can also explore the general benefits and consequences of positive and nega-tive feelings—what it means to experience too little or too much of one or the other. For example, people who are highly anxious might benefit not only from experiencing anxiety less, but also from identifying what purpose it has served in their lives. Does it keep them vigilant, prepared for distress and loss? They can explore how they might use it more strategically. People who struggle with bipolar disorder might explore the danger of manic ecstasy and experiment with developing more serenity, more low-key joy.

Education about the negativity bias and the power of negative emotions is equally critical. Often people believe that negative feelings are bad, perhaps leading to suppression or anxiety. Understanding that the negative affective system is more reactive and responsive to its environment, that negative emotions take longer to metabolize, and that they command more of our cognitive resources—i.e., "bad is stronger than good"—often helps people feel less overwhelmed by and experience more equanimity about their negative emotional experiences (Baumeister, Bratslavsky, Finkenauer, & Vohs, 2001).

Strategies for Developing Awareness of and Regulation of Emotion

Part of increasing our understanding of our emotions involves increasing our awareness of and capacity to *regulate* emotions. The first part of this includes what we listed above, learning more about feelings in general. The second involves helping our clients develop and increase awareness of their own emotions so that they do not feel overwhelmed by or at the mercy of these feelings. This includes learning to tolerate emotions that they may find unpleasant but that have therapeutic utility—such as grief which allows us to express and manage loss, or anger which alerts us to injustice. It also includes discerning where and how they experience their emotions—where in their body do they locate their feelings and what is that sensation? Using mandalas or outlines of figures can facilitate this process. Developing more awareness of these emotions and creating some distance between the experiencing self and the observing self often increases the ability to tolerate unpleasant sensations.

Making art helps regulate affect in other ways. It provides a positive distraction from unpleasant feelings (Drake, Coleman, & Winner, 2011; Drake & Winner, 2012). Artmaking such as painting, using mandalas, or working in clay can also reduce distress and anxiety (Kimport & Hartzell, 2015; Kongkasuwan et al., 2015; Sandmire et al., 2015, Cohen, Barnes, & Rankin, 1995). Physical indicators support this finding, such as research with children which determined that drawing mandalas induced the relaxation response, as evidenced by reduced heart rate and peripheral skin temperature (DeLue, 1999). Expressive activity also balances the excitement evoked by the vivid sensory qualities of art media. The activation of reward circuitry in the brain allows for the simultaneous expression and regulation of strong affect (Hass-Cohen, 2016; Czamanski-Cohen & Weihs, 2016).

Mindfulness

Art therapy has also been combined with *mindfulness*, a practice which is effective both in producing positive affect and reducing emotional reactivity (Monti et al., 2006; Peterson, 2013; Rappaport, 2013). Mindfulness derives from Buddhist traditions of cultivating an observing self that notices sensation and thought without judgment. Jon Kabat-Zinn (1991) and Richard Davidson (2010) are credited most with translating and applying mindfulness to Western psychology.

Cultivating mindfulness involves noticing what we are experiencing physically, emotionally, and mentally (such as physical sensations, feelings, and thoughts) and any input we are taking in from our environment (such as sound, temperature, and smells). Although one is instructed to engage in this without judgments, they tend to arise nevertheless. When they do, one is instructed to note and gently put them aside, returning back to observing, and so on. The overarching goal is to develop an observing self that can attend to but that maintains a neutral stance toward input, negative and positive. Practicing mindfulness can help clients manage stress and tolerate unpleasant affect. It has also been shown to significantly decrease emotional reactivity and to increase feelings of equanimity (Victorson et al., 2015).

Mindfulness has been particularly effective in Dialectical Behavioral Treatment (DBT), an approach which seeks to regulate overwhelming affect (Lineham, 1993). Incorporating art therapy with DBT can help promote identification and acceptance of negative emotional states in the service of emotional regulation (Heckwolf, Bergland, & Mouratidis, 2014; Huckvale & Learmonth, 2009). Drass created a DBT art therapy program using activities such as making "wise mind books" and "distress-tolerance baskets" (2015, p. 169).

Positive Reappraisal

Other techniques can be useful to develop more control over one's affective experience. For example, *positive reappraisal* is a coping strategy which involves transforming our interpretations of a situation so as to lessen its negative emotional impact (Sears, Stanton, & Danoff-Burg, 2003)—i.e., putting a positive spin on stressful situations. It is both facilitated by and generates positive emotions—mediated by the broadening and shifting of perception. We will explore this further elsewhere, when we look at the interplay between feelings, perception, and beliefs.

The synergistic benefits of positive emotion and the art therapy process also figure elsewhere in the PERMA model, as we will explore in upcoming chapters. For example, they foster creativity and induce a sense of engagement which can produce experiences of mastery, pride, and accomplishment. And, as we have mentioned, positive emotions facilitate social interaction, the formation of trust and the building of social resources and emotional capital. This facilitates the initial connection and alliance so necessary to successful therapeutic work. Artmaking then fosters empathy. The combined effect of positive emotions and artmaking promotes deeper engagement in the therapeutic process as it unfolds, and commitment to that process in the longer term. In other words, it keeps folks coming back!

Artmaking also highlights strengths and provides more empowering ways of understanding weaknesses and challenges, which further fosters positive emotions. It helps shift perception and meaning, so that negative and positive experiences are no longer polarized and instead their nuances and interdependent complexities can be explored.

Art and positive emotions can also shift cognitive processing so that we become more attuned to what has escaped our awareness. Art and positive emotions help us manage overwhelming negative feelings, recover from trauma and loss more quickly, and cope better in general. Art and positive emotions help us discover positive meaning in the difficulties we have encountered. They allow us to be more mindful and attend to the good that, despite the tremendous challenges that we are facing in this day and age, is alive and well in the world.

We will now delve into the second domain of PERMA, Engagement. We will start this with an exploration of creativity—both because it is so intrinsic to the art therapy process and also because it emerges so fluidly from the synergistic effect of expression, positive emotion, and connection which are inherent to art therapy.

Discussion Questions

1   What positive emotions do you see early in treatment? Later?
2   What benefits do you perceive in the negative emotions you experience?
3   What tools do you use to help yourself and your clients regulate their emotions?
4   What is your positivity ratio?

CHAPTER **6**

Creativity

When we ask clients who have booked one of our creativity workshops what they are hoping to get out of the experience, not surprisingly they often report that they want to be "more creative." Just as frequently, when we ask them what that would look like, they have a rather fuzzy idea of what creativity means. Usually they want to be "freer" and "more artistic" because they believe they are too "left-brained" and/or "conventional."

What really is creativity? Is it a certain kind of innate talent or intelligence with which we are more or less endowed? Creating something original? Using our "right-brain" more? Thinking outside the box? Being more artistic, or spontaneous and imaginative?

Although creativity is considered to be a central dynamic in art therapy, we, ourselves, realized *we* didn't really have a good answer for what this essential element—*creativity*—was. Like our clients, most of our assumptions about this fundamental attribute were intuitive. Despite being art therapists and practicing artists, we knew very little about how to define and describe creativity and its role in the art therapy process. We recognized that we really needed to get a better handle on creativity, especially because, from a strength-based perspective, it may be one of the most powerful tools that art therapists utilize for healing.

Creativity is another challenging topic to unpack because it is so vast and so intricately interwoven into every aspect of our civilization. You could even say that it defines civilization! You can get a master's degree in "Creativity Studies" at universities across the world. There is an entire trans-disciplinary field of creativity research and study that integrates art, science, technology, education, politics, commerce, healthcare, and so on. Almost everything we do involves tools, technological devices, and/or systems of approaching the complexities of human life that were invented and made by human beings.

What Is Creativity?

We generally think of creativity as making something "new"—imagining, producing, or designing something that did not exist before. Creativity is also defined as originality, innovation, and ingenuity. Freud (1957a), whose ground-breaking psychoanalytic theories were themselves exemplary of creativity, linked creative activity to childhood play and emphasized the importance of both in healthy psychological functioning. Art was viewed as a way to transform unacceptable thoughts into socially acceptable ones. He viewed the artist as using creativity to first escape and then to find a way back to reality "by making use of his special gifts to mold his phantasies into truths of a new kind, which are valued by men as precious reflections of reality" (Freud, 1955, p. 224).

Winnicott (1971), a pediatric doctor and psychoanalyst who championed the importance of play in psychological health, believed that creativity emerges during formative stages in infancy. The sense of safety and wellbeing provided by getting our basic needs met, termed the *holding environment*, provided a *transitional space* for a child to begin separating from their mother and safely experiment with the world. Winnicott (1971) described how toys become *transitional objects*, which a child, in their first act of creativity, infuses with comforting associations of a reassuring mother-figure.

Playing with transitional objects helps infants learn how to differentiate between *self* and *other*: "There is a direct development between transitional phenomena to playing, and from playing to shared playing, and from this to cultural experiences" (Winnicott, 1971, p. 51). The arts, literature, and ritual all arise from the imaginative realm of play.

Humanists such as Rollo May were also interested in creativity. May believed that creativity was an expression of "normal people in the act of actualizing themselves" and that it represented "the highest degree of emotional health" (1975, p. 40). Maslow thought that fostering creativity could generate "a new kind of human being who is comfortable with change, who enjoys change, who is able to improvise, who is able to face [new situations] with confidence, strength and courage" (1971, p. 58).

Creativity in Positive Psychology

Creativity is a complex interplay of neurophysiological, cognitive, and motivational processes (Baas et al., 2008). In the domain of positive psychology, it is defined as the strength of producing an original thought or inquiry that is adaptive and appropriate to the circumstance (Peterson & Seligman, 2004). Creativity involves cognitive fluency, flexibility, and divergent thinking which generates novel and culturally relevant ideas, sometimes accompanied by moments of insight and exclamations of "Eureka!" (Csíkszentmihályi, 1996; Dietrich, 2004b). We can all think of many fascinating creative geniuses— Einstein, Austin, Carver, Kahlo, Jobs, etc. However, for our purposes, we are most interested in everyday creativity—the kind that you find in witty conversations, a striking snapshot on Instagram, the imaginative play-acting of children, decorative icing on a cake, stylish combinations that make a fashionable outfit, or a crafty fix for a household appliance on the fritz.

Creativity in Context

The context of creativity is important—people can come up with original thoughts that are not appropriate or useful to the situation. An extreme example of this might be the tangential thoughts verbalized by people experiencing psychosis—although they demonstrate unique combinations of words, their meanings are so idiosyncratic that they are incomprehensible to others. We typically do not view these "original" associations as creative because they are so peculiar. However, if these ideas can be channeled into something that is culturally accepted and understood, such as artwork, we intuit that although it may be odd, it is approachable and possibly even interesting and appealing. So creativity is in some sense *culturally constructed* (Abuhamdeh & Csíkszentmihályi, 2014).

Creativity and Development

Research shows that creativity continues to evolve over our lifespan (Csíkszentmihályi, 1996; Simonton, 1990). For example, most art educators and art therapists are familiar with Viktor Lowenfeld's work. In a seminal textbook, Lowenfeld (1957) described stages in children's artistic development from the earliest *uncontrolled scribbles* to the graphic style characteristic of adolescent years. Cross-cultural studies have substantiated this progression, if not at the exact ages Lowenfeld described (Alter-Muri, 2002). Others have discussed creativity in advanced age, finding that although there are cognitive declines over the lifespan, creativity can actually boost functioning in the elderly and some people experience the *swan-song* phenomenon, a late-life resurgence of creativity (Simonton, 1990).

Positive Emotions and Creativity

As we discussed in Chapter 5, one of the outstanding benefits of having more positive emotions—feeling better, experiencing more love, gratitude, humor and joy in life—is that they boost creativity. Baas, De Dreu, and Nijstad (2008) conducted a meta-analysis which covered 25 years of creativity research with a total of over 7,000 research participants. They found that positive emotions and mood actually activated new ideas—that is, creativity was enhanced by happiness. Notably, the researchers found that negative moods were associated with lower creativity and less cognitive flexibility.

Positive emotions such as joy and interest promote play, which increases flexibility and responsiveness (Burdette & Whitaker, 2005). Snyder and Lopez (2002) suggested that people who are experiencing positive emotions often use heuristic thinking and holistic processing. In other words, people who are in a good mood are more likely to have richer associations, to make more links among the ideas they already have, and to be more intuitive, flexible, expansive, divergent, and original in their thinking (Isen, 2004; Lyubomirsky, King, &

Diener, 2005). This cognitive broadening is the gateway to creativity. These results support some of the humanist theories of creativity, such as those generated by Maslow (1971) and Rogers (1951), who theorized that love, joy, and other positive emotions were associated with increased creativity.

> A new painting, poem, scientific achievement, or philosophical understanding increases the number of islands of the visible in the ocean of the unknown. These new islands eventually form those thick archipelagos that are [our] various cultures. (Arieti, 1976, p. 5)

Creativity and Flow

Of course, the intrinsic motivation found in the state of flow, of being fully absorbed and engaged by what we are doing, also produces positive emotions. This is why people enjoy artmaking and crafting, as well as other creative activities (Collier, 2011). Csíkszentmihályi writes that creativity holds intrinsic rewards such as "the excitement of discovery, the satisfaction of solving a problem, and the joy of shaping sounds, words, or colors into new forms." (2014, p. 240). Art therapists want to share this kind of experience with others—that sense of being completely focused and engaged in what we are doing. We will explore this element of engagement in much greater depth in the next chapter.

Creativity and PERMA

Creativity is linked to the domains of PERMA in multiple ways. Positive emotions (P) foster creative thinking, which often lead to engagement and flow (E), and when this results in the generation of ideas and actual artifacts, promotes feelings of accomplishment and pride (A), which contributes to sense of meaning and purpose (M), motivation and achievement (A), and when shared with and witnessed by others (R) lead to even more positive emotions (P), and so on. So let's explore the creative process and visit the "islands" that Arieti so poetically described.

The Creative Process

Ernst Kris (1952, cited by Arieti, 1976) thought that the process of creativity involved regression in service to the ego. In essence, the conscious mind shaped material it had *scooped up* from the preconscious—content that was not exactly at the forefront of one's mind but was easily accessible. Arieti defined the creative process as an encounter with the irrational which, through a mysterious transformation, resulted in a new creative product. He called this process the *magic synthesis*.

*Wallas' Model of Creativity: Preparation, Incubation, Illumination,
and Verification*

PREPARATION

Wallas (1926) was one of the first to outline the stages that produce the alchemical process of creativity: preparation, incubation, illumination, and verification. In the preparation stage, we get ready to work by taking in information and warming up. In a very practical sense, the preparation phase can involve assembling the art materials or organizing space to work. Think of this as stretching the canvas or sharpening the pencils. But preparation also involves a psychological state of receptivity to trying something new, of warming up, of being or becoming open to new ideas and points of view, allowing for vague impressions and half-formed thoughts to bubble up in response to an artistic challenge or an art therapy prompt.

INCUBATION

The incubation stage is wonderfully named—sometimes we need a proper amount of nesting and gestation before we generate something new! Incubation refers to nursing and protecting a tiny little seed of an idea. Even though incubation might not look like much to outsiders, it's important because as we do this, we become more engaged and involved in the process. This non-verbal, diffuse simmering stage allows ideas to percolate below our conscious awareness. Although it can look like procrastination or fooling around—behavior that is not always welcomed in a culture that values focused productivity—Biswas-Diener suggest that this may in fact be incubating (personal communication)!

Clients sometimes need to "marinate" in the art studio, to let the creative juices sink in and flavor the therapeutic engagement. This is particularly critical in more studio-based art therapy encounters but we could argue it's relevant in all art therapy settings. Meandering around the studio, playing with the art materials in relaxed manner, shuffling through magazines can be a key part of incubation and allows for divergent thinking to take place subconsciously. "Free from rational direction, ideas can combine and pursue each other every which way" (Csíkszentmihályi, 1996, p. 102).

ILLUMINATION

During the illumination phase, after we've been fiddling around a bit with the art supplies, suddenly an idea pops up from this fertile ground. This is the very satisfying "A-ha" moment that many creative folks know well. An idea appears as if by magic or we see a composition take shape in our artwork. This occurs "when a subconscious connection between ideas fits so well that it is forced to pop out into awareness, like a cork held underwater breaking out into the air after it is released" (Csíkszentmihályi, 1996, p. 104). At this stage, an art therapist might use their technical training to offer instruction with the art media—what type of adhesive to use, how to mix colors without making everything turning into mud, or how to support an extension on a sculpture.

> I don't have a clue. Ideas are simply starting points. I can rarely set them down as they come to my mind. As soon as I start to work, others well up in my pen. To know what you're going to draw, you have to begin drawing . . . When I find myself facing a blank page, that's always going through my head. What I capture in spite of myself interests me more than my own ideas. (Picasso, as quoted in Brassaï, 1999)

VERIFICATION

Lastly, the verification phase is where we properly finish the piece—we might trim some edges, step back from our art work and refine some of the details, or edit a manuscript. This stage entails deductive reasoning. It is the place for revisions and changes. In verification, *convergent* thinking narrows alternatives and aids discernment; final artistic choices are made and alterations are completed to get things *just right*. Here we fit our new ideas together just so. We literally and figuratively "frame" the piece.

Verification involves social aspects—response and feedback to the work from one's peers. In the art world, this might be done during a critique or a gallery show, situating the creative product within the larger culture. In art therapy, we often have some sort of processing time—some variation of "show-and-tell" during which the work is viewed and reflected upon, a process we'll revisit in other chapters. Below we include some tips for art therapists (or anyone) to promote each stage of the creative process, to allow the magical synthesis of creativity to unfold.

Tips for Fostering Creativity in Each Stage of the Creative Process

Preparation

- Provide an orderly and enriched studio space, with stimulating images and ideas to prompt creativity.
- Lay art supplies out in plain view to induce visual stimulation and entice engagement.
- If possible, provide clients opportunities to physically prep art materials.

(continued)

(continued)

- Provide warm-up exercises that can prime positivity and set the state for stage for creativity.
- Support an attitude of openness and the exploration of new and divergent ideas, thoughts, and images.

Incubation

- Advocate time for sleep and contemplation, to allow dreams and daydreams to develop.
- Provide opportunities for nonverbal thinking, be it doodles on the back of a napkin or rough sketches in a journal.
- Take a walk, or do some easy stretching to activate embodied knowledge.
- Experiment with materials.

Illumination

- When necessary, provide encouragement, instruction, materials to overcome technical difficulties.
- Celebrate and enthuse! When things go well in the creative process, pay just as much attention as when things don't.
- Be available, ask questions, show interest in all the details.

Verification

- Provide ways to literally frame or stage the work.
- If relevant and appropriate, create opportunities to display artwork; have artists consider such issues as titles, lighting, and visual context.
- Enable group discussions which allow for new ideas to arise and provide encouragement for small changes to the final piece.

Art Therapy and Creativity

In art therapy, part of the job of the therapist involves helping people engage in and move through the stages of the creative process (Hinz, 2009; Lusebrink, 1990). It is understood that art therapists should have a thorough understanding of the properties of different media so that they can strategically utilize those that are most likely to promote creativity with the given population with whom they are working. We refer you to Lisa Hinz's (2009) masterful summary of the Expressive Therapies Continuum for an in-depth discussion of the ways that particular art media and art therapy interventions influence and promote creative expression.

Setting the stage for creative work—whether it is in a hospital bed, on a psychiatric ward, in a school, a retirement facility, a community studio, or even outdoors—is also done when the art therapist creates a warm and supportive emotional space—what Judy Rubin (1978) coined a *framework for freedom*. This physical and psychological place is essential to initiate the creative process and therapeutic work. Art therapists try to make this framework well-suited for the clients' needs, with suitable levels of structure and containment, so that expression is free to blossom.

Like most art therapists, we set the framework for creativity by promoting feelings of psychological safety and comfort. In addition, because anxiety provoked by the thought of making artwork often stalls the incubation and preparation stages and gets in the way of creative magic, most art therapists know that they need to convey to clients that they are not in an art class. There are no grades, their work will not be judged by conventional standards, and we will help them if they get stuck. We also let clients know that they do not have to be an artist or have any particular artistic skills, that this is a process of experimentation and an opportunity to learn something new about themselves. Doing a quick demonstration of how to use some of the different materials and having the clients explore the ones they are most drawn to often helps them feel more open to exploration.

Growth and Fixed Mindset

To access our best creative thoughts, we want to be willing to explore, to be open to new ideas, and welcome divergent thinking. In short, we want to have a *mindset* which welcomes creativity. Carol Dweck (2006), a leading positive psychologist, developed the concept of mindsets. She explains that our beliefs about intelligence and talent impact how we learn. Do we believe we are born smart (or not)? Or instead that we *become* smart through hard work? If we think that intelligence and talent are fixed traits—either you have them or you don't—that we are born with a particular measure of talent and intelligence that can't change, then we tend to assume that as soon as things get challenging or that we make mistakes, it must mean we are *not smart*. When we have this *fixed mindset*, we believe failure is bad and should be avoided at all costs.

On the other hand, if we have a *growth mindset*, we are more resilient to failure, and, when we encounter setbacks, we persist. We know that struggle is a part of process, i.e. it doesn't always have to be easy to be worthwhile, that mistakes are okay, and intelligence is not a fixed attribute, but rather that it develops through perseverance and grit (Dweck, 2006). Encouraging a growth mindset fosters the willingness to engage in activities that may not guarantee "success" but that provide opportunities for learning and pave the way for creative experimentation.

Warming Up to Creativity

We can promote a growth mindset from the get-go with interventions that increase positive emotions such as those we explored in the previous chapter. Inducing positive emotions can initiate the preparation stage of the creative process. It can provide the willingness to engage in activity (versus opting to passively observe), as well as help overcome anxiety about doing something new and possibly unfamiliar or feeling pressure to make something that is "pretty." This can include warm-up activities such as the "Three Good Things" exercise, savoring daily experiences, remembering "golden" moments when we felt joy or peace, or anticipating things towards which we are looking forward.

Warm-up activities designed to boost positive emotions and foster the creative process can be tailored to account for the particular needs of the clients. Allowing more time, if we have that luxury, such as in an open-studio or an extended workshop, can also promote creativity by providing plenty of opportunity to sit in the preparation and incubation phases of the creative process. We can encourage participants to *just be* in the space—walk around the studio, shuffle through papers, pick up art supplies, or sort through magazine images or stencils. Really welcoming this pondering time allows for a gentle warm-up that acclimates them to the setting, the art supplies, and the art process.

Encouraging experimentation and "making mistakes" can be also an effective way to promote engagement, to help them get into the absorbed state that is known as *flow*. As we will discuss in the next chapter, flow further promotes creativity by making people more relaxed and expansive. When people are in flow, they naturally move from the preparation into the incubation stage of creativity.

We also recommend using clients' unique strengths to promote creativity. For example, if some clients' strengths include heart-centered ones like kindness and generosity, one way to warm them up to making art is to have them create something that is pro-social, such as a gift. In this way, we leverage their strengths to ease them into the creative process.

Other Warm-ups to Creativity

We also use simple structured rituals that help move us from inactivity to activity. These can be quite basic and have very concrete and tangible goals. Just engaging playfully in the process, as art therapists know well, is sometimes more important than creating a product. It may be helpful if the result of the activity does not have a high degree of importance or value. Lightening up the pressure to produce something tends, counterintuitively, to help folks actually do so.

We often have them test out materials before "starting." We have pieces of scrap paper available for people to experiment with different media. If we are doing sculpture or building forms, we have some of those materials, even if only in small quantities, available right from the start for them to touch and manipulate. This serves as a tactile warm-up.

We also include simple writing prompts, such as a short Gratitude List, or free or *spill writing*, in which clients write anything that's on their mind for 3 minutes without pausing. (We'll say, "If you don't know what to write, write 'I don't know what to write, this is silly, nothing comes to mind, this art therapist is nuts!', etc., until something eventually does—the idea is to keep writing the whole time to let the hand movement jog your brain"). We might have them write about someone they admire or who has had an impact in their life.

Other warm-up exercises we've used include taking a piece of paper and using every color of markers, pens, or watercolors, to make a pattern from repeated lines or shapes. We also employ Elinor Ulman's technique of swinging the arms in exaggerated circles as if one is painting or drawing on a large piece of paper or canvas (Ulman & Dachinger, 1996)—also fun to do with glow sticks or sparklers. Movement and music are always helpful because they engage other senses. Another warm-up can be having clients "do a collage of things that you enjoy and then do a painting of your collage." We also use coloring sheets, copying them two or three times and coloring them in with either different art materials or different marks and colors.

Is Coloring Creativity?

Coloring books have been criticized for being pre-packaged "stereotyped" imagery—"craftsy" in the worst sense of the word. Because the imagery does not derive from the artist's imagination, it is not considered creative or "self-expression". In fact, it has been suggested that it actively *stifles* creativity. However, just as magazine collage or stencils are not "original" imagery and yet the way they are combined involves artistic choices, so too do coloring images provide opportunities for personalized expression. This includes not only choice of imagery, but also of materials, as well as the use of color, contrast, shading, line quality, texture, emphasis, etc.—all of the elements that go into any piece of artwork.

This can be seen in the images colored by two clients, Carmela and Edmund, in long-term psychiatric care. Both used the same page from *The Anti-Coloring Book* (Striker & Kimmel, 1984), which combines pre-drawn images with prompts that invite creative responses. They chose a picture of a fairy with the title "What do you need a fairy godmother to do for you?" The differences in their responses (Carmela's in Figure 6.1, Edmund's in Figure 6.2), both in content and style, require little explanation.

(continued)

(continued)

We consider coloring sheets as simply another "medium" that resides on the more controlled end of the Expressive Therapies continuum. For example, we frequently provide coloring images as options for people who are psychotic and who benefit from concrete, reality-oriented tasks, or who are very anxious and find it containing and relaxing, or who are manic and need something that is very structured upon which to focus. Which image they choose, the visual elements they emphasize, and their verbal associations are usually just as rich as those that emerge with other art media.

Clients are often very pleased with their coloring images, proudly showing them to others or hanging them up because the images are comforting and hopeful. For example, David, also in long-term psychiatric care, carefully applied glitter to a simple coloring image of a leopard (Figure 6.3). He liked it so much that he hung it in his room to brighten his spirits.

Warm-ups in Corporate Workshops and Continuing Education

In our corporate and continuing education workshops, we often warm up clients with simple and concrete cognitive activities that have a positive focus. For example, we might hand out written descriptions of strengths, positive emotions, or values and have them check off ones with which they identify. Although this activity appears more "cognitive" in that it involves writing, the content is emotionally evocative and, as we have noted, the warm-up process has already begun just by having art supplies strategically and evocatively placed on the tables.

Often the attendees will have noted the art materials when they come into the room with comments that either reflect anxiety or excitement ("Oh! How fun! We get to play!" or "We're back in kindergarten, are we going to be graded?"). After reading over and check-marking their list, we offer small 4½ inch circular paper or 4x2-inch shipping tags with the suggestion to make a symbol of a strength/value that resonates for them or a positive emotion they would like to experience more at work.

Before we start the artmaking process, we might provide an example of a value/strength/feeling that most people can grasp, such as spirituality or love, and have them report what color and shape/symbol comes to mind when they think about that quality. This activates both the visual centers of the brain as well as higher process symbolic thinking. For spirituality, we often get yellow and purple along with crosses, yin yang, Star of David, circles, and clouds. However, we might also hear brown for the earth, green for growth, or black for the transcendent night sky. For love, we usually hear red and pink along with hearts, hands, connecting rings, and circles. But, again, we might also hear associations like orange for dynamic warmth or a tree for their family.

We also provide multicolor plastic stencils (realistic images of people, animals, transportation, shapes, plants, letters, etc.) which can be used as drawing aids. Even if they do not use them, tactile engagement with the stencils and the visual stimulation of looking at the images can serve as further warm-ups. For those of you familiar with Kagin and Lusebrink's (1978) work in media properties and task instruction, you may have identified that we are warming up people to being creative with more structured activities and controlled media. In corporate settings, the clients often need the containment of cognitive-symbolic tasks and materials that lean more towards the resistive end of the media properties continuum, such as markers, pencils, and stencils to warm up to the creative process.

Just like in short-term clinical settings, these workshops are often very time-limited and in office spaces where more studio-based projects such as those using paints, glue, glitter, and clay may not be possible. In addition, unlike clinical settings, the attendees are in professional relationships where certain boundaries are important to maintain and high degrees of emotional vulnerability may not be appropriate. However, surprisingly, if the clients are properly warmed up, even in these brief and potential-laden encounters they invariably become much more expressive than they believed they could and they are able to reveal parts of themselves that they might otherwise have refrained from sharing. This helps promote the building of more trust and personal commitment among co-workers (as we will explore further in Chapter 9, on relationships).

We note here that, because these are not high-intensity groups, such as immersive encounter workshops designed to dramatically open up clients for deep work, we need to frame the interventions and keep the focus on the participants' professional identity (Huet, 2011). This includes subtly reminding them that although the work we are doing evokes personal associations and, at times, strong feelings, they are at work among their professional peers (and perhaps their supervisors). As we will discuss in Chapter 13, we use our therapeutic training to contain the sharing such that the attendees are not overly exposed or emotionally vulnerable.

Creativity's Enemy: The Inner Critic

Sometimes, even if we are creative and artistic, we feel blocked or stuck. We just can't get started. Many of us also struggle with an inner voice that chatters a low-grade stream of discouraging negativity which dampens our creativity. For some it might just be related to their creative endeavors, but for others it is running all the time. In the world of creativity, this voice has been christened the *Inner Critic* (Hunt, 2004), but we've heard other evocative names, such as the Wicked Witch, that captures the nature of this personality. When our Inner Critic gets out of balance, turning from a helpful and friendly editor into a harsh censor, our creativity tends to shut down. We freeze, instead of loosening up and letting in new ideas.

Although we may assign nefarious intent to our Inner Critics (a client once described her Inner Critic as trying to "suck the joy" out of her life), we suspect that they are generally well meaning if not a bit misguided. We can *reframe* these creatures by identifying what purpose they are trying to serve (Lambert, Graham, Fincham, & Stillman, 2009). Our Inner Critic often wants to protect us from embarrassment or failure, and to avoid frustration and disappointment. However, in doing so, it keeps us from experimenting with new ideas, and from the learning that comes with trial and error. It also keeps us from having fun!

The Inner Critic is often caught up in perfectionism and performance. It is governed by the negativity bias, which, as we identified before, fixates on what might go wrong before we can contemplate what might work go well. Worse, often this inner editor is left over from unfinished business from childhood and is rooted in a place of shame. However, the happiest people accept that striving for perfection is a loser's bet and adopting a more devil-may-care attitude about performance will be more gratifying (Biswas-Diener & Kashdan, 2013).

How to Harness the Inner Critic and Inviting an Inner Muse

If the Inner Critic does mean us well and wants to help us, how would we harness this aspect of ourselves without letting it inhibit our experimental, creative, and fun-loving self? We can dialogue with it to determine what its intentions are. Then we can work on transforming the Inner Critic into a helpful and effective consultant who can offer clarity on what we like, what we don't, guidance about next steps, and clear direction for moving forward. We can also identify an Inner Muse that might compliment the Inner Critic.

Befriending Your Inner Critic

- Name the Inner Critic (You can take it even further and develop a persona or character for the Inner Critic. You can assign a gender, personality, style of dress, manner of speech, etc.).
- Dialogue with the Inner Critic (ask him/her questions like "What purpose do you serve?" "What are you trying to accomplish?" "How would you like to help me?" "How can I help you?!").
- Make a symbol, draw a portrait, or make a figure/sculpture of your Inner Critic (Trout, 2009).
- Make symbols for the strengths your Inner Critic represents (self-protection, judicious restraint, avoiding failure, good judgment).

- Make a symbol, draw a portrait, or make a figure/sculpture of your Inner Muse.
- Make symbols for the strengths your Inner Muse represents (creativity, appreciation of beauty, curiosity, playfulness).
- Picture your Inner Critic and your Inner Muse collaborating toward something you to want accomplish.

Everyday Creativity

We also encourage highlighting the value of everyday or "soft" creativity, in which we use this strength to make the world a tiny bit better, day by day. In other words, we exercise small acts of artful creativity more often: e.g., doodle more; sketch out a problem; draw your morning coffee; draw *with* your morning coffee (i.e., use your coffee as the medium and your spoon as the "brush"); take "art notes" at lectures and meetings; ask yourself a question and answer it with art; make stick figures of the people (and creatures) in your life and personalize them with details and designs.

Be wild; that is how to clear the river. The river does not flow in polluted, we manage that. The river does not dry up, we block it. If we want to allow it its freedom, we have to allow our ideational lives to be let loose, to stream, letting anything come, initially censoring nothing. That is creative life. It is made up of divine paradox. To create one must be willing to be stone stupid, to sit upon a throne on top of a jackass and spill rubies from one's mouth. Then the river will flow, then we can stand in the stream of it raining down. (Pinkola Estés, 1992, p. 343)

Art Therapy Brings to Positive Psychology the Use of Creativity in the Service of Healing

We would say that in a Venn diagram that combines art therapy and positive psychology, creativity is definitely in the section that overlaps. Positive psychology brings to art therapy a deepened knowledge and interest in creativity, a strength that we as human beings, with the challenges we are facing in the world today, need if we are to successfully make our way into the future (Lombardo, 2011). Creativity brings us new dimensions of *lived experience*—firsthand knowledge that we gain through direct engagement in our lives. This includes anything from the swirling design the barista crowns on Gioia's vanilla latte, to pithy observations of sharp-witted comics, handy solutions to household problems, or decorating a pleasing living space.

On the other hand, art therapy brings to positive psychology a profession which, for most of the last century, has utilized an individual's creative strengths in the service of health and healing. Creativity is art therapy's home turf. What art therapists do requires more than verbal counseling skills—it involves channeling the power of the creative process to foster emotional expression, engagement, self-reflection, communication, insight, and connection. Art therapists are thoroughly trained to have a broad knowledge of art materials and techniques so that they can optimally match particular creative pursuits with their clients' developmental and therapeutic needs at any given moment.

Engaging in the art process, especially with art media and interventions that are matched to respective clients, naturally promotes imaginative exploration and the experimental world of play. It induces engagement and flow, which, in and of itself, is healing but which also encourages in-depth therapeutic work—it opens people up. They become more receptive to self-reflection and vulnerability.

In addition, doing art work naturally promotes feelings of satisfaction, accomplishment, and pride. Sometimes this might come just from finding that they were able to engage in a process toward which they had trepidation—doing artwork. However, and perhaps even more significantly, because the art process allows them to *literally* "create"—to make an object that they can see, touch, and feel—a sense of achievement also comes from generating something which before *did not exist*. Then, because this "thing" that was made is a tangible object *outside* of the self that was, nevertheless, *made by the self*, it can provide a new way of seeing and perceiving the self (an aspect of the art therapy process that we will delve into in greater detail in Chapter 11 on meaning and perception).

In summary, art therapy contributes significantly and uniquely to PERMA and wellbeing by so effectively harnessing the creative process and all of its attendant benefits. This includes curiosity and exploration, positive emotions, experiences of engagement and flow, feelings of pride and accomplishment, and the creation of tangible works of art which can be used to explore and shift perceptions. We will now move on from creativity to an examination of flow, the state of being deeply absorbed and engaged which emerges naturally when we jump into the creative process.

Discussion Questions

1   Do you think of yourself as "creative"?
2   Do you warm yourself up to *be* creative?
3   Do you identify an Inner Critic when you're engaging in creative work? What would your Inner Critic and Inner Muse say to each other?
4   What kinds of everyday creativity do you see in other people around you?

CHAPTER 7

Flow

As art therapists, many of us have encountered the following—the art process is in full swing, the client/participants are deeply engrossed in their artwork, and we are faced with a dilemma. Do we interrupt the artmaking to review the artwork or do we let them stay absorbed for as long as possible? Although we fundamentally understand the value of both—often there are time constraints which force us to choose one over the other.

Because of the importance of community building and the insight that can be generated from exploring the associations to the imagery for insight, we often opt for processing the artwork at the expense of pursuing the deep state of focused concentration that engaging in artmaking can produce. On the other hand, with a group that has already had the chance to do some insight-oriented work together, we may be able to let the intense concentration that so frequently permeates the studio persist. If we and our clients are lucky and we have the time, we can do both.

That state of intense concentration, of *effortless attention*, is called *flow*. Like creativity, flow falls under the Engagement in life domain of Seligman's (2011) model of PERMA. Creativity often precipitates flow—when creativity generates experimentation, more often than not it leads to flow. In art therapy, we actively use creativity to promote flow, especially because the deep focus that emerges during flow states induces physiological changes which are both healing and restorative. This also triggers the upward spiral of positive emotion, broadening of awareness, and building of resources that boosts wellbeing and happiness.

What Is Flow?

What exactly is flow? First we'll illustrate with an example which may sound familiar because it captures elements of what is happening in art therapy studios throughout the world. In some of our longer workshops, in which we have the luxury of doing artwork for more than the therapy hour, we often conduct a brief visualization such as a body scan, a love-kindness meditation, or an "illuminated path." We then ease folks into the art process while we turn on some "chill-out" instrumental music. Once we've gotten group members settled into the *incubating* phase of the art process, we, ourselves, also create artwork, both to join in the experience and to model the process (Lachman-Chapin, 1987).

As folks begin to make aesthetic choices about what media, colors, marks, or images will capture whatever they are feeling or the visualization evoked—an illuminated path, love-kindness, body sensations at that moment—a sense of focused attention manifests in the group, a particular energy that is peppered by occasional questions about the materials or requests to another group member to pass some supplies. People are deeply immersed in their artwork, heads bent and fully absorbed while music plays softly in the background. The atmosphere has palpably shifted, like a rushing river settling into a gently babbling brook. This is what is known as flow.

Flow is the state we achieve when we are fully immersed and absorbed in an activity that is *autotelic*—we do it for no other reason than it is intrinsically engaging and rewarding. Flow occurs when we are faced with a challenge that we are skilled enough to master but which requires enough effort that we do not get bored (Csíkszentmihályi, 1991). During flow, we often feel acutely aware of ourselves while at the same time experiencing a lack of self-consciousness. We are fully attending to what we are doing—present in the here and now. We may have a sense of time either expanding or contracting—it may feel like hours went by in minutes, or that what was just minutes felt like a lifetime.

Flow can manifest in many different areas of our lives—in our office organizing our files, on the computer designing code, in the shop taking apart an engine, in the yard gardening, in the den composing a poem, or on the track running a race. Many people who have hobbies, who are athletes, or who are naturally creative experience frequent encounters with this sense of deep concentration.

Although people who have been in flow might report that it felt relaxing, flow is different from simply feeling good. In fact, individuals in flow are often so engrossed, they are not aware of feeling any particular emotions at all until the activity is almost complete. At that point, positive feelings such as joy or pride may emerge.

Characteristics of Flow

• Effortless attention—intense and focused concentration
• Merging of action and awareness
• Loss of self-consciousness
• Sense of control
• Change in the phenomenological experience of time—usually, a feeling that time speeds up or slows down
• Autotelic, an activity done for its own reward, or the fun of it

History of Flow

Csíkszentmihályi, one of the fathers of positive psychology, is best known for advancing the concept of flow. He initially became curious about flow in the 1960s while studying artists—he wondered why they kept doing art so single-mindedly (Getzels & Csíkszentmihályi, 1976). Csíkszentmihályi developed "flow" theory to explain this state of consciousness—taking the expression from what people voiced when they described the experience—that it felt like "being in the flow." In sports, this is sometimes termed being *in the zone*. Csíkszentmihályi determined that humans, on some level, appeared to be most fulfilled when they experienced this kind of highly focused absorption. It didn't involve so much feeling good, in fact it often involved intense concentration and effort, but it made them feel engaged and alive!

Research on Flow

There is now a substantial body of research on flow with a wide range of populations (Moneta, 2004; Collins, Sarkisian, & Winner, 2009; Csíkszentmihályi, 1997a). Closely associated psychological constructs include intrinsic motivation (Deci & Ryan, 1985), peak experiences (Maslow, 1971), and "openness to experience," one of the Big 5 personality traits (George & Zhou, 2001). Not surprisingly, creative people often experience flow (Csíkszentmihályi, 1996), and flow has been theoretically and empirically linked to happiness and positive emotions (Csíkszentmihályi, 1997a; Rogatko, 2009).

The Neuroscience of Flow

If you are into the neuroscience of art therapy, you are in for a treat! Gioia, in her doctoral work, studied the neurological and biological aspects of flow in order to make it as understandable as possible to those of us who are not neuroscientists. We present some of this research below with fair warning—this section can be challenging to read—so if you're not interested (which, however cool the brain mechanics may be to those of you who are more scientifically minded, may leave some others of you cross-eyed and dazed), we won't hold it against you if you skip to the Applications section of the chapter.

Attention

We are now going to bring our attention back to attention. Flow is often considered to be synonymous with *optimal* or *effortless* attention. However, perhaps we need to define attention more specifically. Attention is generally understood to be a cognitive process in the brain which enables focus to be directed toward some aspect of the environment (inner or outer) while disregarding other stimuli (Anderson, 2004). The metaphor of a spotlight is often used. Being able to sort through stimuli, determine what is relevant, and focus on that variable is critical to our survival (Nakamura & Csíkszentmihályi, 2002). Attention is also central to experiencing focused states of consciousness like flow or meditation. When our attention is effortless, we feel the mesmerizing effect of flow as irrelevant thoughts and perceptions are screened out and we become absorbed by the task at hand.

Neurological Activity During the Artmaking Process

The physical activity of artmaking involves complex brain/body processes. Research done by Chávez-Eakle and colleagues (Chávez-Eakle, Graff-Guerrero, García-Reyna, Vaugier, & Cruz-Fuentes, 2007) found a correlation between the creative process and specific brain activity including the following: assimilation of sensory information, motor learning, emotional reaction, and integration of cognition and emotion, as well as affect and meaning. Additionally, Lusebrink (2010) theorized that visual expression in art therapy involves sensory information processing in the occipital, temporal, and parietal lobes. This information is then transmitted through neural networks, along with important emotional input from the limbic area to the prefrontal cortex (Fuster, as cited in Lusebrink, 2010).

Clearly, there is a great deal of mental activity involved in the creation of art. How is it, then, that the experience of flow in artmaking can feel effortless? Our friend, art therapist Tiffanie Brumfield, once compared making art to "taking a refreshing nap." It often feels that way, as if the brain has both been fully alert and engaged but that it had also had a deep and revitalizing rest.

To explain this paradoxical quality, Dietrich developed a model, the *Transient Hypofrontality Theory* (Dietrich & Stoll, 2010; Dietrich, 2003), which differentiates the role of the explicit and the implicit information systems in the flow process. The explicit information system involves higher-order cognitive processes in regions of the brain which act to acquire, represent, and implement knowledge. This knowledge is accessible to conscious awareness and can be expressed through verbal processes (Dietrich, 2004a; Dietrich & Stoll, 2010).

In contrast, implicit information processing is a more ancient evolutionary system. Sometimes referred to as the *emotional brain*, this system holds experience-based knowledge. It is nonverbal and inaccessible to conscious awareness—what we commonly call the *unconscious*. Implicit information processing explains how we often naturally know how to do things but, when asked to describe what we did, we cannot articulate it. Knowledge in the implicit system is hidden from view and must be discovered through active processes. For this unconscious material to be revealed, we must "*perform or execute* implicit knowledge, which allows the explicit system to observe it and extract essential components" (Deitrich & Stoll, 2010, Kindle Location 2138-40; emphasis added).

So, to understand what's happening in flow, we need to understand that there is a complex interaction between the explicit and implicit information processing systems in the brain. The characteristics which define the phenomenological experience of flow—distorted sense of time, lack of worry, reduced awareness of the self, and effortless attention—can all be recognized as consequences of the explicit system fading "offline" (in the prefrontal cortex and the anterior cingulate cortex) and the implicit, unconscious system stepping in to direct behavior. The prefrontal cortex is in charge of cognitive activities such as time awareness, worry about failure, and other tasks related to self-consciousness. Dietrich (2004a) states that during flow, executive attention is the only prefrontal cortex functioning still active—there is a selective disengagement of all other higher functions while resources are diverted toward the task at hand. This creates that unique sense that we are concentrating without trying at all.

Applications of Flow to Art Therapy

Because creativity, flow, and improved wellbeing have been empirically linked, the study of flow clearly has implications for art therapy. One of the most healing components of the art therapy process is the deep relaxation and absorption that we and our clients experience when we enter a state of flow. Coming back to Tiffanie's quip, when we are in flow, although we don't actually take a nap, it feels that way.

Flow and the Relaxation Response

Herbert Benson, the world-renowned mind/body expert, coined the term the *relaxation response* to describe the physiologic changes in the body, such as lowered heart rate, blood pressure, breathing rate, and metabolic rate found when we are in a state of calm and at ease (Benson, Greenwood, & Klemchuk, 1975). He asserted that crafts and repetitive, rhythmic activities such as knitting can evoke the relaxation response—they reduce stress by "breaking the train of everyday thought" (Benson, 2009, p. 141).

As mentioned in the chapter on positive emotions, initial research indicates that the focused absorption of artmaking can activate the parasympathetic nervous systems which induces the relaxation response (Collier, 2011; Croghan, 2013; DeLue, 1999; Kuchta, 2008). For example, in a study of women who engaged in sewing on a regular basis, psychologist Robert Reiner determined that doing crafts is incompatible with negative states such as anger, worry, obsessions, and anxiety. He concluded that craft-making distracts from everyday pressures and promotes concentration on the here-and-now (Robert Reiner, personal communication, May 13, 2016).

Other Kinds of Flow

Being in flow and doing artwork does not necessarily produce a meditative state. Imagine a busy art studio full of highly energized 12-year olds creating a giant city out of cardboard boxes—high levels of flow but likely not much calm relaxation! Because they are experiencing effortless attention, immersion in the moment, a lack of self-consciousness, and a skill/challenge balance, this is still flow. In either meditative or more active experiences of flow, the implicit system is in charge—there is effortless attention and a lack of self-consciousness. The explicit system—tracking time and higher order cognitive functions—are still predominantly off-line.

Coming In and Out of Flow

At any given moment, artists may be more or less in flow, as the interaction between their skills and the challenge of the environment alternately affects the mobilization of the explicit and implicit systems. As artists experience visual, motor, and other sensory input through interaction with the art materials, their attentional focus is spotlighted on *both* external environmental stimuli—color, shape, and texture of the art material—*and* internal stimuli—thoughts, feelings, impressions.

When our explicit information processing system comes fully back "online," so to speak, we are often surprised by what we've created. In fact, when asked, we might say at first that we don't know what we've made and we just "went with the flow," because while *in* flow, the down-regulation of the prefrontal cortex limits this kind of cognitive processing. Many of us have had this experience. Now we have the explanation for why time rushed by, we didn't worry, and the artmaking process was so enjoyable!

Benefits of Flow

It has been demonstrated that many people find the qualitative experience of flow life-enhancing (Csíkszentmihályi, 1996). Reynolds and Prior (2006) suggested that being in flow can lead to optimal wellbeing due to associated feelings of accomplishment, control, and autonomy. In their qualitative study of women artists with cancer, they noted beneficial factors such as reduced feelings of helplessness and increased self-confidence. The intense concentration these women experienced in flow was found to banish intrusive fears and concerns about cancer—at least, for a period of time. Ullen and colleagues (Ullen, de Manzano, Theorell, & Harmat, 2010) confirmed that positive flow-inducing experiences distracts people from negative and painful stimuli. By providing healthy diversion, flow helps us to regulate our emotions.

Furthermore, Seligman (2002a) suggested that, like experiencing positive emotions, flow states build emotional capital for the future. Research has shown that flow states are linked to the upward spirals of positive emotions that increase wellbeing (Fredrickson, 2004; Fredrickson & Joiner, 2002; Rogatko, 2009). Recent work in neuroscience related to the affective plasticity of the brain supports the possibility of beneficial links between meditation, flow processes, and neurological growth and development.

Benefits of Flow in Art Therapy

Recent art therapy research is establishing the benefits of flow in art therapy. For example, Lee (2009), in a qualitative study of immigrant Korean children with adjustment difficulties, found that flow helped them escape boredom, loneliness, and anxiety. Both engagement with the process and with the researcher herself were found to facilitate flow. Art therapy researcher Hovick (2014) found that a simple physical warm-up to artmaking reduced feelings of self-consciousness and enhanced the intrinsically rewarding qualities of the experience. Burkewitz's 2014 study, "Coming to the Studio, Going with the Flow," measured in a small sample responses to engaging in six painting sessions. Over the course of one month, the artists reached higher levels of flourishing as evidenced by increased positive affect and reduced negative affect (Burkewitz, 2014). Overall, these studies support the idea that flow in art therapy is therapeutic both through distraction from anxiety and through active engagement.

The science of flow during the artmaking process provides empirical support for the *art-as-therapy* approach (Kramer, 1971)—that just the act of making art is healing. However, rather than framing it as sublimation, flow theory helps explain the mechanisms at play when we are deeply engaged in the creative process. Artmaking channels anxiety, transforms chaotic energy, and promotes concentration. Art activities that produce absorption and deep focus, such as coloring, drawing mandalas, working with clay, painting, beading, and knitting can be very effective in inducing experiences of flow. As Kaplan states, "when art making partakes of the characteristics of 'flow', it provides the kind of optimal experience that produces feelings of psychological growth and makes life in general more worth living" (2000, p. 76).

Warming Up to Flow

Not surprisingly, as art therapists we suggest that doing art is a natural way for people to activate everyday creativity and experience flow. Some people are blessed to be able to naturally and effortlessly jump into activities in which they experience flow—art, writing, running—but others may find that, even though they know what gets them into flow, they rarely get around to doing it. If you are that second group, you may have wondered, "If I enjoy doing this so much (painting, hiking, gardening), why don't I do it more?!" There may even be a part of you that actively resists doing it. And you may have bemusedly asked yourself, "Why would I avoid doing something that, when I actually start doing it, feels so good?!"

Csíkszentmihályi (1991) tells us that for many people, getting into flow requires an initial effort that may at first feel uncomfortable. He explains that one of the reasons that people often end up choosing sedentary but less rewarding activities such as watching TV or passively sitting around, is that these activities *appear* to provide opportunities for rest and relaxation. However, what they *actually* tend to do is drain our energy and leave us feeling depleted and listless—they do not provide the invigoration that flow activities induce. Although Csíkszentmihályi does not discourage people from indulging occasionally in what, these days, we might call "vegging out," he says that we need to create habits that overcome our more passive tendencies and help us work through the initial resistance that keeps us from activating experiences of flow.

There are varying levels of the flow experience. A person's experience of flow—the depth of relaxation and absorption they achieve—may be more or less engrossing depending upon their skills and abilities. Art therapists can presume that flow has been being achieved when their clients appear focused and lack self-consciousness; they describe the artmaking experience as having either gone by quickly or as having felt like it had lasted much longer than they'd realized; and they say they found it surprisingly worthwhile.

For some people, increased structure may be required for flow—whether in the form of an art directive (e.g., "use these watercolors to paint"), or a theme-based directive (e.g., "draw something for which you are grateful"), or any combination of the two (Hinz, 2009). We use warm-up activities such as those we outlined in the chapter on creativity—short writing prompts, simple drawing tasks using small paper, and/or guided meditations. A clear directive or guided activity in art therapy may produce more flow, or, as Rubin would say, a *framework for freedom*. It provides the semblance of structure. This can also be done through instruction on specific art supplies or techniques (e.g., collage, cutting paper, mixing paints) that is initially structured but often becomes more open-ended.

Because each individual had different artistic skills, some need heightened complexity to maintain the flow state. For instance, in an all-day workshop we ran at Smith Center using Altoid Tins boxes to makes shrines to love and forgiveness, one participant, a former student of ours, Valerie P. searched the Internet during a break to find out how to fold an origami paper crane (Figure 7.1). This challenge, self-initiated, stretched her artistic skills, suggesting that she intuitively understood that this could increase her experience of flow. On the other hand, another participant, who was getting frustrated trying to affix beads to her tin, clearly needed technical support from the facilitators. This helped her remain in flow instead of becoming overwhelmed by the challenge presented by the art materials.

Most art therapists intuitively encourage flow states when they are choosing art media and prompts/directives. At times, clear instructions and technical support will facilitate flow, at other times, open-ended exploration and experimentation will be best. Regardless, applying aspects of flow theory to art therapy can greatly influence our working understanding of how art therapy functions. This includes the ability to quickly assess artistic skill and signature strengths and to suggest corresponding tasks that provide challenge while limiting anxiety.

Flow and Timing

Both Gioia and Rebecca are lucky enough to work in settings where having enough time is a given. Most of our workshops run from 1½–5 hours. Having an environment with the time, space, and support conducive to incubate, to experiment, and to make mistakes is critical in facilitating moments of flow. Given that the skill/challenge balance can change at any moment, the timing of art therapy interventions can impact the degree to which individuals stay in flow.

If clients are deeply in flow during the time allotted for artmaking—i.e., they are deeply engaged with the art materials, focused, less verbal—and this time runs out, the art therapist has a choice to make. Should she extend the artmaking process and sacrifice part or all of the verbal discussion period—particularly as participants often need at least a few minutes to gear up to verbal processing (transitioning from more implicit to explicit information processing)—or interrupt the flow experience for the sake of moving into discussion? Both of these experiences are critical to the therapy process. This is a conundrum not easily resolved and one which we defer to the clinical judgment of the therapist at that given moment. On the other hand, people can also enter flow by engaging in conversations that evoke group flow, which we discuss below.

Flow and Music

Art therapists can also promote the experience of flow through environmental elements such as music and lighting (Chilton, 2013; Hinz, 2009). One secret weapon that Gioia uses to induce flow in the art therapy studio is down-tempo "lounge" rhythms. These "chill-out" tunes tend to have tempos between 80–110 beats per minute, and thus may induce a physiological relaxation response. They are also characterized by un-syncopated ensemble rhythms, R&B-influenced vocal samples, chorale patterning, a repetitive chorus, ambient synth textures, use of modal harmonies, and slow-moving bass lines. Artists such as *Nightmares on Wax, Thievery Corporation, Bonobo*, and *B-Tribe* epitomize this style.

Factors to Consider in Order to Evoke Flow in Art Therapy

- Quantity of time
- Amount of privacy
- Need for physical and emotional safety
- Room to work, lighting, table space, possibility for messy materials
- Artistic preferences
- Art media qualities and participant's skill/challenge balance
- Art media qualities and the group leader's skill/challenge balance
- Relevance/accessibility of the directive
- Type and volume of music
- Relational connections with the therapist or the group

Social Flow and Mirror Neurons

Positive psychologist Charles Walker (2010), in his research with college students, discovered that people often experience more flow when in social groups. This is clearly relevant to our work as art therapists because so many of us work with groups. Also compelling is research on mirror neurons (Gallese, Eagle, & Migone, 2007). Recall the description of flow in our art therapy workshops where, together with our clients, we as facilitators engaged in the art process. In doing so, we instinctively understand and resonate with the movements that others in the group are making as they work on their pieces (Hass-Cohen, 2016). We are both psychologically and physically attuned at such times.

Even if we do not ourselves actually make the same gesture, as we watch one another draw, our brain's neurons can mirror and essentially learn that behavior. Therefore, the skill/challenge balance so critical to flow may be mediated by the new learning happening through the mirror motor neuron system. This is relevant for art therapists who wish to increase their clients' experiences of flow. In other words, making artwork alongside our clients may increase flow through activation of the mirror neuron system (see Franklin, 2010, for example). Further research in this area will likely enhance our ability to provide experiences of flow in art therapy groups and dyads.

Flow and Strengths

As we will discuss in the next chapter, Seligman (2011) maintains that we enter a flow state when we use our highest strengths, aspects of ourselves that are core to who we are and what we value. Engaging in activities that are congruent with but which also stretch our strengths and abilities should naturally promote flow. This should be no surprise when we consider that flow is so closely linked to skill/challenge balance.

It may also explain why many of us, therapists and art therapists, experience flow in our work. Although most of us grasp that what we do is not easy, and many people in our lives often exclaim that they could never do what we do, to us it often feels effortless. When we are in the throes of our work, we are generally completely focused and engaged in ways that are completely congruent with our interests, strengths, and abilities. So, let us next dive more deeply into the next element of Engagement—into character strengths and how we can use those to induce flow and increase wellbeing.

Discussion Questions

1   What activities put you into a state of flow?
2   What do you do to warm yourself up to flow?
3   What takes you out of flow?
4   What techniques do you use to warm up your clients to flow?

CHAPTER 8

Strengths

We often ask our clients, "What is your 'super power'—a quality for which you are known, that you feel is core to who you are as a person?" Often, there is a pause as they search in their minds for characteristics that define them. Clients sometimes say that they are much more in touch with their weaknesses than with their positive attributes. If they really struggle and simply cannot think of anything positive about themselves, we ask them to think about something that family members or friends appreciate about them, or what they are known for among their friends, at work, or in their communities. We also give out lists of strengths and have folks pick out the qualities with which they identify most.

Struggling to recognize and label our strengths is not uncommon—research has actually confirmed this phenomenon (Linley & Harrington, 2006a). The negativity bias may partially explain this oversight. We may be more naturally attuned to our weaknesses and how they are causing problems for us than on ways in which we are performing well. We may also feel that there is more room for growth in addressing our weaknesses than our strengths (Biswas-Diener, Kashdan, & Minhas, 2011).

In addition, there may be an inherent *strengths blindness* (Niemiec, 2013) that results from a tendency to interweave our strengths with our personal values such that they are more likely to be viewed as "the right thing to do" rather than as unique characteristics. We may also overlook the uniqueness of our strengths because we tend to overestimate the similarities we share with others. For example, we might not identify that we, ourselves, are particularly kind or honest because we might presume that these are not strengths but rather ways that everyone should naturally behave.

As we have noted, historically the mental health professions, particularly in the US, have focused more on remediating deficits than on developing strengths. Although trying to improve upon our deficiencies may intuitively make sense— if there is a problem, we should focus on correcting it—positive psychologists have suggested that pathology may result as much from deficits in strengths as from weakness. Recent research shows that focusing on strengths may be as healing, if not *more* healing, as trying to compensate for deficiencies (Wood, Linley,

Maltby, Kashdan, & Hurling, 2011). It is not that our weaknesses disappear, they simply lose their prominence. When they are no longer the primary focus, positive qualities may emerge and flourish.

Robert Biswas-Diener (2011) likens weaknesses to the water sloshing around in the baseboard of a sailboat—we might notice it but hey, we're sailing, it's to be expected! However, if too much water gathers we have to bail it out, or if there's a leak, plug it so that we don't sink. If there's a breach in the hull, we might have to take more extreme measures and dock the boat for repairs. Nevertheless, even when our boat is perfectly intact, if we want to move, *our strengths are our sails*. We need them to propel us forward!

Operating from our strengths is another form of Engagement, the E in PERMA. Using our strengths makes us feel energized and fills us with authenticity. Operating from our strengths has properties similar to flow—it is so rewarding in and of itself that it makes us feel vital and alive, on top of our game. This is what positive psychologists call optimal functioning—what Seligman (2002a) calls "the engaged life."

Benefits of Focusing on Strengths

Although it may be self-evident, it deserves to be underscored that emphasizing strengths in treatment is critical—for multiple reasons. Therapy outcomes improve when therapists are primed to focus on clients' strengths. For example, with Cognitive Behavioral Therapy, better results were seen when treatment gravitated around strengths rather than deficits (Cheavens, Strunk, Lazarus, & Goldstein, 2012). In other research, people who used strengths more frequently experienced reduced stress and depression, as well as increased self-esteem and greater subjective and psychological well-being (Proctor, Tsukayama, Wood, Maltby, Eades, & Linley, 2011; Seligman, Steen, Park, & Peterson, 2005; Wood et al., 2011).

Similar research found that people who use their strengths were more likely to achieve their goals (Linley, 2015; Linley, Nielsen, Gillett, & Biswas-Diener, 2010). Focusing on strengths early in treatment also encourages buy-in into the therapy process—it engenders motivation and hope and, as a result, clients are more likely to persevere with treatment (Conoley, Padula, Payton, & Daniels, 1994). In addition, by making the lives of our clients more satisfying and fulfilling, amplification of strengths may buffer against recurrence of psychiatric symptoms.

Focusing on strengths is also correlated with more effective recovery from illness (Peterson, Park, & Seligman, 2006) and with fostering resilience and promoting perception of psychological growth in the aftermath of adversity. When clients are able to identify the qualities that have helped them surmount their challenges, they experience empowerment from and appreciation for their capacity to survive. On the one hand, this acknowledges existing loss or trauma; but it also it expands beyond identifying primarily with having been a victim into positive identification with their resilience (Wolin & Wolin, 1993).

Focusing on strengths may also alter negative stereotypes of psychotherapists as aloof authority figures psychoanalyzing the troubled in an attempt to untwist their distorted thinking and restore their broken relationships. Instead, therapists might be seen as collaborators helping resilient people activate their strengths, skills, talents, and abilities to face challenges and improve the quality of their lives.

What Are Strengths?

Strengths have been defined in several different ways:

- That which helps a person cope with life (Smith, 2006)
- Critical survival skills that allow people to right themselves (Masten & Coatsworth, 1998)
- A combination of natural talents, knowledge, and skills (Buckingham & Clifton, 2001)
- A capacity for feeling, thinking, and behaving in a way that allows optimal functioning in the pursuit of valued outcomes (Linley & Harrington, 2006b)
- The psychological ingredients, processes, or mechanisms that define morally valued virtues (Peterson & Seligman, 2004).

Most psychologists view strengths through the lens of classic trait theory. Like other elements of personality, strengths are considered to have a strong genetic component. Although they appear be relatively fixed and stable across the lifetime, they may not be consistent in all domains of a person's life. For example, there is some suggestion that strengths may be influenced by situational factors—an individual may exhibit certain strengths in particular situations and not in others. There is also evidence that certain strengths, such as modesty or independent thinking, may emerge and be valued more in some cultures than in others.

The Shift to Focusing on Strengths

That strengths are worthy of attention is nothing new to the realm of mental health. For example, the very popular Myers-Briggs Type Indicator (MBTI) applied Jungian theory to identifying 16 different personality profiles (Myers, 1998). The MBTI suggests that people have basic styles of operating in the world that manifest in a preference towards one end on a continuum of opposing tendencies. People are usually either more extroverted (E) or introverted (I), i.e., they tend to get re-energized either by engaging with others or by spending time alone. Both reflect equally healthy by very different ways of operating in the world. Others characteristics include thinking (T) or feeling (F), sensing (S) or intuiting (N), and perceiving (P) or judging (J).

The assumption is that when people know which of the 16 possible personality combinations that they most identify with, such as ENFP which Gioia and

Rebecca both ascribe to, they will be better able to understand their preferences and aptitudes, and modify life choices accordingly. Although these personality types are not considered to reflect strengths, per se, they are thought to reveal the operating style in which the person will be most energized and effective.

In the 1990s, psychologist Daniel Goleman (1995) contributed substantially to discourse on strengths when he suggested that some people are endowed with interpersonal strengths—*emotional intelligence*—that emerge above and beyond measures of cognitive intelligence. Howard Gardner (2011) also proposed that we expand our notions of intelligence, which in the past had looked predominantly at intellectual aptitude, to consider multiple intelligences, such as linguistic, musical, logical-mathematical, spatial, bodily/kinesthetic, and interpersonal and intrapersonal intelligences.

The notion of a *Strengths-Based Approach* in therapy emerged in the 1990s from the field of social work. Saleebey (1996) articulated this direction when he noticed that the traditional processes in which clients were assessed involved elaborate identification of presenting problems, environmental stressors, and psychiatric symptoms. He observed attention to strengths was usually only cursory. Saleebey proposed that, in assessing and treating clients, social workers use a more holistic approach that incorporated their clients' unique strengths and abilities and that identified resources within themselves and in their environment.

Saleebey (1996) outlined a useful comparison of a strengths-based versus pathology-based approach which we've paraphrased below:

- The comparison is possibility-focused vs. problem-focused.
- A person's *behavior* is viewed as the problem vs. the *person* is viewed as the problem.
- Counseling is a collaborative process vs. the therapist interprets and fixes the client.
- Individuals, families, and communities are viewed as the experts on their lives vs. only professionals are experts.
- Focus is on what is functioning and right about the person vs. the medical model which focuses on what is wrong or abnormal.
- Therapy builds on strengths vs. therapy reduces symptoms.

Different Models of Strengths

One of the hallmarks of positive psychology is the call for strengths to receive more articulation, theoretical framing, and scientific inquiry. Peterson and Seligman (2004) were so passionate about the importance of strengths in well-being that they assembled an exhaustive and detailed compilation of core strengths and positive qualities that have consistently emerged throughout history and across all cultures. They classified these qualities into six virtue domains under which fall 24 character strengths with concrete definitions for each.

They give examples of paragons throughout history who seem to personify each strength and of ways that it has appeared in different cultures. And finally, they offer strategies for assessing each strength and specific interventions for cultivating that quality.

Although not exhaustive, *Character Strengths and Virtues* is significant in its attempt to provide a detailed *taxonomy* for the language of strengths (Peterson & Seligman, 2004), a clear vocabulary for describing these attributes. In order to be included, each quality had to meet certain criteria. For example, it had to be morally valued in its own right, it could not be a quality that diminished other people, and it had to emerge universally in most cultures. Seligman (2011) states that these 24 strengths underpin the five elements of PERMA, that utilizing our highest strengths not only provides an avenue for engagement and flow, it also leads to more positive emotions, meaning, accomplishment, and better interpersonal relationships. Smith-Jones (2014) expanded on the *VIA Inventory of Strengths* by adding economic and financial strengths, as well as survival skills and kinesthetic strengths.

Other well-articulated models of strengths have also been developed. Donald Clifton and his colleague Marcus Buckingham at the Gallup Institute have conducted extensive global research in this realm. In the *Clifton Strengths Finder* (Buckingham & Clifton, 2001) they outlined 34 *talents* that people manifest. They suggested that strengths emerge when talent is combined with effort and investment. Another model which we will discuss below, the *Realise2* (Linley & Dovey, 2012), outlines four domains in which strengths manifest.

How to Practice Using Strengths

"What gets you through when times are tough?" We have used this directive with all sorts of clients in all sorts of settings—with cancer patients in all-day retreats, on inpatient psychiatric units with people who are in crisis, and with resort guests who are looking for balance and insight. Regardless of which population, more often than not our clients identify more with their vulnerabilities and much less with their strengths. And if they do have some idea of their strengths, they are often not clearly defined. We have found in clinical settings, strengths are usually more anecdotally noted and circumstantially described. They are rarely a significant component of treatment planning and goal setting.

Assessing and Identifying Key Strengths

Research suggests that identifying strengths, in and of itself, has been associated with increased happiness and decreased depression (Seligman, Steen, Park, & Peterson, 2005). We see this when our clients discover aspects of themselves they may have been unaware of or that they had overlooked. In doing so, they clearly find greater personal satisfaction, self-awareness, and self-esteem.

Specific strengths assessments can be used to capture positive qualities. The *VIA* corresponds directly to Seligman and Peterson's *Character Strengths and Virtues* (Peterson & Park, 2009; Peterson & Seligman, 2004). Others mentioned before, such as the *Realise2* and the *Clifton Strengths Finder* have been used most in corporate settings to help high-functioning individuals maximize their careers; however, they offer useful paradigms for clinical work as well. Both the *VIA* and the *Clifton Strengths Finder* have been adapted for children (Rath & Reckmayer, 2009). Other assessments such as the *Behavioral and Emotional Rating Scale* (Epstein & Sharma, 1998) and *Multiple Intelligences Developmental Assessment Scales* (Shearer, 1996) are also useful tools for identifying strengths in children.

Developing and Regulating Strengths

Although just identifying and using our strengths improves wellbeing, positive psychologists suggest that we need to fine-tune our strategies even more if we want to truly optimize the value of applying a strengths-based model (Biswas-Diener, Kashdan, & Minhas, 2011; Rashid, 2014; Linley, 2015). A more nuanced approach to doing so might look at how strengths can emerge differently depending on context (some strengths might appear in some situations around certain people but remain underutilized in other circumstances), regulating the use of strengths in proportion to situational demands, and taking into account the effect their use has on us and on others. In other words, using "the right strengths, in the right amount, in the right situation" (Robert Biswas-Diener, personal communication, May, 2010).

Although strengths have been seen as fairly fixed attributes, in fact they often emerge more or less depending on the situation. We may be very courageous when we are protecting someone who is being bullied, but shy and nervous when we have to go on stage. We also want to discern when and how much to use a strength. For example, it may not be appropriate to use the strength of humor with someone who has just suffered a loss, yet it may be just the right thing to help lift someone's spirits when they are down. In clinical work, humor can also serve as a useful catalyst to help clients overcome hesitation or resistance and warm them up to the therapy process (Ricks, Hancock, Goodrich, & Evans, 2014).

Energizing Strengths and Learned Behaviors

We also want to differentiate between strengths that are empowering and engaging versus learned *behaviors*—areas where we perform well but which drain our energy (Linley & Dovey, 2012). British psychologist Alex Linley and his colleagues created the *Realise2* [sic], a model with 60 characteristics which fall into four categories: Realized Strengths, Unrealized Strengths, Learned Behaviors, and Weaknesses. They provide instructions for addressing the different domains. *Realized strengths* are those that we know we have. We should use them more. *Unrealized strengths* are those we are not aware of and, once identified, we should also use more. *Learned behaviors* are skills which we possess but which, when we apply them, deplete us. We should use them less. *Weaknesses* are areas where we don't perform well and rob us of energy. We should use these as little as possible.

In our work, often the most revelatory moments come when people identify that they are spending a lot of time engaging in learned behaviors—doing things that they are good at but do not enjoy. They may be very proficient at these tasks and people depend upon them to fulfill those responsibilities, but doing so leaves them depleted and disengaged. This explained Gioia's insight that, although she had what others might consider to be the "ideal job"—getting paid well to work with elementary school children, little documentation required, long vacations, etc.—she was restless and bored. She realized that she much preferred working with adolescents and people struggling with drug and alcohol addiction. Even though these folks were often defiant and full of pathos, it felt like a calling—they inspired and fully engaged her and provided the kind of skill/challenge balance that allowed her to experience flow.

In Gioia's case, she was able to remove herself from a situation which called upon more learned behaviors than it did opportunities to employ more energizing strengths. Many of our clients may not be able to extract themselves from situations that require frequent use of learned strengths, such as unavoidable job responsibilities or caring for a family member who has special needs. At these times, one may couple a learned strength, or even a weakness, with a more stimulating *realized* strength that keeps us motivated enough to labor through a difficult but necessary and meaningful task.

Using our strengths to compensate for weaknesses is particularly relevant if we have innate vulnerabilities that challenge our happiness. For example, as we have mentioned previously, having a genetic propensity for traits associated with neuroticism—emotional sensitivity, negative mood, anxiety, excessive worrying—or struggling with a physical or mental illness that is not curable and perhaps even terminal, can interfere significantly with happiness and wellbeing. In these cases, we certainly do not want to ignore our weaknesses. However, positive psychologists suggest that rather than attempting to "fix" these challenges, which in some cases may be an exercise in futility, we should use our strengths to manage them. Although we certainly want to be *aware* of our vulnerabilities so that we can more effectively compensate for them, we don't want to devote all of our energy on trying to change them (Biswas-Diener, 2011). For example, Rebecca, after recognizing that she met most of the criteria for neuroticism as well as having chronic pain, uses her strength of self-regulation to get regular exercise and extra sleep when she is feeling particularly anxious or physically uncomfortable.

We can also compensate for areas in which we are challenged by partnering with other people whose strengths complement ours. For example, we have been able to apply this in our joint writing projects. Although Rebecca writes very well, she struggles with starting our books and articles. Fortunately, Gioia—who is innovative and full of ideas and energy—will often generate initial content and pass it over to Rebecca who goes from there. In this way we moderate our weaknesses and learned behaviors with each other's strengths.

Overuse of Strengths

Chris Peterson suggested that we might even view weaknesses and mental illness vis-à-vis strengths. He defined each of the 24 *Character Strengths and Virtues* with relation to its qualities, its opposite, its absence, and its overuse (Seligman, 2014), suggesting that pathology could be seen through these criteria. For example, the qualities of courage are bravery, persistence, authenticity, and vitality. Its opposites are cowardice, helplessness, deceit, and lifelessness. Its absence emerges as fright, laziness, insincerity, and restraint. Its excess is foolhardiness, obsessiveness, righteousness, and hyperactivity. For love, its qualities are intimacy, kindness, and social intelligence. Its opposites are loneliness, cruelty, and self-deception. Its absence manifests as isolation, emotional detachment, indifference, and obtuseness, and its excess is emotional promiscuity and intrusiveness.

We might see this in our clinical work when our clients say that they are "honest to a fault," but struggle with interpersonal relationships because others experience them as harsh or critical. Or that they have a "big heart," but complain "I care *too* much!" suggesting a need for establishing boundaries when practicing their capacity to love. Generosity, if exercised without restraint, may lead to feeling taken advantage of and resentment. Being cautious and measured may be a hazard when spontaneity and quick action are needed. Being logical and efficient may seem insensitive when sympathy and compassion are in order. Those of us in mental health might recognize that being overly caring may foster dependence in others and leave us emotionally exhausted, especially if we tend to others without addressing our own needs (we will return to the topic of self-care in Chapter 13).

Strengths Constellations

Linley (2015) suggests that we can enhance strengths by combining qualities that complement each other. For example, we might join *Strengths of Being*, which includes authenticity, personal responsibility, self-awareness, and service-orientation with *Strengths of Relating*, which include compassion, emotional awareness, empathic connection, and rapport building (Linley & Dovey, 2012). Diener (2003) also notes that one might be endowed in certain domains, such as social intelligence, but less so in others, such as straightforwardness. In addition, some clusters of strengths may preclude others. For example, honesty and authenticity might be less compatible with diplomacy and agreeableness.

Strengths Spotters

We can also cultivate being "strengths spotters"—building awareness not only of our own strengths but other people's outstanding qualities and skills (Whitney, Trosten-Bloom, & Rader, 2010). For example, Biswas-Diener suggests learning from our spouses, friends, and colleagues their underlying values and what they are passionate about:

> When do you hear their voice rise or speed up? What seems to activate and empower them? Try keeping an eye out for uncharted strengths over the rest of the week. Pay attention to the way your friends and colleagues use their time, what they do when they are alone, how they interact with one another. (2013, p. 87)

Becoming *strengths spotters* can help us build and solidify connections by making us more appreciative of others. Therapists are often blessed to have this quality in the repertoire of strengths that engage and energize them.

Cultural Sensitivity

Strengths are often presumed to manifest within the individual; however, they are also heavily influenced by cultural factors. For example, although Peterson and Seligman's (2004) *Character Strengths and Virtues* includes qualities that appear to emerge across all cultures, some may be more or less valued in different parts of the world and within certain social groups. For example, humility and temperance may be more prized in Eastern cultures, self-expression and assertiveness more in Western cultures. Individualism may hold more value than collectivism in some cultures. Attuning to these influences is critical in adopting a strengths-based approach.

How to Use Strengths

- Identify your strengths.
- Identify strengths that deplete you—use them less.
- Identify strengths that energize you—use them more.
- Regulate strengths, utilize them judiciously.
- Identify how certain strengths impact others and when they are most functional.
- Identify strengths of others.
- Complement your strengths and weaknesses with others' strengths and weaknesses.

Art Therapy and Strengths

Although most art therapists would identify themselves as operating from a strengths-based paradigm and we often tout art therapy's capacity to highlight strengths, we don't always have concrete strategies for applying a strengths-based art therapy practice. In the following section, we will outline how we apply strengths in a *positive art therapy* approach. This includes suggestions for assessing and using strengths with clients. We also describe what art therapy uniquely contributes to the realm of strengths and ways that this can be further promoted. We revisit strengths in Chapter 9 as they impact relationships and the supervision of art therapy students and practitioners and again in Chapter 13, where we provide suggestions for applying a strengths-based model to our work in corporate settings and additional tools for bringing strengths into the training, practice, and development of therapists.

Assessing for Strengths in Artwork and the Art Process

We start this discussion with a focus on art therapy assessment because, whether or not we agree that art therapists should conduct formal assessments, we naturally form impressions about our clients based on their interactions with the art materials and the artwork they create (Betts, 2012). In addition, if we work in clinical settings, we are often asked to report what artwork communicates about our clients and whether we like it or not, efforts to secure mental health licensure has compelled graduate art therapy programs to require Assessment and Diagnosis in their degree.

In addition, because treatment as we know it is often geared toward addressing *presenting problems,* art therapists are often forced to provide clinical input which fits *DSM* criteria. To the credit of our profession, several art therapy assessments such as the "Diagnostic Drawing Series" (DDS) (Cohen, Mills, & Kijak, 1994) and the "Person Picking an Apple from a Tree" (PPAT) (Gantt, 1990) and the "Formal Elements Art Therapy Scale" (FEATS) (Gantt, 2009) have effectively correlated visual elements with psychiatric diagnoses. However, few of the most commonly used art therapy evaluations have articulated parallels between graphic content and strengths.

For example, in the case of the DDS, although Mills suggests that, through its administration, "one can and should see client strengths" (2011, p. 404), there is a presumption that strengths are evident, de facto, by the *absence* of pathology. The same can be said for the FEATS. Gantt and Tabone (2011) describes some attributes which can be found in normal drawings—e.g., that the imagery is logical, well integrated, and has a reasonable amount of detail, and colors appear to be appropriate to the subject matter. Although one might infer that qualities such as "integrated" reflect strengths, Gantt does not provide any *explicit* descriptions of how strengths manifest in imagery.

This makes sense when we consider the context within which these assessments emerged. The FEATS grew out of Linda Gantt and Paula Howie's efforts to correlate precise visual elements with specific diagnoses in the *DSM* (Gantt & Tabone, 2011). The DDS was developed during the early 1980s "to help ensure our survival within the increasingly embattled and competitive health care environment" (Cohen, Mills, & Kijak, 1994, p. 109). It was designed to lend legitimacy to the art therapy field and improve the "clinical acumen" of art therapists "within institutions that emphasize intake, triage, diagnosis, treatment and discharge planning" (p. 105).

Let us be clear, we do not wish in any way to disparage these or any other attempts made on the part of dedicated art therapists to empirically validate art therapy's capacity to increase insight into our clients. We have no critique of the DDS or the FEATS, other than suggesting that these tools, as might be expected at the time they were formulated, focused more on identifying pathology than on showcasing client strengths. However, we do suggest that, in order for us to have a more balanced picture of our clients, we would benefit by engaging in the same process for systematically matching visual content with strengths as have been used to ascertain evidence of symptomatology.

The Integrative Method

In fact, we are tremendously indebted to innovators such as Cohen, Mills, Gantt, and Tabone who created systematic ways of correlating the formal elements in artwork to their meaning. For example, Cohen was influenced by Janie Rhyne. Recall that Rhyne (2001a, 2001b) outlined a gestalt approach to art therapy, based on Rudolph Arnheim's proposition that visual expression is an *isomorphic* representation of psychological dynamics—that visual elements in imagery are external manifestations of internal processes (Cohen & Cox, 1995). Cohen collaborated with Carol Cox (1995), one of our mentors at George Washington University, in developing what they called the *Integrative Method* for understanding the structure of visual imagery and the process whereby it was made.

Although they focus mostly on the artwork of survivors of severe childhood trauma and clients with dissociative disorders, it provides basic tools that can be applied with all art therapy clients. Cohen and Cox suggest that "the art process, the art product, and the practice of art therapy all have isomorphism at their core" (1995, p. 2), i.e., imagery and the process with which it was created enables us to infer the internal state of the creator:

> Once the isomorphic relationship between an artist and an art production is acknowledged, one may begin to elaborate on the meaning in terms of its psychological implications. In the *isomorphic mirror*, all aspects of the art-making process and product reflect the artist's inner life. (Cohen & Cox, 1996, p. 2)

Related is the notion that, in perception, the mind rapidly takes pieces of information from its visual field and forms a *gestalt*—a global impression of what it sees. Similarly, Gantt and Tabone (2011) maintain that, when looking at art work, we naturally engage in *pattern matching*, whereby we decipher visual cues in such a way that we experience an intuitive sense of what a picture might mean.

Cox and Cohen's (1995) integrative method includes developing visual literacy (looking at the visual elements in the art form), the process whereby it was made, and the content and symbolic meaning of the imagery. They provide the language for describing and understanding the information that is communicated through these avenues. We suggest that just as these strategies have been used to reveal psychiatric diagnosis, they also provide rich metaphorical pathways for articulating strengths.

The Building Blocks of Visual Imagery

Cohen and Cox refer to Donis Dondis's *Primer in Visual Literacy* (1974), a resource from the world of art criticism which provides the tools to "read" and understand visual content in imagery. Dondis, who was also influenced by Arnheim's ideas about visual perception, likens developing literacy in visual analysis to learning a language. She suggests that understanding the components and composition of art can be taught in the same way that one would teach the fundamentals of grammar and syntax.

The building blocks of visual form are comprised of elements such as line, shape, form, color, texture, space, and value. How these components are combined structurally helps convey their meaning (Dondis, 1974). This includes aspects such as the number, arrangement, and scale of elements, the clarity of presentation, the interrelationship of images, and the use of special effects and color. Subsets of these categories consist of features such as pattern, emphasis, variety, unity, balance, rhythm, style, movement, proportion, negative/positive space, focus, direction, attention to detail, simplicity, complexity, intensity, juxtaposition, figure-to-figure and figure-to-ground relationships, perspective, depth, and developmental level.

In addition to including the elements of visual form, Cohen and Cox also incorporated aspects of the *Expressive Therapies Continuum* (Kagin & Lusebrink, 1978) into their model. They suggest that media properties—particularly their range of fluid to resistive qualities—and the tools used to create the artwork were important factors to consider.

Using Visual Literacy to Identify Strengths

Just as we would with evidence of pathology, when using visual literacy to identify strengths we engage first in a detailed description of the formal elements. We then ask how do the visual elements serve as metaphors for the client and their situation? Do the elements and patterns in the imagery reflect the clients' competencies and resources in their lives and, if so, how? What is successful in the art work? What visual elements lead to that impression?

We have seen countless illustrations of this in our work with clients with thought disorders. For example, Figure 8.1 by Frederick, a patient in long-term care for chronic schizophrenia, contains clear elements of thought disorder—e.g., word inclusion, unusual "patchwork" in the coloring of the animals, and impoverished representation of the human form. However, the strengths evident in the image—e.g., deliberate mark-making, attention to detail, bright colors, interaction between the animals in the image, and a literal invitation to "come in"—clearly outweigh any evidence of pathology. In addition, although he used stencils to outline the animals, suggesting that he might generally benefit from some structure, he was able to construct a coherent composition independently, suggesting both cognitive organization and imagination.

We have heard protests that the assessment process should be impartial—that it should be used to learn *any and all* information possible about the client, not necessarily that which is "bad" or "good". We agree and suggest that using visual literacy, because it is a process of observation, is a useful method for managing *judgment* and *interpretation* of the imagery. In essence, it is a practice in mindfulness. However, as we have mentioned, because of the negativity bias, as clinicians, we are often more naturally inclined to notice evidence of pathology. Therefore, we often need to consciously focus on evidence of strengths—to *attend to the good*.

The Art Process as a Reflection of Client Engagement and Strengths

Frances Kaplan (2012) suggests that observing how clients *engage* in the art process, not just their imagery, may be one of the most relevant ways that we can use art to learn more about our clients. When observing process, we ask questions such as, "How quickly do they warm up to the art process? Do they become more expressive or less expressive? Do they become more relaxed or more agitated? Are they able to dialogue with the artwork, to gain insight from the imagery, and/or to engage in exploration with others about their image?"

We also notice behavioral elements, such as level of investment, effort, energy, physical vitality, creativity, ingenuity, imagination, ability to focus, and tolerance for frustration. For example, Anna, an inpatient client who presented with disorganized/pressured speech and manic behaviors, created a succession of "images" which shows signs of thought disorder—word inclusion, concrete and loose associations, and flight of ideas (Figure 8.2)—in between bouts of intrusively disrupting other group members. In order to help her focus, Rebecca suggested she draw what was important in her life. Anna responded immediately, sitting quietly and intently for several minutes to create Figure 8.3, a picture of her son just after he was born. Her ability focus despite her manic state when the subject matter was deeply meaningful to her reflected some degree of reality-orientation, coherence, and capacity for attachment.

We also recommend that art therapists replicate their clients' artwork—a practice taught to us by Carol Cox which she credits to Bernard Levy (personal communication, 2016)—to get an empathic "dip" into the process through which the artist underwent when they were making their piece. Using the same kind of material, mark-making, color, composition, form, detail, etc. often gives us additional insight into their strengths.

Working with Meaning

The final phase of Cohen and Cox's (1995) integrative model includes a multi-level approach to determining meaning in the artwork. They refer to Kreitler and Kreitler's proposition that multiple related and contrasting meanings can be contained in a single image. This presupposes that no single element in the art work can encompass its full meaning—that all of the elements that go into its making—the imagery, the process, the content of the imagery, and the associations—must be integrated into a "network of meaning" (1972, p. 3).

When looking at meaning through a strengths-based lens, we might ask questions such as "What does the imagery suggest about the artist's preferences, values, beliefs, relational capabilities, etc.? What about their verbal associations relate to the visual elements of the imagery? How do they respond to exploring the metaphors that are suggested in the visual elements of the art work? What discrepancies and congruencies emerge between the imagery and the verbal associations to it? What insight does the artist infer from these comparisons?" Again, we will delve further into exploration of meaning-making in Chapter 10.

Working with Our Clients Using Visual Literacy

Cohen and Cox (1995) suggest that art functions not only as a vehicle for communication with the therapist, but also as a means of *self-communication* and *self-revelation* for the artist. Cohen, Barnes, and Rankin provide illustrations of this process in their workbook, *Managing Traumatic Stress Through Art*. For example, they have clients describe the line quality of their images using objective terms such as straight or curved and subjective terms such as dynamic or lyrical—to notice what is most visually striking in their images and "think, write, and talk" about these impressions (1995, p. 135). Just as we suggest that this process of visual analysis can be used by therapists to observe strengths, they can also be used by *clients* to attune to their strengths.

In addition, as many art therapists operating from a client-centered approach intuitively know, if we equip our clients with the skills to learn about themselves through their artwork, they will be better able to gain insight through their *own* observations rather than feeling like it is being omnisciently imposed upon them. This may not only defuse their tendency to feel that their artwork is being "analyzed," but it may also put the client squarely in the driver's seat. We often start this reflective process by suggesting that, as Jung (1965) believed, art work is *a message from the self to the self*. If they were to attune to that message, what would it be?

When we empower clients with the language of visual literacy—i.e., we give them the tools to reflect upon their artwork and explore the meanings and metaphorical parallels these visual elements and their approach to doing art might hold—they are often surprised that it reflects much more than they had realized. Often they initially dismiss their artwork as childish and simplistic and assume that most of the visual effects are accidental or unintentional. However, after they explore the visual choices that they either consciously or unconsciously made, they often experience a significant shift in their perception and appreciation of their artwork. They frequently like it much better "even if it doesn't belong in a museum." They realize that their style of expressing themselves—their choice of art materials, of color, texture, symbols, etc.—is a unique and personal signature. They appreciate more fully that, however humble their art work may be, it eloquently illustrates essential aspects of their core nature—positive, negative, and neutral—and their ways of seeing the world.

In a group process, participants can be also coached to give feedback to their peers based on the specific visual elements that they see in each other's artwork (always with the permission of the respective artist). Sometimes it can be surprising how quickly group members grasp and are able to communicate qualities about the artwork—that it is either expansive or contained, bright or muted, abstract or representational, has a central focal point or has many different points of interest, is geometric or organic—and to query each other about how that might reflect who they are.

This not only educates participants about the potential of art to express unique qualities of the various members, but just as it does in individual work, it can minimize the impression that the therapist is the only person equipped to "interpret" the imagery. In addition, when the artists receiving this kind of input from their peers, it often gives them a more appreciative glimpse of themselves through the eyes of others.

Positive Art Therapy Assessment

Donna Betts (2012) recommends we adopt a positive approach to art therapy assessment in working with our clients. This includes: 1) integrating multiple sources of information and determining how they apply meaningfully to the individual's life; 2) working collaboratively with clients; 3) viewing the outcomes of assessments and the actual assessment process in the context of the therapeutic relationship, and 4) incorporating client strengths and resources into the clinical picture.

Betts (2012) suggests that we can modify positive psychology assessments to include an art therapy component, e.g., a four-part matrix developed by Snyder and colleagues (Snyder, Ritschel, Rand, & Berg, 2006) for cataloguing clients' internal and external assets and weaknesses. Betts observed that this matrix naturally lends itself to visual representation. Clients might make artwork mapping out a quadrant for each, thus providing a more detailed impression of the clients' internal and environmental resources and challenges.

We might also adapt other tools: e.g., illustrating bio-psychosocial assessments to visually depict physical, psychological, social, and spiritual assets; responding with imagery to interventions from solution-focused therapy such as asking clients who are struggling "What if a miracle happened?" (Walter & Peller, 1992); depicting what it will look like when the presenting problem improved or exceptions when it was better and what contributed to making it so, or mapping "the people who support and help you in your life" (Bannink, 2014). We can look to the results of strengths assessments such as those mentioned above to explore how specific strengths such as the capacity to love and be loved, spirituality, social justice, love of learning, or tenacity emerge in visual imagery or in the process of making it.

Both Betts (2012) and Scheinberg (2012) suggest that art therapy assessment should place particular emphasis on measuring hope. Although hope is classified as an emotion, it can also be a strength/character trait with which one is more or less endowed, a coping style, and/or a cognitive mindset. Hope is comprised of elements such as motivation and goal-directed activity, agency, and pathways. Agency is the belief in our capacity to affect our environment. Pathways are the means that we believe we have available to achieve our goals and alternative routes if the initial ones are obstructed. Hope is critical not only because it is considered to be an essential buffer against hardship, but because it effectively predicts psychological adjustment, health outcomes, and resiliency (Snyder, 2000).

Lest we ourselves be guilty of focusing more on weaknesses than strengths, we recognize that many art therapy assessments *do* provide concrete indicators of strengths. Most notable is the Rawley Silver Drawing Test (Silver, 2002) which provides language for positive manifestations of categories such as emotional content, self-image, humor, and cognitive skills, i.e., the ability to select, combine, and represent. The first three categories are rated on a scale of 1–5. For example, on the humor scale, humor that disparages others gets a low score and humor that is playful or reflects resilience gets a high score. In the emotional content scale, strongly negative themes such suicidal ideation and stress get low scores and positive themes such as caring relationships get high scores.

Other art therapy evaluations have also been recognized for highlighting strengths. For example, the PPAT clearly illustrates problem-solving skills (Gantt 1990). The "Bird's Nest Drawing" (Kaiser, 1996) assesses social attachment, connection, and love. The "Draw-a-Person-in-the-Rain" task has been used to measure hope (Rose, Elkis-Abuhoff, Goldblatt, & Miller, 2012). The "Bridge Drawing" (Hays & Lyons, 1981) explores developmental growth, meaning, motivation, and future-orientation.

Art Therapy Interventions and Strengths

Although we believe that art therapy assessments would benefit from linking visual imagery and the artmaking process with more specific strengths models (Betts, 2012; Chilton & Wilkinson, 2009), we also know that most art therapists utilize interventions which naturally pull for strengths. For example, even directives as simple as representing oneself as an animal or a tree will reveal strengths and assets—e.g., with a tree we look at its roots, branches, foliage, fruit, any creatures living in or around it, etc. In fact, there are so many art therapy directives that mine for strengths that we could not begin to include them all. We point out a few below and more in Appendix A.

Cohen, Barnes, and Rankin suggest that clients do artwork about their level of functioning—when they are not doing well, when they are at their "level best," and what factors contribute to the latter. They provide a list of strengths and have clients choose ones which have helped them cope, e.g., "asking for help when needed" or "sense of humor" (1995, p. 123).

Scheinberg (2016, in personal communication) incorporates a psycho-educational approach to strengths. She has noticed that, in order for her clients to be aware of and maximize the benefits of using their strengths, it helps if they have descriptions of what those qualities might be (she uses handouts of the *VIA*) and an understanding of their positive impact on wellbeing. After holding a discussion, she has clients complete a strengths mandala which includes *current strengths*—those they feel they are already actively employing—and *working strengths*—qualities they would like to develop more.

Because so many of our clients have shaped their identity around their weaknesses and the problems they have encountered, we also provide concrete tools to identify more of their assets and strengths. Along with the *VIA*, we also use Booth and Sleeman's (2007) "Strengths in a Box," 150 cards of strengths that fall into 4 different *suits*—heart, head, hands, or spirit—and that include qualities such as "determined," "punctual" and "team player".

We often use these cards as a warm-up for "Spirit Dolls to Honor Strengths and Resilience," one of the workshops we hold for people have been affected by a life-threatening illness. After the participants identify cards that resonate for them, they wrap a small message to their strengths in the interior of a doll they make out of wire and fabric. A variation of this might be to have clients draw or form a symbol for the strength card(s) they chose. Art therapists can also make their own set of strengths cards that are relevant to the clients with whom they work. Even better, have their clients make a set for themselves!

In our clinical work, we focus on strengths right at the start of treatment to build rapport (Rashid, 2014). This means essentially employing solution-based strategies (Saleebey, 1996) such as mining for the strengths and resources that have helped clients survive and thrive despite the adversities they have faced. We also present the potential for art to provide unique insights into aspects of themselves of which they may or may not have been aware. We educate our clients in the language of visual literacy and apply those tools with their artwork and, if they are in a group, with others' artwork to help them gain information about themselves and transform their perceptions of themselves and their situations (as we will explore further in Chapter 11 on meaning and perception). We apply these strategies in almost all of our work, regardless of the directive, setting, or population.

What Art Therapy Brings to the Realm of Strengths

Just as art therapy can benefit from adopting a positive psychology approach that focuses more on identifying, developing, and refining the use of strengths, the world of positive psychology would be greatly enhanced by art therapy's capacity to reveal and highlight positive characteristics. As we in the art therapy field have always known, art can showcase strengths in ways that verbal strategies alone cannot. The visual elements in the artwork provide rich evidence of qualities that might not emerge as eloquently, *if at all*, through other forms of expression. The way artists engage with art materials and their associations to their imagery also offers rich metaphorical illustrations of their style of approaching and interacting with the world. Combined, this provides a way for us to see our clients and for our clients to see themselves and others that is unique, compelling, and empowering.

We move now from exploring the realm of Engagement, the E in PERMA—creativity, flow, and strengths—to looking at Meaning, the M, and examining the way that art can help us identify our values and illustrate what gives our lives meaning and purpose.

Discussion Questions

1   What are your top signature strengths? Which strengths energize and which deplete you?
2   What strengths do you frequently see in your clients? Your co-workers?
3   How can art therapy assessments help you to understand your clients' strengths better?
4   What ways do strengths emerge in the way your clients engage in the art process?

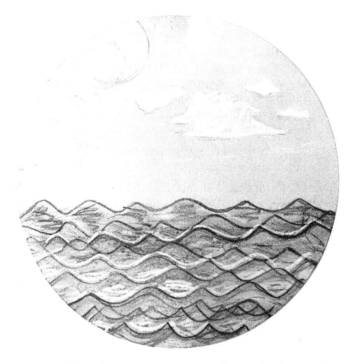

Figure 5.1 Having clients depict a positive emotion they would like to feel more often helps them visualize and experience those emotions. For example, by illustrating serenity, Lamont, a client with substance dependence, was able to access feelings of "low-key joy" (p. 75).

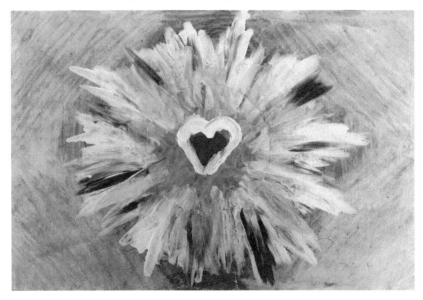

Figure 5.2 Kristin, another client with substance dependence, drew a small heart with oil pastels to illustrate "love". Combining the creative process with visualization led her to more fluid media and to extend radiating lines from the heart onto larger paper, literally illustrating the "broaden-and-build" effect of positive emotions (p. 75).

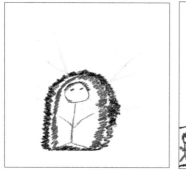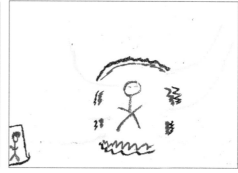

Figures 5.3 and 5.4 Laura, a woman with a history of childhood sexual abuse, spontaneously represented the depression and pain she was struggling with by surrounding a stick figure with red and black scribbled lines (5.3). She explained that the yellow arrows bouncing off of this "shell" meant that "no good can get in or out." When asked what it would look like "if the good got in," Laura recreated the image (5.4) so that the black and red marks "let the good flow through" (p. 78).

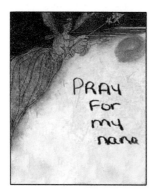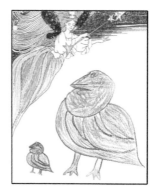

Figures 6.1 and 6.2 Coloring images provide concrete structure and opportunities for reality-orientation and grounding for clients who are anxious, agitated, manic, psychotic, and/or disorganized. For example, two patients in long-term psychiatric care, Carmela (Figure 6.1) and Edmund (Figure 6.2) chose the same coloring sheet in an open studio art therapy group. The differences in their creative responses to the same image of a Fairy Godmother are self-evident (p. 91).

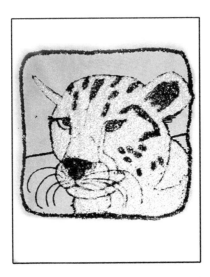

Figure 6.3 David, also in long-term psychiatric care, carefully filled a coloring sheet of a leopard with glitter. The glue under each color of glitter needed to dry before another color of glitter could be applied, requiring patience and planning. He was so pleased with his image that he hung it up in his room to brighten his spirits (p. 92).

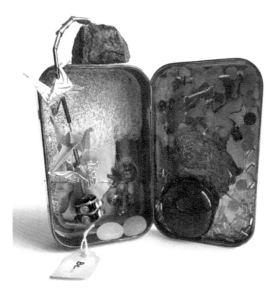

Figure 7.1 Art therapy activities induce flow by providing enough challenge to engage but not overwhelm clients. For some clients, that means simpler, structured tasks and more technical support; for others, more complexity. During an all-day workshop for clients and caregivers affected by cancer, one participant, Valerie P., maintained a deeply absorbed state of flow by researching online the intricacies of folding an origami crane, adding it to a detailed "miniature shrine to love and forgiveness" (p. 104).

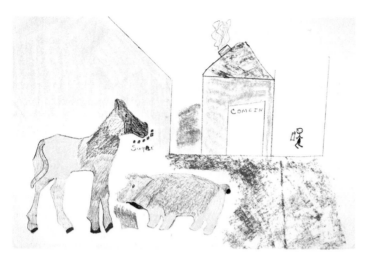

Figure 8.1 Frederick, in long-term inpatient care for schizophrenia, made imagery that reflected thought disorder—word inclusion, unusual "patchwork" in the coloring of the animals, and impoverished representation of the human form. However, the deliberate mark-making, attention to detail, bright colors, interaction between the animals in the image, and the literal invitation to "come in" clearly outweigh any evidence of pathology (p. 120).

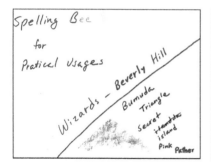 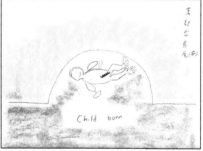

Figures 8.2 and 8.3 Anna, an inpatient client who presented with disorganized/pressured speech and intrusive behaviors, created a rapid succession of images which showed signs of thought disorder—word inclusion, concrete, loose associations, and flight of ideas (Figure 8.2, Anna, "Spelling bee"). To help channel her mania, she was encouraged to depict what was important in her life. With quiet deliberation, Anna drew "A child born" (Figure 8.3), demonstrating that, despite her manic state, when the subject matter was deeply meaningful to her, she showed the ability to focus, indicating some measure of reality-orientation and capacity for attachment (p. 120).

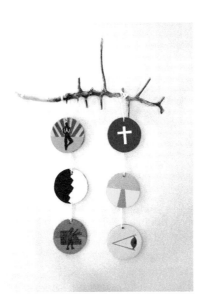

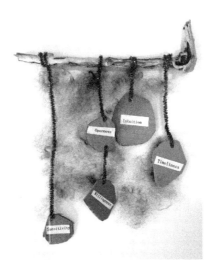

Figures 10.1 and 10.2 We often explore meaning and purpose by providing a list of values (see Appendix D) and having clients make artwork about those which they resonate with most. Jack, a client in drug and alcohol treatment, created a "values wall hanging" of cut-paper collages to represent Balance, Faith, Industriousness, and Vision (Figure 10.1). Lamont (who drew Figure 5.1) created a wall hanging using cut cardboard and blue unspun wool to symbolize his commitment to Openness, Intuition, Sensitivity, and Willingness (Figure 10.2) (p. 161).

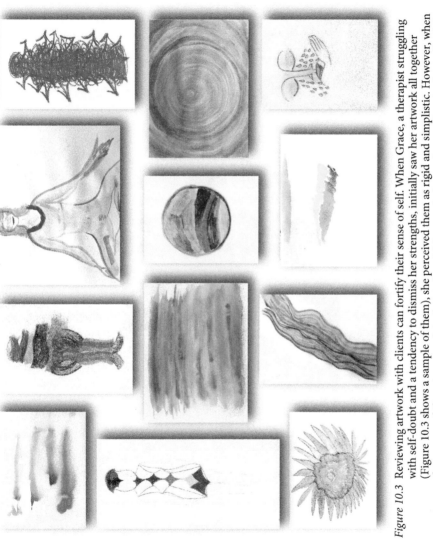

Figure 10.3 Reviewing artwork with clients can fortify their sense of self. When Grace, a therapist struggling with self-doubt and a tendency to dismiss her strengths, initially saw her artwork all together (Figure 10.3 shows a sample of them), she perceived them as rigid and simplistic. However, when she compared them to artwork in the studio which were darker and more chaotic, she realized that hers were brighter and more fluid. She was surprised by the continuity of visual themes, e.g., warmth, movement, power, and immediacy (p. 163).

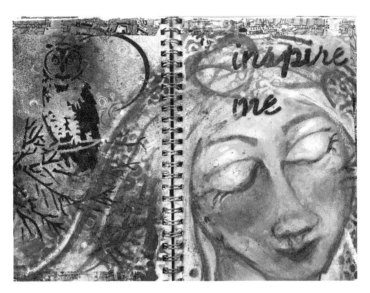

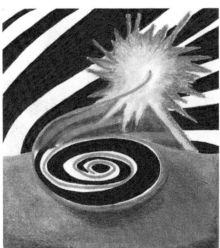

Figures 11.1 and 11.2 During a workshop with cancer patients on "Celebrating Resilience," we, the authors, made artwork alongside group members. Gioia's image (Figure 11.1), served both to celebrate getting her PhD and to invite new ideas. Rebecca's (Figure 11.2), a healing path leading to a hopeful sun, represented her relief that her sister's health was finally improving. Group members commented that Rebecca's image looked like "a fuse exploding." Initially, Rebecca worried this might mean she was about to "explode," however, when she observed visual elements such as the upward spiral and the rich colors, she contemplated more positive meanings—it might instead be a spark of celebratory energy! The intriguing characters in Gioia's image also suggested deeper meanings which, through techniques such as having parts of the characters dialogue with each other or storytelling, she could choose to explore (pps. 167–187).

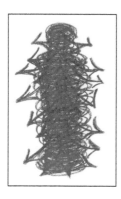 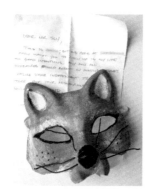

Figures 11.3 and 11.4 In Figure 11.3, Grace, (who reviewed her artwork in Figure 10.3), depicted a sense of violation she experienced when people invaded her personal space. When she saw the image's visual appeal, she concluded that setting boundaries/expressing her anger could be "elegant" (p. 183). In Figure 11.4, dialoguing/role reversing with imagery can often reveal positive meaning. For example, Joshua depicted his addiction in a mask of a fox, Mr. Sly. When he role-reversed with Mr. Sly, Joshua recognized the self-determination he represented and the need to direct this strength toward more positive outcomes (p. 185).

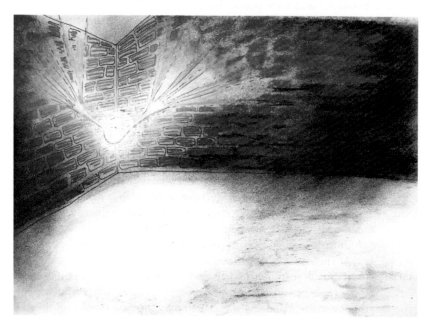

Figure 13.1 Art therapy students and clinicians can explore how they perceive their role by depicting themselves "as a source of light." Art therapist Eileen M. saw herself as a "light in a brick room" (Figure 13.1), explaining that although it was sometimes difficult to stay "lit" when she confronted the "wall of darkness" and emptiness she saw in her clients, rather than trying to tear the wall down, she wanted to help illuminate it (p. 212).

CHAPTER 9

Relationships

In the workshops that we run at Smith Center for people affected by cancer—patients, caregivers, and therapists—we usually have about ten people, mostly women of ages ranging from their twenties to their seventies. We warm up with a simple drawing activity such as a small mandala of three things that went well that morning. This kind of soft beginning accommodates both the early birds and the late arrivals.

After about 15 minutes of quiet artmaking, we pull our chairs into a circle with our mandalas and have people introduce themselves. We ask them to share what brought them to the workshop and something about their three good things. Because many of the participants are caring for someone who has cancer or are ill themselves, we propose that they disclose only what is comfortable at that moment. However, they are often quite open—almost immediately sharing what they are going through, even commenting that they are surprised they are doing so that quickly among a group of strangers. As they talk, heads nod empathically and there is even laughter when they mention light blessings such as finding a parking space, as well as more profound appreciations—that they still had some hair despite chemo or they got to cuddle with their favorite creatures that morning.

We also share *our* blessings, modeling that we are there as participants as much as facilitators. We follow introductions with either a discussion about some aspect of wellbeing—positive emotions, strengths, resilience—or some form of meditation, such as love-kindness or a body scan. Then we present whatever art process we'll engage in—e.g., altered books, spirit dolls, or small "shrine" boxes. The art supplies are laid out for them; traditional art materials as well as objects of all sorts, from shells and feathers to coins and bottle caps.

Because they are usually already warmed up to each other and the art process—they've made mandalas and shared why they are there, and they've seen the delightful selection of materials waiting for them—they usually jump right into making art. And then, for a few quiet and focused hours, the group experiences communal flow. A spirit of quiet camaraderie fills the room as afternoon light pours in from the courtyard garden. Occasionally, technical complexities provide interesting artistic challenges. Although we are there to help, just as often other group members offer effective solutions.

During the group process, we simultaneously engage in making our own artwork and carefully attune to each other and to the participants. We pause whenever we sense that someone might need focused attention—cutting wire for someone with hand tremors or helping someone gather supplies.

With about an hour left for processing, we pull ourselves out of the deep engagement of flow (usually with light prompting from Rebecca while Gioia grumbles about not wanting to stop), in order to give each person an opportunity to speak about her small treasure. During the closing discussion, it becomes clear that group members have connected with each other through making the art together and sharing not only about the losses that brought them there but also the joys and strengths that their imagery expresses.

As we led more of these workshops, we began to notice that not only was the artwork eloquently communicating what was most important to each person, but equally powerful was the way these expressions were witnessed by the group. The combination of the two was profoundly moving for them. In order to deepen these connections, we began supplying envelopes upon which each group member wrote her name. After each person shared about her work, others wrote/ sketched on small slips of paper messages of hope and encouragement (signed or anonymous) and tucked these messages into the artist's envelope to peruse later.

We found that this not only gave the participants a concrete memory of how they had touched each other, but it also shifted the tendency for sharing to be directed toward us as facilitators. It captured that other participants were equally interested and affected by each other and their artwork. It gave them feedback about the impact they had had on their peers and a chance to practice love-kindness towards each other. The envelopes were often incorporated into the art, tucked inside altered books or art journals or attached to a spirit doll. When the artist went through their messages later, they served as reminders of the empathy and appreciation they felt for each other.

Other People Matter

When people talk about what makes them happy it's usually their relationships. Although relationships were not initially included in Seligman's Three Paths to Happiness, he consistently received feedback that the pleasant life, the engaged life, and the meaningful life were essentially *meaningless* without relationships. For example, Seligman's buddy Chris Peterson became famously known for insisting that "Other people matter!" and that any talk of happiness needed to take that into account. So Seligman added the R to PERMA and perhaps it is no accident that relationships end up smack dab in the middle— they are the lynchpin of flourishing.

According to positive psychologists Reis and Gable (2003), good relationships with others are *the most important* source of life satisfaction and emotional wellbeing. Ryff (1989) identified interpersonal connections as a core element of psychological wellbeing. People who have good friends and positive relationships are happier and happier people have more friends. This has important downstream consequences: "Nurturing, supportive contact with others, a sense of belonging or mattering to others, and participation in social groups have been tied to a broad array of mental health and health benefits" (Taylor, 2011, p. 207). Social support induces hormonal changes that boost brain health and protect us against heart disease and other immune-related disorders, leading to increased overall health and longevity.

In addition, as research has verified, not only are relationships gratifying, they are critical to our survival (Cozolino, 2014). This confirms what humanists suggested—that people are propelled as much by social needs as by more primitive drives. In addition, we know that interpersonal connectedness and support is incredibly important to resilience (Everly, McCormack, & Strouse, 2012). In the face of adversity, a secure relationship with a caregiver can make all the difference in the world.

Positive Relationships

Although we will touch on what we know from psychology-as-usual about relationships, as we proceed, we will spend more time on theory and research emerging in positive psychology that is adding to our understanding of relationships, particularly what fosters *positive* relationships. We explore implications of this work for art therapy as well as how art therapy uniquely contributes to improving relationships.

Keyes (2003), in his model of flourishing, suggested that people who have positive relationships exhibit interpersonal characteristics such as acceptance and actualization. In positive relationships, be it with family, friends, teachers, colleagues, mentors, neighbors, acquaintances, or others in our communities, we feel cared for, safe, and connected. Supportive relationships are fundamental to wellbeing—humans need each other!

However, because interpersonal dynamics can be so complex, we could just as easily say, "it's complicated." Although people usually identify that their relationships are the most meaningful area of their lives, they also report that they are the source of some of their greatest frustration, distress, and dissatisfaction. Even in some of our most intimate relationships, we may feel misunderstood, disconnected, and isolated.

Psychology-as-usual has focused predominantly on those aspect of relationships—the role that loneliness, resentment, ambivalence, criticism, blame, hostility, jealousy, co-dependency, poor communication, social isolation, and insecure attachment play in interpersonal dynamics. This makes sense when we consider the impact these have on the individual and on relationships. In addition, because of the dominance of the negativity bias, even minor negative interpersonal exchanges can override positive ones. This is why conflict can cause such distress to the parties involved and why, as with any suffering, we in the helping professions are motivated to help alleviate that distress.

However, as a result, much less attention has been paid to what characterizes *positive relationships* and what makes them thrive. Positive psychology is interested in not only how we can *decrease negativity* but also how we can *increase positivity* in relationships. Even though, at first blush, it is a subtle differentiation, it is again a shift from "fixing what's wrong" to "building what's strong."

Positive psychologists suggest that just as we need to balance the greater impact of negative emotions with a higher ratio of positive emotions, so too do we need to counter negative experiences in relationships with a higher ratio of positive experiences. Lambert and colleagues (Lambert, Fincham, Gwinn, & Ajayi, 2011) propose the metaphor of a savings account for relationships—steady deposits of positive experiences create a balance of healthy emotional capital that buffers the relationship against the impact of negative experiences. For those who are less partial to equating relationship dynamics to financial transactions, we might instead think of a reservoir which is either draining or being filled.

We can increase the positivity cache in our reservoirs through several strategies: increasing positive emotions in relationships, capitalizing on positive events, boosting love and gratitude, practicing mindfulness in relationships, finding the good in negative experiences, spotting strengths, exploring values and beliefs, and attending to the good. Because it is the foundation of the work that we do as therapists, we preface this exploration with a look at the therapeutic relationship. We start there because not only is positivity vital to relationships in general, it is fundamental to establishing a strong therapeutic alliance.

Positivity in the Therapeutic Relationship: The Therapeutic Alliance

Regardless of the therapist's orientation, it is now established that a strong therapeutic alliance is a universal component of effective therapy (Lambert & Barley, 2001). In other words, the *therapeutic relationship matters*. It is the foundation for any work that proceeds. However, although the curative nature of the therapeutic alliance is now implicitly understood, practical tools for generating it are often not explicitly taught (Seligman, 2011). In addition, when there is training in this area, it tends to focus more on helping *clients* experience more trust and safety in the relationship, rather than also helping *therapists* bond more with their clients. Now this is where it gets really complicated! How one approaches the therapist's relationship with their clients differs dramatically depending on the role they believe that relationship plays in therapy.

Transference and Countertransference

For example, in psychodynamic treatment, therapists are encouraged to maintain a neutral stance upon which clients project their feelings, commonly known as transference (Freud, 1958). In this paradigm, we experience individuals we are currently in relationship with as if they were significant figures from our childhood. Therapists are presumed to experience similar feelings—countertransference—in response.

Transference and countertransference are understood to be very useful for identifying dynamics within the psyche of each respective participant and in the therapeutic relationship. However, there is the presumption that properly managing the transference/countertransference dynamic includes not only identifying feelings that derive from past relationships but also *separating* them from current relationships, putting them in their relevant place in time and context, and resolving the developmental concerns that they reflect. In addition, although therapists may *consciously* recognize that transference and countertransference are unavoidable and even helpful, often they *unconsciously* believe that there is something shameful about feelings that arise between therapist and client, especially their own. As a result, transference and countertransference are often perceived to be something that should be avoided or contained.

It turns out that Freud, to his credit, was on to something—research has revealed that transference and countertransference *is* a reliable, measurable phenomenon. However, whereas psychodynamic theory suggests that its development is rooted in unresolved conflict, social psychologists Andersen and Berk determined that the transference/countertransference dynamic is "a normal, nonpathological process, occurring both inside and outside psychotherapy, following basic rules of social information processing" (1998, p. 81). People *do* relate to others by using what they have learned about other people they've known in the past. Our "significant-other representations"—that is to say our internalized memories, beliefs, and feelings about our relationships with special people in our lives—are unconsciously operating in our current relationships.

It is thought that most people generally experience a *mix* of realistic and transference reactions to others in their lives (Gelso, 2002). Therefore, we can assume that not only is it doubtful that therapists would be neutral toward their clients—but even less likely that they'd be unencumbered by their own past relationships. In essence, it's impossible *not* to be! In a positive psychology framework, we want to move beyond analyzing these relationships to actively harnessing this dynamic. From the start of treatment, we want to promote *positive* transference and countertransference. We want to foster positive feelings between ourselves and our clients especially at the beginning, when it is essential that not only do our clients experience more hope, sense of connection, and trust, but that *we do too*.

Unconditional Positive Regard

In contrast to Freud's "blank slate," humanists suggested that therapists should convey a genuine and caring presence—let's call this a "warm slate." For example, Carl Rogers (1951) suggested that therapists cultivate an attitude of *unconditional positive regard* toward their clients. This *person-centered* approach involves conveying authentic appreciation toward our clients for who they are.

Although providing unconditional positive regard toward our clients is a noble intention, it is something that we often take for granted, as if it should be effortless and incidental. After all, we are simply supplying an understanding ear. Therapists are often teased (both by themselves and others) that they get paid to "just sit and listen" or jokingly parodied for their banal support—for sympathetically mirroring to their clients, "What I hear you saying is . . ." or gently deflecting requests for advice with "What do *you* think?"

Wouldn't it be great if it were that simple and easy! However, from a positive psychology perspective, we might point out that not only is empathic listening one of the best things that psychotherapy has to offer, in fact, it is one of the *most* challenging things therapists do. Showing compassion and good will toward clients is no small feat. It can actually be quite difficult given that we, just like our clients, are often coming to the relationship "cold." Just as we might not instantly feel safe and welcoming to a stranger on the street, we might also not necessarily feel empathy and warmth toward our clients right off the bat.

In addition, similar to the psychodynamic model, unconditional positive regard is taken to mean that, as therapists, we accept our clients without bias. This may be difficult to do, especially if they have engaged in behaviors that we do not condone. Rogers addressed this by clarifying that it meant approaching our clients with the belief that each client has "vast resources for self-understanding, for altering her or his self-concept, attitudes, and self-directed behavior" (1978, p. 7). By carefully attuning to what our clients value and are trying to achieve, we can then be instrumental in creating a climate that supports this psychological growth.

Yet again, although most of us would unfailingly agree that this is a worthy position, it is something else to maintain such an open-minded and optimistic attitude. At any given moment, as we will talk about in more detail in Chapter 9, on meaning and perception, we, just like our clients, are experiencing a multitude of unconscious biases and judgments that are influencing what we believe about our clients and their capacity for growth and change. Therefore, just as we want to actively warm up to our clients, so too do we need to engage in strategies that help us identify our own beliefs about therapy and to see our clients more clearly.

Compassion and Empathy

Compassion is the ability to understand the difficulties we and others have experienced without judgment, while at the same time feeling motivated to relieve their suffering. Empathy is a component of compassion—it is the "process by which positive and negative emotions are shared, without losing sight of whose feelings belong to whom" (Decety & Meyer, 2008). Most approaches to building an effective therapeutic alliance include the assumption that the therapist cultivates empathy both toward and in their clients. Rogers (1975) described it as accurately sensing the feelings and personal meanings being experienced by our clients and communicating this understanding to them.

Brain science describes empathy as involving three separate processes: 1) *emotional simulation*—evoking an emotion through imagination; 2) *perspective-taking*—envisioning another person's point of view; and 3) *emotion-regulation*—modulating emotions through various strategies (Elliott, Bohart, Watson, & Greenberg, 2011). It includes imagining the perspective of their clients and accurately mirroring their clients' experiences while simultaneously regulating their own emotional state. This is where, as therapists, we offer supportive comments, body language and facial expressions to communicate that we "get it." Therapists' ability to demonstrate empathy and compassion is fundamental to helping clients feel like they are being understood (Elliott et al., 2011).

Intersubjectivity

Although the term intersubjectivity smacks of jargon, at its simplest, it means that "reality" is a *jointly* constructed experience. We aren't isolated individuals encased in our own private universe. We overlap. Think of a Venn diagram: each person represented by a circle with intersubjectivity as the space in between. This is important because a therapeutic alliance is *co-created*. Both the therapist's and the client's mental and emotional state shape that shared space. Therefore, we want to be conscious of what we contribute to that dynamic. Furthermore, we believe that we can not only be active agents in what energy we channel into the therapeutic relationship but also that it will be more productive if we shift the intersubjective space to be more *positive*.

Strategies for Building Positive Relationships

We've been talking about the traits that characterize the therapeutic relationship, particularly those that build a strong therapeutic alliance. Fortunately, therapists are often naturally endowed with these qualities—self-awareness, insight, empathy, and compassion. In fact, these are frequently the strengths that led them to the helping professions in the first place. However, just because we might be blessed with these attributes does not mean that we inherently know how to create and foster a therapeutic alliance. Doing so entails specific skills. Think of the therapeutic alliance as a muscle, something that we can and want to strengthen through conscious activity.

In a positive psychology approach, we build that muscle using the same techniques that we use for increasing positivity in relationships in general. In a positive art therapy approach, we interweave those efforts with art therapy principles and discover how they are mutually complementary.

Positive Art Therapy and Positive Relationships

Does art therapy boost positivity in relationships? Absolutely! Humans connect with each other through art. Artmaking, rituals, and ceremonies articulate, express, and reinforce our sense of who we are and where we come from. It is both literally and figuratively one of the foundations upon which communities, cultures, and civilizations are built!

Art illustrates the human experience in a language that crosses cultures, time, and space. Human beings fundamentally understand visual imagery, regardless of its origin. Art bears the unique signature of the artist and reveals what how they see the world. Art taps into parts of ourselves that we cannot consciously access, personal and universal—what Jung (1986) called the *collective unconscious*. In groups, as people reflect on their imagery, they identify patterns that emerge in between and among the group members. This heightens the sense of shared humanity, the experience of universality that is so critical to the therapeutic process (Yalom, 1995). This is why *art therapy* is far more than simply making art alone—it includes the heightened sense of identification and connection that emerges from witnessing and sharing art together.

Art is a way of communicating that speaks beyond words. It makes visible what cannot otherwise be seen and cuts through the need for translation and interpretation. It gives us a picture of our minds and our internal landscape. It maps the inter- and intrapersonal terrain of our relationships. It reveals the dynamics and flavor of our relationships—social networks, connections, disconnections, conflict, power differentials, our place in culture and society, intimacies.

Art not only expresses our thoughts, feelings, and concerns, but it gives us a unique perspective on those things. It is a way of learning something *new and different* about ourselves and others. It reveals what we value and what matters most to us. And, as we will discuss further in the next chapter, it cuts to the core of what gives our lives meaning and purpose.

Art becomes manifest in the world, an object separate from its maker upon which, from a distance, we can reflect. This is one of art therapy's greatest assets—that artwork literally gives us a different perspective and, as a result of this externalization, we as the viewer experience a shift in our perceptions. This happens whether we are the therapist, the artist him- or herself, or another group member.

Art, at its simplest, offers something exceptional to the R in PERMA. Making art together jumpstarts connections! Broadly speaking, it both creates and commemorates human culture and civilization. It taps into the collective pool of experience and knowledge that we all share as humans. It provides a short cut to communicating, instantly relating what might be time-consuming or even impossible to articulate in words. It reveals and strengthens our common humanity while also illustrating what is personally relevant and meaningful to us as individuals. It shows who we are and what we value. This not only helps us learn something about ourselves, but also gives others a chance to get to know us in a way that they could not have otherwise. We see ourselves differently. Others see us differently. And, when we are looking at their artwork, we see them differently. Art enables "an empathic participation in the lives of others" (Barone & Eisner, 2012, p. 9).

We can enhance these inherent strengths by incorporating principles and strategies from positive psychology that further build relationships. A *positive art therapy* approach uses art to do just that, to build the connection "muscle" by increasing positive emotions, practicing mindfulness, finding the benefit in negative emotions and experiences, capitalizing on strengths, exploring values and beliefs, and attending to the good. As we proceed, we will interweave these positive psychology strategies with art therapy concepts and define how they are mutually complementary.

Positive Emotions as Warm-up to Therapy

We launch this discussion with positive emotions because not only do we consider them to be one of the most essential components in positive art therapy, but also in positive relationships. We cannot underscore this enough! From the get-go, we are very consciously and strategically inducing positive emotions into the therapeutic encounter. When we say this in trainings, we are often met with consternation and dismay. People think we are either repressing negativity in the service of superficial positivity, glazing over our clients' distress because we can't tolerate suffering, or colluding with their defenses—criticisms that are also leveled against positive psychology in general.

This is far from the case. Whether in group or individual work, we always begin with attuning to what our clients are initially presenting—answers to the question "what brought you here and why now?" Often therapy is a response to some sort of stressor that has become uncomfortable or painful enough to warrant outside assistance.

Therapy is a risky venture and, to take on that challenge, our clients need to feel safe. This is fundamental to most models of psychotherapy. Acknowledging the reasons that they came to us, willingly or not (many of our clients have been involuntarily hospitalized or court-ordered to treatment), and responding empathically to their distress is critical to building initial safety. In a positive psychology approach, we also begin with this line of inquiry—both in order to get a sense of the clients' main concerns and to develop trust. However, we do not dwell there. As we discussed in Chapter 5, on positive emotions, we shift fairly soon to exploring what it would look like "if it were better."

Often, when people are contemplating their situation improved, they start off "in the problem." They usually voice that they are hoping for a reduction or resolution of the stressor they are facing (less loneliness, depression, strife, anxiety, etc.). Again, if we consider the negativity bias, this makes sense. When we're suffering, it dominates our attention. We are focused on wanting it to stop.

In order to counter this tendency, we want to visualize not just what we are moving away from but also what we are moving *toward*—be it more love and enjoyment in our relationships, more recognition in our work, more energy, etc. As we have described, clearly articulating and visualizing "better," by default, induces the positive emotions that accompany that imagined state.

Experiencing positive emotion is critical at the start of therapy because clients need, on some level, to have hope. Then *we*, as therapists, by witnessing our clients visualize positive states, experience that hope as well. This is intersubjectivity. Evoking feelings of hope in *both* parties accelerates the therapeutic alliance and promotes feelings of safety, support, and love: "Powerful therapeutic bonds are built by deeply discussing positive emotions and experiences" (Rashid, 2014, p. 26).

In summary, at the very early stages of building the therapeutic alliance, we capitalize on Fredrickson's (1996) *Broaden and Build* theory. We do so first by responding empathically to our clients' distress. This makes them feel safer and is the first step in forming that alliance. When they feel safer, they are able to consider not only their challenges but also other perspectives—their attentional field is broadened. Introducing positive emotions allows the therapist to feel hope and a sense of possibility as well. It makes them feel better about their work, which in turn makes *them* feel more optimistic and willing, and broadens *their* attentional field, all of which improves the therapeutic dynamic. Strategically incorporating positive emotions early on favorably grounds the intersubjective space in a foundation of positivity.

Questions to Warm Up Positive Emotions in Therapeutic Relationships

- What would it look like if it were better? Are there times when it has been? (Visualizes possibilities, identifies exceptions, illuminates what people value and what makes them feel good).
- What's working and what's going well in general, or if the person is struggling with a difficult situation, in that dynamic? (Gives hope and empowerment).
- What were three good things—routine or extraordinary—that happened today, and why? (Introduces humor and builds comradery).

As described above, the first strategy we employ in building a therapeutic alliance is creating a harbor for our clients to safely express their feelings and voice their concerns. The second strategy involves fostering both in them and in ourselves a sense of connection and hope. How and when we interweave the art process into these first steps depends on the situation. Generally speaking, we believe that not only do we need to warm up our clients to the therapeutic relationship, we also need to prime them for creative expression.

As we discussed in the chapters on creativity (Chapter 6) and flow (Chapter 7), many of our clients are eager to make art and we, as art therapists, often pride ourselves that doing art can be "less threatening" than talk therapy. On the other hand, it is equally true that many others, especially adults and especially in groups, are very intimidated at the prospect of doing art— perhaps because it is the first time they've done so in years, or because of negative experiences with art in their childhood, or anxiety about being judged by others. Therefore, when we are introducing artmaking into the mix, their *relationship to art* is a variable. In addition, regardless of their excitement and degree of comfort with artmaking, people need some warm-up to the creative process.

This is where it gets complex. For example, even if artmaking provokes negative emotions like fear or anxiety which might *reduce* receptivity to engaging in novel behaviors, the visual stimulation of art supplies is waking up other parts of the brain. Just seeing clay, colored pencils, markers, and/ or paints serves as warm-up to the artmaking process. Engaging in kinesthetic activity—picking up pastels or kneading clay—further warms us up to the therapeutic process. The art supplies promote emotional arousal and expression, which facilitates the release of oxytocin, the brain's natural reward hormone (Hass-Cohen, 2016).

This alleviates stress and increases feelings of safety, pro-social behaviors, and therapeutic bonding. In other words, participating in artmaking, *regardless of one's feelings about doing so*, often makes people feel better and helps them connect. Engaging sensorimotor stimulation and kinesthetic activity naturally encourage curiosity and play. This helps regulate anxiety and makes us willing to take on risks with and in front of others (Panksepp & Biven, 2012).

In addition, we generally find that with whomever we work, artmaking invites inclusion. Even when folks are initially sheepish about showing their artwork, that, in and of itself, connects them to others and to their shared humanity. We further boost connection by helping them identify aspects of their imagery that communicate universally—colors, shapes, line quality, symbols, etc.

USING POSITIVE EMOTIONS AND ART THERAPY TO DEEPEN RELATIONSHIPS

Positive emotions, particularly ones like hope, sense of connection, and curiosity, play a prominent role not only at the beginning but at all stages of the therapeutic relationship. Emotions like compassion, forgiveness, kindness, gratitude, pride, and inspiration fuel the work of therapy. Because of their curative nature, we want to keep infusing the intersubjective space between therapist and client with these emotions.

In addition, we want to educate clients about the impact of positive emotions on relationships in general. Although we tend to think of emotions, positive or negative, as experienced within the individual, they are more often than not interpersonal in nature. Positive emotions like amusement, gratitude, and love are usually generated *between* people. Even "intellectual" feelings such as curiosity and interest are often produced in dyads, groups, or teams.

Just as positive emotions have significant impact on the individual, so too do they on relationships. They help us connect with others, building the relational networks that we need to survive. Our relationships are also a core source of meaning in life and feeling connected to others improves wellbeing. This in turn leads to more social affiliation, mutual assistance, and resilience, further boosting positive emotions and generating Fredrickson's *upward spiral of positivity*.

Not surprisingly, positive relationships in general are characterized by higher ratios of positive emotions (Gottman, 1999). In fact, Gottman, a leading researcher in what makes relationships successful, identified that relationships do not suffer as much from strong negative affect as from *the absence of positive affect*. Relationships are most likely to thrive at a ratio of 5:1 positive to negative exchanges. With this in mind, we continue to engage in strategies that intentionally and consciously induce positivity in the therapeutic relationship and in all of our relationships in general.

Capitalizing In related research, positive psychologists have identified that not only are supportive relationships tremendously important in times of trouble, they may be even more vital when things *go well* (Gable, Gonzaga, & Strachman, 2006). For example, psychologist Shelly Gable, in her article "Will You Be There for Me When Things Go Right?", discovered that active and constructive responses to *good* news ("Wow, that good thing happened?! Tell me more!") also called *capitalizing*, play a key role in positive relationships. This supplements research which revealed that lack of responsiveness and disinterest are damaging to relationships (Gottman & Silver, 2015). In other words, Gable identified that *indifference to positive news* can be just as damaging to relationships as indifference to bad news.

As therapists, we want to offer this kind of celebratory "support" when things go well. *Kvelling* (the opposite of *kvetching* or complaining) small triumphs is not only helpful during the formation of the therapeutic alliance but also throughout the duration of therapy. This includes highlighting progress and exploring what has helped our clients experience those changes. Comparing art imagery from different stages of treatment often graphically illustrates improvements—artwork may appear brighter, more organized, or more expressive. Recognizing and acknowledging these changes solidifies the therapeutic relationship and foster a shared sense of hope.

Love Therapists often avoid exploring "love" in the therapeutic relationship for fear of blurring boundaries and creating misunderstandings. There is often concern that feelings of love might lead down a slippery slope to enmeshment or inappropriate sexual behavior. Clearly it is unethical and harmful to engage in exploitive relationships with our clients, as the Art Therapy Credentials Board and most mental health ethical codes state in no uncertain terms. Indeed, most discussions of love in the literature refer to clients' erotic or romantic thoughts and feelings towards their therapist or vice versa (Sonne & Jochai, 2014).

However, here we are talking about a *different* kind of love. We are referring to what therapists otherwise know as attachment, attunement, resonance, interactive reciprocity, intimacy, empathy, compassion, etc. (Chilton, 2014; Bentzen, 2015; Moon, 2008)—clinical terms for what is, at its simplest, love. Fredrickson (2013) defines love as a *momentary upwelling* of three interwoven events: "first, a sharing of one or more positive emotions between you and another; second, a synchrony between your and the other person's biochemistry and behaviors; and third, a reflected motive to invest in each other's well-being that brings mutual care" (p. 17).

We suggest that these occur often in the therapeutic relationship. As we synch up emotionally and physically with our clients—leaning in, making eye contact, doing art—positive emotions like hope, gratitude, and amusement arise. These moments of shared compassion, humor, and physical alignment fuel connection and willingness to engage. This *positivity resonance* engenders coherent heart rhythms which in turn evoke feelings of security and well-being (McCraty & Childre, 2004). Both clients and therapist experience *love* that neither exploits nor violates professional boundaries. Instead it is evidence of healthy attachment.

Love, in this sense of the word, can even emerge in a single session or in fleeting encounters like the workshops we described at the beginning of the chapter. In such exchanges, not only do we feel love toward our clients, and they toward us, but they feel it toward each other. Because art therapy synchronizes us bio-behaviorally through the physiological kinesthetic experience of artmaking and play, it boosts positive emotions and inspires feelings of belonging and connection. The shared imagery that emerges further promotes this kind of rapid bonding. Love thrives in art therapy!

In the therapeutic relationship and with dyads, groups, and teams, any strategies that encourage collaboration can help promote this kind of love—murals, group projects, appreciations, etc. If there is not enough safety yet, we can generalize using interventions such as love-kindness meditation, identifying someone important to us, or making gifts for others.

Positive Emotions and Race

As we will discuss in Chapter 11 on meaning and perception, we all have a range of unconscious biases—short cuts that our minds take in order to avoid being overwhelmed by the vast array of information that we are being inundated with internally and externally at any given moment. One of these is our *Own-Race Bias* (ORB), the tendency for people to distinguish facial differences in people of their own race more quickly than those of other races—a bias which is ubiquitous to *all* racial groups. Hence, the colloquial expression "they all look the same to me!"

There is speculation that this occurs for two reasons. First, racial characteristics are the first cue humans perceive when sorting through distinguishing variables, e.g., gender or age. Second, we perceive cross-race faces less *holistically* than our own (Rhodes, Brake, Tan, & Taylor, 1989), i.e., we see them more as "objects" than as "people." Barbara Fredrickson and Kareem Johnson conducted research into the effects of positive emotions on ORB which provides encouraging direction for bridging racial gaps. In their research with White college students, they determined that humor and joy "eliminated differences in recognition of Black and White faces" (Johnson & Fredrickson, 2005, p. 879).

Art therapists can indirectly address this by boosting positive emotions in the art studio and creating a safe and nurturing environment for clients to get to know one another. Engaging collaboratively in art-making further promotes positive connections. Witnessing each others' artwork evokes feeling of empathy and universality which can bridge the distance that separates us from people we perceive to be "other."

We can also harness the *broadening effect* of positive emotions to address themes more specific to cultural and ethnic identity. For example, "where I come from and who are 'my people' are" both highlights and celebrates differences. As the National Coalition Building Institute proclaims, "Real pride welcomes diversity!"

Gratitude Gratitude, another positive emotion that often emerges organically in relationships, is strongly linked to wellbeing, relationship building, and prosocial outcomes (Wood, Froh, & Geraghty, 2010; Bartlett & DeSteno, 2006; Tsang, 2006). Research also suggests that when we experience gratitude, we feel supported, more connected, and motivated to bond further with those toward whom we felt grateful (Algoe & Stanton, 2012; Kok et al., 2013). In art therapy, gratitude often emerges spontaneously when clients see the colorful array of pastels, papers, and paints that are at their disposal—they frequently say that they feel like they are being served "a buffet" of art supplies.

Appreciations also inspire gratitude. Artwork about someone who has been kind to us or who had a positive impact on our lives, thanksgiving murals and acknowledgment messages help express and reinforce gratitude. In addition, because people who feel gratitude feel closer to others around them, when we explore gratitude in therapy, even if it is directed toward people outside the therapeutic encounter, it strengthens the therapeutic alliance and, in groups, builds cohesion.

Mindfulness and Art Therapy in Relationships

Although we strongly believe that positivity is critical to relationships, both in and out of therapy, it is important to explore *all* interpersonal dynamics, regardless of their positive or negative valence. Because positive emotions and artmaking early in the therapy process helps expand our perceptions, we can combine these to examine our relationships in a more receptive state. The artwork externalizes representation of both our conscious and unconscious thoughts and feelings, giving us opportunities to explore them with more detachment. Artwork can challenge the innate perceptual blinders and cognitive distortions that we all share. By giving us a much fuller—and we might even say *more accurate*—"picture," art gives us profound insight into what we believe and feel about our relationships.

This can be especially useful when we are working with couples, families, partners, friends, groups, or professional teams. Even in one brief encounter, artwork provides new and surprising perspectives on interpersonal dynamics. For example, Rebecca provides a consult entitled "Positive Partnerships" at the resort where she works. If the relationship being addressed is generally stable and clients are there "to learn something new," Rebecca uses directives such as "what matters to you most" or "what you value in your relationship." If there are stressors, she might have them make symbols for what it would look like if things were to improve, or for strengths they perceive in their relationship despite their challenges.

The participants are then encouraged to "mindfully" observe the concrete elements they see in each other's artwork using the language of visual literacy (outlined in Chapter 8 on strengths). This helps them move beyond their preconceived ideas of what the art "should" look like, theirs or others, and what they intended to depict—to mindfully notice *what is actually there*.

As they do, they begin to grasp the metaphors the imagery conveys and to "see" themselves and each other more clearly. If their imagery is very similar—color, composition, imagery, symbols—they often find it comforting that it reveals underlying commonalities and shared values. If it is very different—quality of line, placement or organization of elements, degree of abstraction or representation—they often experience a rush of comprehension that, just as they had suspected, they really *are* coming from different perspectives! However, they also usually experience relief that those differences are less threatening than they had previously thought.

Invariably, as the discussion proceeds, those who initially noticed more similarities begin to identify subtle differences that then inform the dialogue. Those that were struck by their differences begin to notice commonalities, metaphors for areas where there is unity in the relationship. Inevitably, they perceive more positive aspects in the relationship and see each other more appreciatively. Such directives are also effective in groups and teams when the participants notice how eloquently simple imagery reveals positive aspects about the artist and their relationship to the group.

Not only does looking at the art work vis-à-vis its visual elements allow our clients see themselves and others differently, it helps us as therapists get a glimpse of our clients that we could not get in any other way. This is critical because, at its simplest, it is *perspective-taking*, fundamental to empathy. Using the analogy of walking in someone else's shoes, seeing clients' artwork helps therapists slide nimbly into the slippers, sneakers, pumps, oxfords, or boots of their clients. If it is with couples, families, teams, or groups, seeing the artwork helps other group members get into those shoes. This is what art therapists fundamentally understand about art therapy—what we see in therapy sessions but also later if we share artwork in treatment planning meetings. We witness the flash of comprehension that occurs when our co-workers see the clients' art. Suddenly, they too step into those shoes.

Finally, because artwork introduces clients to aspects of *themselves* in ways that words alone cannot, they are able to step into different sets of their *own* shoes, to see *themselves* differently. As we will discuss in the chapter on meaning and perception (Chapter 11), we might have them explore the relationship between these different parts of the self. This promotes *self-compassion*, which includes being more accepting of ourselves and recognizing that our life experiences come from a shared humanity, which, however imperfect, is worthy of esteem (Neff, 2003).

ART THERAPY TECHNIQUES TO MINDFULLY EXPLORE RELATIONSHIPS

Response Art In response art, an art therapist makes art in response to a client's artwork, with the goal of creating meaning or increasing empathy (Fish, 2012). Sometimes this artwork is shared with clients as "a strategy that can enhance the therapeutic alliance by reflecting internalized, embodied, resonant material back to the client" (Franklin, 2010, p. 164). Levy's technique of replicating the artwork (Cox, 2016, personal communication) serves as another form of "response" art, a way to empathically connect with our clients.

Gioia used response art in her doctoral research and found that when she shared her imagery with the research participants, they voiced that it made them feel "witnessed" and "mirrored," that the artwork tangibly reflected her empathy for their experience (Chilton, 2014, p. 190). They felt not only deeply understood, but that her response art *amplified* and gave them a fresh perspective on what their own artwork was addressing.

Joint Artmaking   In joint artmaking, two or more people collaborate to create a work of art. This might include the art therapist and a client or multiple clients working together, such as in a mural. Members of a group can also each start a round-robin project that is passed around until everyone has contributed. A similar intervention might have individuals creating separate pieces which are assembled together as a whole, such as a quilt, or pie-shaped segments of a mandala. These collaborations often generate humor and joviality which promotes connection. Navigating the complexities of working together also reveals interpersonal dynamics among group members and within the therapeutic relationship, as well as in the broader scope of their lives, which can then be explored.

Social Atoms   Originally developed by J. L. Moreno (1947), social atoms are diagrams of social networks. The directions are simple: place a symbol for yourself anywhere on a page, and then map symbols for people (or creatures) in your life in order of closeness/intimacy. Variations can be used to explore current, past, or future relationships. Social atoms are great tools for expanding awareness about and giving us new insight into our relationships—they can reveal boundaries or the need for them, as well as who we'd like to be closer to and from whom we might want some distance.

Finding the Benefit in Negative Emotions and Experiences

Gottman (1999) identified that one of the most common myths about successful relationships is that they are conflict free. Other misconceptions include: if you have to work at communication the relationship is in trouble; conflicts must be resolved if a relationship is to survive; or, if you seek therapy for your relationship, it is probably too late. In fact, conflict is not only inevitable in all relationships, it can be productive.

Conflict provides opportunities to understand other people's expectations, preferences, and needs better. Fundamental interpersonal requirements include physical wellbeing, autonomy *and* interdependence (e.g., respect, love, community), integrity, play, celebration, and spiritual connection. Conflict usually originates when some of those needs have not been met. Addressing that can help to ameliorate the conflict (Burton, 1990). In this way, conflict can mark turning points in a relationship, moments which inspire collaborative problem-solving and deeper levels of commitment (Braiker & Kelley, 1979).

In addition, just as avoidance and suppression of negative emotions are damaging to individuals, so too are they to relationships. *Avoiding* conflict is more detrimental than addressing it. Negative emotions are often *useful* in relationships. For example, anger alerts us that some form of transgression has taken place—perhaps a boundary has been crossed or a need has not been honored; sadness signals there has been a loss; fear indicates something important is at risk. Research has shown that *appropriate* expression of negative emotions is not only healthy for relationships but essential to helping them thrive (Graham, Huang, Clark, & Helgeson, 2008).

Gottman (1999) identified that relationships characterized by *harmful expressions of negativity* such as high levels of criticism, defensiveness, contempt, and/or stonewalling were most vulnerable. We do not want to avoid conflict or negative emotions in our relationships, but rather find ways to acknowledge and express them productively.

USING ART TO FIND BENEFIT IN NEGATIVE EMOTIONS AND EXPERIENCES

Again, art therapy can be instructive for exploring the dimensions of a relationship, both positive and negative. Even if clients have the conscious intention of depicting a struggle in the relationship, because artistic imagery accesses other parts of consciousness (implicit processing), it will invariably reflect more than that polarized perception. When we help our clients use visual analysis to explore the formal elements and metaphors they suggest, they often see that what was first intended to represent difficulties expresses not only the negative, but also the positive, and all of the in-between.

For example, Rebecca's client Janelle was feeling overwhelmed and frustrated that she had run into "a wall" in her relationship with her son. When she sketched this wall, in chalk pastels, and held the picture at a distance, she was surprised that it was much brighter than it had looked up close. She realized it wasn't solid at all but in fact, was permeable and translucent, and "much more workable" than the barrier that she had perceived in her mind. Four large connection loops she had drawn on the surface of the "wall" also suggested an energetic quality that reflected more movement that she had realized. She recognized that this was a general trend in her life—she often felt discouraged and deflated by her relationships but when she did artwork about them, the overall imagery was always brighter and more dynamic than she expected.

We can use these techniques not only with present concerns but also old wounds—betrayal, resentment, or trauma—which may overshadow our relationships. As we will explore in Chapter 11, because artwork accesses hidden parts of consciousness, it can transform memories that were hurtful or traumatic, unlocking them so they are no longer fragmented flashes of memory frozen in time. It provides distance from and gives a much fuller version of those events and our role in them. This detachment promotes integration of those memories and the creation of new, more empowering narratives. It paves the way to acceptance and forgiveness of others and, perhaps most importantly, of ourselves.

Not only is using artwork to look at dynamics helpful in individual work with clients, it can be even more useful when it includes relevant parties, especially if they have some investment in trying to bring healing to the relationship. It allows them to simultaneously express their emotions and get a unique glimpse into the way the other parties perceive the situation. The visual language they use introduces the metaphors that then become the means through which to improve communication and rebuild the relationship.

Summary of Positive Art Therapy and Emotions in Relationships

To go back to the analogy of relationships as savings accounts or reservoirs, it isn't that we want to avoid negative experiences, it's that we want to balance the drain they create by increasing the number of deposits or filling the well of positivity. We want to promote the broadening and building potential of positive emotions very early in the therapeutic dynamic to increase our clients' and our own willingness to engage with each other and shift how we perceive our relationships. We also explore the benefits of negative emotions and conflict. And finally, we harness the undoing effect of positive emotions—the capacity of feelings such as love, compassion, gratitude, curiosity, and humor to help relationships cope in the midst of difficulties, to recover more quickly from stress and negative events, and to provide all of the benefits that come from meaningfully connecting with others (Fredrickson, 1998; Kok et al., 2013).

Strengths in Relationships

Like most therapists, art therapists are naturally inclined to promote trust in the therapeutic relationship by supportively exploring the distress that compelled our clients to seek treatment. Although this is important, compelling clinical research has identified that compared to a treatment-as-usual, problem-focused approach, when therapists spent five minutes before sessions focusing on their patients' *strengths*, therapeutic bonding and therapy outcomes—symptom reduction and goal attainment—improved (Flückiger & Grosse Holtforth, 2008). In short, in order to grow and reap the benefits of a strong therapeutic alliance, we want to focus more on strengths than on problems.

This can be challenging though, as it not only subverts the medical model but often the expectations our clients bring to therapy. It also requires some skill to simultaneously acknowledge pain and suffering while delicately shifting focus to our clients' strengths and what has helped them survive. To do so, we do not ignore "the problem"; however, as we explored in the chapter on strengths (Chapter 8), we also begin to explore the intra- and interpersonal resources that have helped them thus far (Betts, 2011). In fact, relationships in and of themselves are a form of strength. They grow out of what Park and Peterson (2010) called the "heart" strengths—gratitude, love, kindness, teamwork, forgiveness, etc.

STRENGTHS SPOTTING

In the treatment center where Gioia works, she often uses *strengths spotting* to help groups bond. After providing a list of strengths, she passes out index cards on which group members identify a strength they have, a strength they admire in others, and a strength of the person sitting to their left. Even with relative strangers, people often quickly "get" each other's strengths! They are usually able to pinpoint some quality—thoughtful, prompt, funny, fashionable—that they admire about that person.

The most significant shift in mood and energy happens when they share that strength with their peer. Following up, Gioia asks the recipients if their neighbor got it right. Laughter usually ensues as they more often than not confirm what the other said. Sharing these strengths increases the love, support, and sense of universality critical in building group cohesion.

We also use strengths to explore relationships when we teach positive art therapy to graduate art therapy students. Initially, when we taught about strengths, we used an assignment developed by Chris Peterson in which the students take the VIA Strengths survey and observe their signature strengths "in action." They are also instructed to record their reflections on using one of their strengths in a new and different way for a week.

As we read their observations, we were impressed by the depth of learning taking place and the impact it was having on their perceptions of themselves. However, we noticed that because we were the professors, we were the only ones that got to read all of the "*A-ha!*" moments that they were experiencing. In addition, we also observed that although the assignment helped them learn more about *their own* strengths, it did not inspire much observation of *others'* strengths.

We addressed this by using the online electronic platform to have the students read and respond to a peer's paper. Using questions from *appreciative inquiry*, a method of systematically focusing on what is working well (Cooperrider & Srivastva, 1987), we asked them to write an open letter to the author identifying what they found valuable and what strengths stood out as they read it. Surprisingly, the students did more than was required—they avidly read and responded to many of the papers, sometimes all of them! They reported that doing so gave them deeper insights into each other's strengths and made them feel more connected to each other. They also identified that it made them much more aware of the strengths of other people in their lives, both friends and strangers.

When the role of relationships began to take on more prominence in positive psychology, leading Seligman to shift his wellbeing model to include the R in PERMA, we realized that *we* needed to focus more on social connection. To further develop our students' strengths-spotting skills, we decided that, instead of an assignment devoted to their identifying their *own* strengths, we would have them celebrate "Strengths in My Community." This included creating symbols for a strength they noted in: 1) a friend or family member; 2) an art therapy colleague, teacher, or supervisor; and 3) an art therapy client. Witnessing the wide range of strengths that they observed in people from such diverse areas in their lives further enriched their strengths-spotting skills.

APPRECIATIVE INQUIRY

As we mentioned before, we can build relationships in art therapy clinical supervision using strengths spotting and *appreciative inquiry* (Fialkov & Haddad, 2012). For example, instead of focusing most on problems our students are experiencing in their clinical development or clients they find challenging, we build on ways that they are successfully navigating their work. We might ask: "When have you felt that your practice of art therapy has been at its best? When have you felt most connected to your clients? What was happening during those moments?" And in turn, we might ask ourselves, "What would it look like if I were to be able to be most helpful for my student? What is going well in the supervisory exchange?"

Gioia and her former student Rachel Schreibman used *poetic inquiry* (writing poems as a research process) to discover what worked in their supervisory relationship (Schreibman & Chilton, 2012). By exploring "exceptional" moments, times when they were most energized by each other, they learned about aspects of the art therapy profession that they valued. Using this approach helped them to appreciate the intersubjective nature of art therapy relationships and to see the importance of positive regard in modeling behaviors, exploring professional boundaries, and finding links between positive emotions and learning.

VISUAL ANALYSIS AND STRENGTHS

When working with clients, as we discussed earlier, employing art therapy interventions that heighten mindful observation of the artistic elements—with the metaphorical messages the latter can imply—often naturally leads to recognizing strengths. We can also purposefully focus on strengths. For example, in individual work, if clients are struggling with or trying to improve a relationship, their artwork often reveals strengths in the relationship they hadn't perceived before. Again, although we may guide them in that process, often the imagery naturally highlights those for them.

We can also do this in dyads, groups, and teams—having them depict the strengths they perceive in each other and in the relationship. We can provide lists of strengths and identify how certain qualities in one person might either frustrate or complement those of others, or how over- or underutilizing some of them affects the relationship. We can explore ways that we might maximize their use to benefit both the individual and the relationship or ways that applying our respective strengths might help us accomplish tasks which we would otherwise, individually, find daunting or draining.

STRENGTHS OF HUMANITY

Recall that helping others not only helps build relationships but also improves wellbeing for the individual. There are countless ways to use art to promote prosocial behaviors starting with simple directives like "Thank you" cards and making gifts for others. These can nudge us out of ourselves and shift the rumination that often dominates anxiety, depression, and pain. For example, on one of the psychiatric units where Rebecca worked, clients made Christmas cards for medical patients in other parts of the hospital. Even though the precipitating circumstances around their own hospitalizations were often traumatic (e.g., suicide attempt, drug overdose, psychotic break), they embraced this project with enthusiasm, wanting to lift the spirits of others whose circumstances they believed were more severe than their own.

Exploring Values and Beliefs

As we discussed in Chapter 8, identifying strengths in ourselves and others often reveals underlying values and beliefs. Focusing on strengths naturally reflects what is important to us. Then, when others know what we value and we know the same about them, it promotes understanding, empathy, and connection (Gottman, 1999). We get a glimpse of what is motivating them and what they are trying to achieve. Even if we do not agree with their opinions or we do not approve of their behaviors, we are better able to acknowledge and even possibly accept differences if we understand what is driving them.

Because artwork so eloquently illustrates our frame of reference and looking at others' artwork allows us to see theirs, it gives us unique access to very personalized expressions of values and beliefs. We might mine directly for this information through interventions such as providing a list of values with instructions to pick 5–10 with which they resonate—first individually and then as a couple/family/team—and then make symbols for those values. We might also use directives such as "What is important and matters in your life" that focus on the present or the *Best Possible Life* to visualize what our relationships could look like in the future.

We can also use any art directives that explore identity, worldviews, passions, dreams, and what gives our lives meaning and purpose—topics which we will explore in more depth in the next chapter. Doing so in tandem with others helps identify differences in values and expectations as well as shared meanings, hopes, and aspirations. Establishing this baseline gives us room for compromise in areas where we disagree. It can help us identify what we see as a deep need, sometimes called a *deal-breaker*, versus a *preference*, something we would like but do not have to have in the relationship. It can also mitigate the damaging effects of conflicts when they arise.

Gottman (1999) proposed that partners increase their understanding of each other by identifying their *Love Maps*, what is important to their *significant other* such as their dreams, worries, hobbies, friends, favorite foods, etc. Just the expression "love map" inspires artistic response! Along those lines, partners can explore how their art represents their collective strengths and values through the challenge of combining their love maps into a single image or a three-dimensional sculpture.

Gottman (1999) also described what he calls *The Sound Relationship House*. In this conceptual structure, love maps serve as the foundation. The floors above include sharing fondness and admiration, turning toward our partners instead of away, keeping a positive perspective, managing conflict, and making life dreams comes true. The top level is creating shared meaning. And finally, the supporting walls of the house are trust and commitment. As you can imagine, the metaphor of a house for our relationships also lends itself well to visual representation. Although Gottman worked mostly with couples, these constructs can apply to other interpersonal relationships—friends, families, work teams, community groups, etc.

Attending to the Good

All of the interventions for promoting positive relationships that we have listed above—combining positive emotions with art therapy to warm up to the process and deepen relationships, capitalizing on positive events, boosting love and gratitude, finding benefits in negative emotions, practicing mindfulness, strengths spotting, and exploring values and beliefs—organically flow into the last strategy: *attending to the good*. We will explore this in much greater detail in Chapter 11 on meaning and perception, but for now, suffice it to say that expanding and shifting what we perceive about our relationships naturally highlights positive elements therein. And through positive interventions and art therapy, we can consciously counter the negativity bias and actively notice what is good in all of our relationships.

Our Friendship

Before we move on, we thought it would be fitting to address our own relationship. Although sometimes we tussle about things, we've been friends for over 25 years. We were cautioned when we started Creative Wellbeing Workshops that it might be the end of our friendship. Earlier in our partnership, we did frequently argue over how to run the business—Rebecca was more frugal and cautious, Gioia more visionary and optimistic. At those times, we tried to step back and use the tools that we were promoting in our work.

When we were cranky with each other, we paused to list three good things. When things got heated, we tried to identify what strengths and values were driving the other person (however frustrating they seemed to be at that moment), or figure out what she was trying to accomplish. And when it seemed as though we had arrived at insurmountable impasses, we tried to remember our collective mission as well as our individual needs, our preferences, what we enjoy, and how we could use our strengths to compliment rather than clash with each other.

Because we have such different presenting styles, in the early years that we worked together we occasionally jostled for the limelight or felt undermined by each other. However, as we learned to play off of and to complement rather than detract from each others' strengths, we became much more unified as a team and we began to enjoy running workshops together much more than doing them alone. As a result, we now collaborate even when we would make more money "flying solo." And because the work that we do together is so much more fun for us, in the long run it is more sustainable.

The feedback we receive also changed. Whereas in the early days, our audiences often preferred one of us over the other, we now hear almost exclusively that one of the highlights of our workshops is the opportunity to work with such different but complementary presenters. Sometimes we have talked about how it may be that our workshops and classes are so well received because we invite the participants into our friendship, widening its circle, and offering them the same respect and warmth we offer each other. They feel the love and positivity between us—the fact that we feel happy to get the opportunity to work together—and it changes the dynamic in the room for the better. In the end, we haven't just survived working together, we not only love each other but we also *like* each other more!

Discussion Questions

1   What are some of the most important relationships in your life?
2   What are some of the strengths and values you see in those relationships?
3   What role has conflict served in those relationships?
4   What are your thoughts about love, humor, or laughter in therapy?

CHAPTER **10**

Meaning and Purpose

When we took the "Approaches to Happiness" questionnaire, it was not surprising that we both scored high on *Meaning*. Being art therapists, we have both been blessed with a clear sense of what we are doing in this world. For us it's very simple—we want to use art to help people have the highest quality of life possible and we want to give and receive love. Corny, maybe, but at our core, this is what we are about. It also seemed fitting that when we took the VIA Strengths Inventories, we had *appreciation of beauty and excellence* and *capacity to love and be loved* in our top five strengths. What gives our lives meaning and purpose seems to be fundamentally intertwined with and to grow out of our strengths and what energizes us.

Within that context, we follow the previous chapters on strengths and relationships with a look at meaning because, in our work talking about these domains more often than not flows organically into discussions about what is most important and what matters to us most. Our strengths and our relationships are inextricably linked to what we value and view as inherently good and right in the world (Peterson, 2006; Peterson & Seligman, 2004). For example, someone who is high in compassion and empathy often values kindness. They might also value social justice, because it involves fighting for the rights of others. Someone who has a love of learning usually values the search for knowledge and discovering how things work. In other words, people often see their strengths as so fundamental to *how life should be* that they do not perceive that those characteristics might be unique to them.

Peterson (2006) further proposed that although *identifying* strengths is important, how we *direct* our strengths is also critical to a live well lived. Seligman, Parks, and Steen (2004) suggest that meaning comes from using our strengths in the service of something larger than ourselves. This includes channeling our energies toward pursuits that satisfy our longing for purpose and our desire to connect meaningfully with others through family, work, community, religion, spirituality, or the search for knowledge. Meaning in life shifts the emphasis from *what feels good* to a given individual to *what is important* to them and others (Steger, Sheline, Merriman, & Kashdan, 2013).

Meaning is central to most approaches to wellbeing. It was critical to Seligman's (2002, 2011) Three Paths to Happiness and now to PERMA. It is also fundamental to Ryff's model of psychological wellbeing and Keyes's model of flourishing (Keyes, 2003; Ryff & Keyes, 1995). It underlies the *eudemonic* approach to wellbeing that suggests that happiness comes from discovering, cultivating, and living in accordance with one's virtues (Peterson, 2006). We could also say that it is a critical component of subjective wellbeing (Diener, 1994) which frames *hedonic wellbeing* within the broader context of a person's perceived satisfaction with the most important domains of their lives.

Meaning and purpose shape our identity and sense of belonging (Seligman, 2011). When we experience the *presence of meaning*, we have an understanding of who we are, we see our place in the world, and we have an overarching sense of purpose. We have answers to the question, "Why am I here?"

Defining Meaning

Before we delve further into the deep and vast realm of meaning, however, we have found it easier to approach *meaning* from two vantage points—*Meaning and Purpose* and *Meaning and Perception*. We refer to meaning and purpose as our overarching beliefs about meaning in life and what purpose it serves. We think of meaning and perception as the process of perceiving and appraising what we experience and the role that beliefs and attention play in forming our impressions of "reality." These two forms of meaning intertwine to form the narrative we weave about our lives: about what has happened to us in the past, what is happening to us now, what we predict will happen to us in the future, why we are here in the first place, and how this all fits into the greater picture of the world around us.

It is difficult to separate the variables that contribute to and the benefits that derive from these two different aspects of meaning. This makes sense when we consider that our fundamental ideas about the meaning of life and our purpose in the world both influence and are influenced by what we believe, what we perceive, what we notice, and how we *make* meaning out of our experiences. Nevertheless, we have found that two constructs have elements that can be differentiated and which, for us, appear to organically emerge from our clinical work. We will attempt to present these two aspects of meaning as clearly as possible and as they relate to the field of art therapy. We start here with meaning and purpose.

Meaning and Purpose

Meaning provides us with the sense that our lives matter, that they make sense, and that they are more than the sum of our minutes, hours, days, and years (Baumeister & Vohs, 2010; Park, 2010). Baumeiser and Vohs (2010) regard meaning as a human need—one of the ways that we impose stability and find order in an otherwise chaotic and ever-changing world. In some ways, we could say that meaning is what we are all striving for—we are trying to make sense of things and find our place in the world.

Victor Frankl was instrumental in putting meaning on the map of psychology in his book, *Man's Search for Meaning*. Frankl (1985) recounted having been held in a concentration camp for three years during which time, as prisoner #119104, he was tortured, forced into slave labor, and wrenched from his wife and his family members, most of whom were killed. Despite being exposed to the depths of depravity to which humans can descend, he also witnessed, both in himself and others, the power of the human spirit to sustain itself and even find meaning in horrifying circumstances. Frankl insisted that the *search for meaning* is a primary force in human experience—that it both derives from and helps protect us against adversity.

Meaning appears to have different components. One is the sense that life, itself, has significance and meaning outside of our own personal existence (Baumeiser, 1991). Meaning also includes the sense that the life we live has some degree of predictability, reliability, and regularity—that there is an order and structure to "reality" upon which we can depend: "Lives may be experienced as meaningful when they are felt to have a significance beyond the trivial or momentary, to have purpose, or to have a coherence that transcends chaos" (King, Hicks, Krull, & Del Gaiso, 2006, p. 180).

Positive psychologist Paul Wong (2011) has devoted himself to the role of meaning in wellbeing. He outlined the four most essential elements of wellbeing—Purpose, Understanding, Responsible action, and Enjoyment—PURE. *Purpose* has to do with life goals and core values. *Understanding* refers to the need to comprehend the world around us and to understand ourselves and others. *Responsible action* refers to the process whereby we balance our own needs and interests with those of others. *Enjoyment* comes from taking pleasure in our experiences and in being alive.

Wong (2011) identified seven *sources* of meaning: happiness, achievement, intimacy, relationship, self-transcendence, self-acceptance, and fairness. Related paths have been identified: positive experiences and the sense that life is pleasant and rewarding; making patterns and connections from life events; being deeply involved in creative activities; meeting challenges and achieving our goals, and belonging to and serving a greater good (Baumeister & Vohs, 2010; Csíkszentmihályi, 1997; Deci & Ryan, 1985; Park, 2011; Seligman, 2011).

Values

Values are a core component of meaning (Wong, 2011). They serve as the foundation for what we think is right—or wrong—in the world. Often our values are so implicit to our ideas about *how things should be* that we are not consciously aware of them. Values have been defined as enduring beliefs that are inextricably linked to our personal and cultural identity. They serve as standards that guide how we select and evaluate the people and institutions we encounter and the actions in which they and we engage (Schwartz, 2012).

Values can be thought of as noun—the worth or meaning that something holds—and as verb—to appreciate or admire something (Peterson, 2006). Values are not only ubiquitous to all cultures, they *define* culture. Cultural or social groups manifest their shared values in distinctive ways through spoken or unspoken codes that regulate how people should behave among themselves or with other groups. These norms create sanctions against deviance and help establish the order that makes life predictable and coherent (Peterson, 2006).

Values are often hierarchical and operate relative to one another—i.e., when we apply them to a given situation, some win out over others. Values are also expressive—they are closely linked to self-identity, social identity, and communal identity. People tend to gravitate toward people who share similar values (Peterson, 2005). For example, perhaps you too believe that art is healing, that it's important to be of service to one's community, that people should be lifelong learners, and so you've naturally gravitated towards this book, which—surprise!—also reflects those values.

Values not only shape our aspirations, they influence how we organize and direct our efforts (Lundgren, Luoma, Dahl, Strosahl, & Melin, 2012). Value-driven goals are more intrinsic and self-concordant, as we will explore in the chapter on accomplishment (Chapter 12). Values form the basis of purpose in life, as we will now examine.

Purpose

Although meaning and purpose are often used synonymously, *purpose* can be differentiated as "a stable and generalized intention to accomplish something that is at once meaningful to the self and of consequence to the world beyond the self" (Damon, Menon, & Cotton Bronk, 2003, p. 121). Purpose relates more closely to the part of meaning that involves our beliefs about our own individual existence and what we are here to accomplish in the world. McKnight and Kashdan (2009) identify purpose as a central, self-organizing life aim.

Fulfilling our purpose entails directing our behaviors towards fulfilling that mission—what in humanist terms would be called self-actualization and the realization of our full potential (Maslow, 1971; Rogers, 1963; Steger et al., 2013). Deci and Ryan (1985) and Ryan and Deci (2000) explore this in their Self-Determination Theory (SDT). They suggest that to be *actualized*, three basic psychological needs must be met: the need for competence and mastery; the need for relatedness, to connect meaningfully with others; and the need for autonomy, to be able to pursue goals that are intrinsically motivating and congruent with "the true self." These needs emerge in *all* cultures, both individualist and collectivist (Sheldon & Elliott, 1999).

Passion

Passion is closely related to purpose and mission. Passions are self-defining activities that we find important, that we love, and in which we invest time and energy (Vallerand, 2008). Some may be relatively superficial and others may be core to our identity. Although most people would identify their purpose as a passion, they wouldn't necessarily identify all of their passions as part of their purpose. For example, an art therapist might identify that her purpose was to help people access the healing benefits of the creative process. On the other hand, she might have a passion for salsa dancing and R&B music, but not believe that these were core to her purpose in life.

Vision and Mission

Vision and mission are constructs that appear more in business and organizational development (Lipton, 1996); however, they also have useful application for exploring meaning in life. *Mission* answers the questions "Why do I exist?" or, before coffee, "Why get out of bed?!" Mission is usually articulated by global, simple, and clear statements that reflect our most essential core values and purpose. For example, as we stated earlier, our mission is to use art to help people and to love and be loved.

Vision reflects the inspiration and desired impact of what we are hoping to accomplish. It serves as an enduring promise and paints a vivid picture that it is both future-based and present-focused, as if it were being realized now. For example, our vision is to see people feeling better through using art and the creative process, feeling more energized and engaged, seeing themselves and others differently, and having more meaning in their lives. Mission and vision provide the content from which to distill specific goals and objectives. Mission and vision are the *who* and the *why*; goals and objectives are the *how* and the *when*.

> "When we have a clear vision, we feel more connected to the world, more alive. The gap between our thought and action, our internal world and external world, vanishes, and we more fully occupy our 'self'. Our everyday choices feed off our vision the way a lantern flame feeds off kerosene" (Butler, 2010, p. xvi). Another metaphor begging for an art response!

Identity

Purpose and meaning are inextricably linked to our identity, who we believe we are at our core. Identity derives from experimenting with various *identity alternatives* and finding those that are most congruent with our values (Marcia, 1993). In other words, we might ask the question "Who am I?" but also, and perhaps even more telling, "Who am I *not*?" Identity crystallizes as we try on what does and does not fit and commit to choices that are congruent with our growing sense of self (Crocetti, Avanzi, Hawk, Fraccaroli, & Meeus, 2013).

Benefits and Challenges of Trying to Find Meaning and Purpose

Purpose and meaning in life are strongly correlated to wellbeing—to life satisfaction, health, increased positive emotions, higher levels of optimism, better self-esteem, fewer psychological problems, and lower mortality (Park, 2011; Steger & Kashdan, 2006). In addition, sense of meaning and purpose appears to help people to recover more quickly from adversity and to buffer against feelings of hopelessness (Graham, Lobel, Glass, & Lokshina, 2008; Lightsey, 2006).

For people who have a *strong sense of purpose*, exploring meaning appears to make them happier (King et al., 2006). However, for those who score *low* on presence of meaning, searching for it is actually *negatively* linked with wellbeing—it appears to *increase* depression and anxiety (Steger et al., 2013). This suggests that we need to approach meaning and purpose delicately, depending on the audience with whom we are working.

On the other hand, if we take an existential approach to meaning, we might welcome and encourage the *angst*—the anxiety and dread—that can arise when we are looking at core issues of meaning and purpose. For example, William James (1929) suggested that people who suffer from and overcome a *crisis of meaning* emerge stronger and more enthusiastic about life than those who never delve into larger questions about their existence in this world. Frankl (1985) believed that it was through encounters with *the existential void* that we find true meaning and transcendence.

Is There Meaning in Life?

Existentialism, a branch of humanist philosophy and psychology, suggests that human existence is the accidental byproduct of the Big Bang eons ago and that life, in and of itself, has no actual, objective meaning. However, because of this *lack* of meaning—this *existential vacuum*—each individual has both the freedom and the responsibility for creating and defining their own unique meaning in life (Frankl, 1985). On the other hand, Heintzelman and King refute the notion that life is inherently meaningless. In fact, they suggest that it is actually "*brimming* with meaning" (2014, p. 563).

King (2012) asserts that, because people report that they experience meaning through social connection, positive experiences, and finding some sense of order and reason—all of which are more common than not in the lives of most people—human experience is actually *inherently imbued* with meaning. She also suggests that meaning is much more mundane and ubiquitous than we think. She points to the fact that most people report that they find meaning more through friends and family than through loftier notions of purpose, significance, and coherence.

Heintzelman and King (2014) propose that because our world is infused with predictable and reliable patterns throughout the natural world, we organically experience a sense of coherence and order—e.g., day follows night follows day, after winter comes spring, we stand on the ground, the sky is above, etc. King (2012) proposes that rather than emphasizing meaning as something that we are either searching for, missing, or needing to create, instead we see meaning as something that we *detect* or *uncover*.

Spirituality and Transpersonal Psychology

Nevertheless, there is an aspect to meaning that is mysterious and unfathomable. It inspires great yearning for connection and transformation. Spirituality and religion derive from the ineffable sense that there is something greater than the humble trappings of human existence. As William James said, there is "a belief in an unseen order, and that our supreme good lies in harmoniously adjusting our self thereto" (1929, p. 59).

Transpersonal psychology grew out of the desire to incorporate these spiritual dimensions into theories of human motivation, human development, the workings of the mind and the practical application of psychotherapy. James (1929) may be one of the earliest psychologists to extensively address the relevance of religion and spirituality to the field of psychology, writing about them in *The Varieties of Religious Experience* (Ryan, 2008). Jung (1966/2014) also explored this realm in his theories about the collective unconscious and his interest in universal myths and symbols.

Assagioli (1959), a contemporary of Freud's, can also be credited with seminal ideas that influenced the transpersonal movement. In correspondences with Freud, Assagiolo proposed that psychoanalysis should go beyond ego development and remediation of distress to include a progressive integration of the personal with the spiritual, a process he called *Psychosynthesis*. Assagioli advocated for using guided imagery, artwork, body work, and meditative practices to inspire creativity and connect us to our common humanity.

Freud said "I am interested only in the basement of the human being." Psychosynthesis is interested in the whole building. We try to build an elevator which will allow a person access to every level of his personality. After all, a building with only a basement is very limited. We want to open up the terrace where you can sunbathe or look at the stars. (Roberto Assagioli, in Keen, 1974, p. 99)

Maslow (1971) was the first to actively identify transpersonal psychology as the "fourth force" in psychology, in contrast to psychoanalysis, behaviorism, and humanism. Transpersonal psychology was an attempt to bring to psychology the spiritual wisdom that could be found in cultures throughout the world— Christian Mysticism, Buddhism, Kaballah, Native American traditions, Catholicism, shamanism, yoga, meditation, altered states of consciousness, and ritual. The transpersonal approach looks at the personal concerns of the individual but contextualizes them within a broader frame of spiritual growth and universal connection. Personal development and the trials and tribulations of human experience serve as pathways through which one connects to spirituality and universal transcendence.

Spirituality and Worldviews

Whether addressing spiritual beliefs or a lack thereof, it is important to explore the worldviews that underpin a person's life. *Worldviews* are fundamental paradigms that people hold about the nature of life and their place in the world (Koltko-Rivera, 2004). Although they are similar to beliefs and values, they are more global and form the foundation of what we believe about, and how we perceive and process "reality," a topic we explore further in the next chapter.

Worldviews serve as the foundation for philosophy, spirituality, and religion. Koltko-Rivera (2004) extensively outlined categories of worldviews which cover pretty much anything that we contemplate as human beings. These include assumptions about human nature and our ability to change, our relationship with the natural world, our relationships with others, how the mind works, what motivates and guides behaviors, good versus evil, our spiritual beliefs, etc.

Art Therapy and Meaning and Purpose

In cultures worldwide, art is an avenue to express our deepest values and to find meaning in life. Lawrence writes, "Art is a way of knowing that is indigenous to all cultures and traditions. Art engages all of our senses and speaks to us in ways that allow us to access knowledge that cannot be expressed in words" (2008, p. 123). Postmodern philosopher Gadamer stated that artistic creations provide "'a spiritual energy that generates order'" (in Innis, 2001, p. 31). In addition, as Dissanayake (1999) identified, we innately use art to make "special"—to celebrate that which we value and find life-affirming.

Jung (1966/2014) suggested that art served as a way to access and reveal all of the layers of consciousness, starting with the personal self and progressively leading to the universal realm of the collective unconscious. Art therapist Bell wrote, "art-making is deeply imbued with transcendent and non-materialistic qualities of human experience [and] opens up an intra-psychic space where spirituality can be acknowledged, explored and understood" (2011, p. 215).

Not surprisingly, meaning and purpose come up in art therapy—if not imme-diately, then at some point in the process—because art naturally communicates what is relevant and meaningful in our lives. Allen (2012) and McNiff (1992) have written about how art helps us uncover and discover *soul truths*, intuitive, embodied knowledge about ourselves and our place in the world. Many other art therapists have explored the ways meaning, purpose, and spirituality arise in their work (Crooks, 2013; Farrelly-Hansen, 2001; Feen-Callgan, 1995; Franklin, Farrelly-Hansen, Marek, Swan-Foster, & Wallingford, 2000; Hiscox & Calisch, 1998).

In the mid-1970s, Roberta Shoemaker-Beal, in her *holistic approach* to art therapy, used art as a form of *active meditation*—dividing mandalas into four quadrants to explore body, mind, emotion, and spirit (Franklin et al., 2000). Shoemaker-Beal maintains that because expressive art allows for deep percep-tual shifts in belief and worldviews, it helps us discover and stay connected to our *entelechy*, a term Jung used to refer to the core of our being (2016, personal communication).

Pat Allen, in her seminal book, *Art is a Way of Knowing*, wrote that a focused practice of artmaking gave her a path through existential despair to find meaning in her life: "My existence was marginal, uncompelling because my feelings, necessary for a sense of meaning, were missing. Artmaking is my way of bringing soul back into my life" (Allen, 1995, no pagination). Allen also alludes to the transpersonal nature of art—its ability to "dissolve boundaries and reveal our interconnectedness with one another, as well as reveal the dig-nity of our uniqueness."

Moon, in *Existential Art Therapy*, writes that art therapists make art with their clients "that is tied to the creative struggle with the core issues of mean-ing, aloneness, freedom, and death" (2016, p. 210). McNiff in *Art as Medicine*, describes how he helps clients develop a sense of purpose and meaning by using "art's regenerative and redemptive aspects in the personal, social and spiritual spheres" (1992, p. 18).

Ellen Horovitz (2002), in her book *Spiritual Art Therapy*, conducts a *Belief Art Therapy Assessment* whereby clients create artwork about what "God means to you" or "What gives you strength and meaning?" She also inquires into the *opposite* of God (Horovitz, 2014). *Spirituality and Art Therapy* (2001), edited by Mimi Farrelly-Hansen, includes input from a range of art therapists on topics including five established spiritual traditions—Christian, Buddhist, Jewish, Yogic, and Celtic—as well as feminism, shamanism, and archetypal psychology to the field of art therapy. In it, Farrelly-Hansen (2001) describes the role that art played in feeding her "spiritual hunger." She also has clients explore their feelings about prayer and faith through art.

Research in art therapy and meaning has also yielded some interesting results. For example, Darewych (2013, 2014) conducted studies with orphans who had been institutionalized and college students using the "Bridge Drawing" (Hays & Lyons, 1981), modified with a path to facilitate more exploration of meaning and purpose. She found that participants who scored higher on "presence of meaning" drew more "sources of life meaning" paths (such as to relationships, careers, or spirituality) than those who scored as having less meaning in their lives (Darewych, 2014).

Czamanski-Cohen (2012), in her research with critically ill patients, determined that artmaking helped them reconnect to parts of themselves that they felt they had lost as a result of their illness. Collie, Bottorff, and Long found similar results. Art provided a safe place for them to explore the existential terror they were experiencing and to recapture a sense of positive identity in the face of existential fears of "annihilation of the self" that came with their cancer (2006, p. 765). It helped activate parts of themselves that had gone dormant and to "put back together" parts they felt had "broken" (p. 765). It also connected them "to the vast creative energy that exists in the 'ether'" (p. 768).

Puig, Lee, Goodwin, and Sherrard (2006) determined that creative arts therapies not only enhanced wellbeing but it helped cancer patients reframe their illness and perceive it as an opportunity for transformation and growth. Reynolds and Prior (2003), in their study of the impact of artmaking on women with chronic illness, found several consistent themes emerged, e.g., revisiting priorities, filling an occupational void, increasing future orientation and feelings of control, and connecting with a positive self-image that was not defined by their cancer. Wood, Molassiotis, and Payne (2011) observed that art therapy provided patients with opportunities to positively *recalibrate* their identity.

Working with Meaning and Purpose in Art Therapy

We find that our clients—be it with the "working well" or with people with significant psychological, emotional, or physical challenges—are often at a loss when they reflect upon the question "Why am I here?" Finding ways to help them tap into what gives their lives meaning is critical. However, because of the anxiety and feelings of emptiness that this can evoke, it's one of the most delicate aspects of our work.

Gioia recalls a time when she tried to explore this with a client before he was ready to do so. She had recently discovered the *Meaning in Life Questionnaire* (MIL) (Steger, Frazier, Oishi, & Kaler, 2006) and decided to see if it would be helpful in intensive inpatient drug treatment. The MIL assesses both the search for and the presence of meaning in life through a process of rating agreement to questions such as "I am looking for something that makes my life feel meaningful" or "My life has a clear sense of purpose."

This proved too much for one of Gioia's clients, who replied "No" to all questions related to *presence of meaning* and "Yes" to all those related to the *search for meaning* and then abruptly left the group. We suspect that he might have been overwhelmed by the angst that the questions can trigger. Gioia has since been very careful about how she uses this tool. "Baby steps" may be advisable when working in this realm.

Positive Emotions

Although pleasure just for its own sake can be antithetical to overall meaning in life, there is substantial evidence that when people feel good, they believe life is more meaningful (Lyubomirsky, 2008; Park, 2010; Ryan & Deci, 2001). Some positive emotions are particularly relevant to *meaning in life*, such as gratitude, equanimity, serenity, and hope. For example, when working with psychiatric inpatient clients who have attempted suicide, we often ask, "What were you hoping to achieve?" Most of the time they respond that they simply wanted some peace. In these cases, suicide seemed like a means to achieve that result—an end to their suffering. With such clients, we ask them to explore that imagined feeling—relief, serenity, happiness—to visualize it in their minds, to feel it in their bodies, and to manifest it in their artwork. This helps counter helplessness and despair.

What Matters to You Most?

An easy way to ascertain what clients find meaningful is to simply ask, "What matters to you most?" This provides a straightforward and yet deeply personal path to help clients identify what is most essential to their lives. In other words, what gives their life meaning may not be so much lofty ideals but rather the mundane and yet profoundly important things that occupy their lives. In this process, we ask them to include elements that characterize their everyday experience—places, people, animals, activities they enjoy, what they do with their time, etc. This helps reveal the fullness of their lives by "finding the sacred in the ordinary" (Franklin et al., 2000, p. 102).

Dark Night of the Soul

A variation of "What matters most?" is the "Dark Night of the Soul." This metaphor is helpful when clients have survived some sort of crisis, adversity, or loss, either because of an external trauma, psychological challenges, or existential concerns. We ask "when you experienced difficult circumstances what gave you hope in the midst of your troubles? What got you through?" The resulting artwork illustrates both their personal strengths and what is most significant and meaningful in their lives. It reveals their resiliency and sources of hope. When that is witnessed by others, positive feelings of affirmation and connection are enhanced.

Strengths

As we mentioned earlier, when we explore strengths with our clients, it often naturally segues into discussions about values. In addition, since meaning often comes from authentically applying ourselves to endeavors that we find engaging (Peterson & Seligman, 2004), it is very useful to find out what we do well and what strengths make us feel most energized.

Strengths Leading to Values

We can segue from strengths to values by having clients identify which ones relate to their core beliefs about how one should conduct oneself ("Of course, you should be kind!", "Of course, you should exercise restraint!"). We can have them recall someone they admire and what traits make them worthy (Peterson, 2006). Using the word admire can defuse polarities like right vs. wrong or good vs. bad.

Identifying Important Values

As mentioned earlier, because values are often implicit, it can be helpful to identify core assumptions about the way life is "supposed" to be and how these govern our choices. (Steger et al., 2013). Playful approaches such as looking at truisms and seeing which ones resonate most can reveal implicit assumptions about values; e.g., "Waste not, want not" versus "*Carpe diem*/Seize the day." These can easily be converted into art directives, e.g., dividing a piece of paper to contrast two opposing ideals.

As we mentioned in the previous chapter, we can provide lists of values and make artwork about those they resonate with most. For example, we have our clients in drug and alcohol treatment do "Values Wall-Hangings." Figure 10.1 was made by Jack, a client whose appreciation for precision and care was evident in the meticulous cut-paper collages he created to depict Balance, Faith, Industriousness, and Vision. Figure 10.2, made by Lamont (who drew "Low-key joy" in Chapter 5), symbolized Openness, Intuition, Sensitivity, and Willingness. He interwove a soft wool throughout the piece in his favorite color, blue, a self-symbol holding the values together.

Congruency of Values

In therapy, we want not only to help people determine what their personal values are, but also whether or not they are operating within them. We also ask whether they are living in accordance with what is truly important to them, what is acceptable in their social and professional lives, and/or what is considered appropriate in the larger context of the culture within which they reside. After identifying how specific values have shaped their decisions, clients can look at how certain values may conflict with each other and how, as a result, decision-making might be more complex and difficult (Steger et al., 2013). We help clients prioritize life goals and identify ways to apply their values such that they experience less ambivalence and increased congruency.

The wall-hanging directive referred to above can be modified to a "Values Mobile." The movement among shapes that are held together by a unifying structure can illustrate the way values interact with each other and how differing values may throw us off and complicate the process of making decisions. Trying to balance the elements in the mobile so that it is more stable can serve as a useful metaphor and provide interesting insights into our attempts to juggle differing values.

We also create "Value Mandalas," a modification of a positive psychology intervention called the "Bull's Eye Inventory" (Lundgren et al., 2012), which looks at how congruent we are with our values in the domains of work/education, relationships, personal growth/health, and leisure and barriers we have encountered in trying to fulfill those aspirations.

In the values mandala, we place a symbol for ourselves at the center. Like a social atom, we place the symbols for our values in their proximity to the self-symbol based upon how essential it is to our core identity. A variation can be to recreate the mandala placing the symbols relative to how much *they actually act upon them*. And finally, we might have them include barriers to enacting their values and motivations to enact them more. Those familiar with Joan Kelloggs's (1978) work on the Great Round might even ascertain where on the bull's eye/mandala different symbols were placed and explore the implications of these choices with their clients.

Identity

Art therapy has long been known as an effective way to develop and express identity. Spaniol (2003) suggests that art therapy strengthens sense of self. Identity serves as a starting place for discovering aspects of the self that tie into values, beliefs, assumptions, worldviews, and meaning and purpose. Hundreds of directives to address this theme have evolved and been passed around the art therapy community over the years (Linesch, 1988; Wadeson, 1980/2010). Below we list many that have become so familiar to the field that their origins are difficult to determine.

SELF-SYMBOLS

Simply asking people to visualize a color and shape to represent themselves can serve as a warm-up to exploring identity. Other art therapy tasks also lend themselves to addressing core identity: self-portraits, masks, paper dolls, superheroes; using one's body in the artmaking process, such as making hand outlines, masks, and body tracings; or experimenting with writing one's initials or name in artful ways (such as a graffiti tag). People also love to draw themselves as animals, houses, trees, weather patterns, bridges, shields, or shrines.

WHO AM I? WHO AM I *NOT*?

Many of our clients struggle with having any sense of their identity at all—to the point that when we ask them to make imagery about themselves (self-symbols, artwork about their strengths, etc.) they are at a loss. We often warm them up to the topic by posing the question, "Who am I *not?*" Having them notice and describe others, and compare and contrast those others with themselves, often provides tangible examples of how they, themselves, are unique. Comparing their imagery to that of others facilitates this process beautifully—this can be in contrast to artwork of others in a group, but also to artwork that is hanging on the wall in the studio. We usually have several pieces on display which are stylistically unique so as to offer clear visual differences with which our clients can compare their own imagery.

Doing artwork about qualities in others whom they admire (or dislike) can help them get a sense of their own characteristics. Additional directives such as folding a page to delineate "likes *vs.* dislikes," "how I see myself *vs.* how others see me," "my private *vs.* public self," and so on, can help people sort out who they are, what they value, and what holds meaning for them. When we discuss the images, we ask if and how the visual elements might reflect their preferences and style of operating in the world.

IDENTITY THROUGH REVIEW OF ARTWORK

If we have the luxury of working longer term with clients, a review of their artwork often reveals recurring self-symbols which reinforce identity, connection to closely held values, and deeper awareness of meaning and purpose in life. These provide tangible markers that can be compared over time (Wadeson, 1980/2010). Recurrent visual imagery and themes underscore a unifying sense of self. This was particularly helpful for a client of Rebecca's, Grace, a therapist herself who had been struggling with profound feelings of emptiness and loneliness since the dissolution of her marriage. She was plagued with doubts about herself and the choices she had made; she was convinced that she had ruined her chances for happiness and that it was now "too late." She had difficulty discerning any of her strengths and frequently trivialized her artwork as trite or childish.

When we laid out a series of images that she had made throughout the time that we had worked together (Figure 10.3), Grace initially dismissed any similarities or themes that emerged other than they looked "tight," "simple," and "disorganized." She was encouraged to mindfully notice other visual qualities and to compare her imagery with artwork in the studio made by other artists. After looking at paintings, sculptures, and drawings that were in sight—some of which were dark and disorganized—she recognized that hers were quite light and fluid. She noted that orange and magenta frequently appeared and that these colors were not only bright but were also warm and dynamic. She also acknowledged that the images had a pleasing symmetry—a few even felt "expansive" and she noticed "energy" was evident in a many of the drawings.

At the end of the session, Grace noted the "continuity" in her artwork—in the stylistic qualities and the themes that reappeared in her imagery: warmth, vibrancy, fluidity, movement, energy, power, spirituality, immediacy. She was surprised at how much she had enjoyed looking over the span of her work and the consistency of visual themes that revealed themselves. She also recognized that, despite how devastating her divorce had been, there was a part of her that was not only still intact but was alive and well.

Worldviews and Beliefs

Worldviews are at the foundation of philosophical, spiritual, and religious values. They cover pretty much anything that we contemplate as human beings and around which we form beliefs (Koltko-Rivera, 2004). Similar to identifying strengths and values, examining worldviews can consist of exploring essential beliefs about what life means and how the world should be. These include assumptions about good and evil, the nature of knowledge, traditions, spirituality, authority, the purpose of life, the planet and the universe, time, and even our stance towards other worldviews.

Questions to Elicit Worldviews

- Human nature: naturally good/naturally evil?
- We can never change/We can always change?
- Is it better to *be* or to *do*?
- What resonates—upholding traditions, living in the present, or planning for the future?
- How should we treat others?

Art therapy, with its capacity for metaphor and symbolic depth, is ideally suited for this kind of exploration. Through storytelling, parable, mythology, and creative endeavors of all kinds, we can examine our beliefs and how they shape our worldviews. This can also help illuminate the spiritual paradigms that are at play in our lives. For example, in Gioia's work with clients in substance abuse recovery, she asks them to use collage on folded paper showing on one side "what you are powerless over" and on the other "what helps you feel empowered." Often images of their disease/addiction—bottles of alcohol or drugs—are contrasted to images representing their support system or a higher power (God or some other spiritual presence). Magazine images of sunsets and starry skies often emerge as representation of the divine and incomprehensible, which begins dialogue about deeply held beliefs.

Helping Others

Aristotle thought that authentic happiness and fulfillment was achieved by loving, rather than in *being loved*. The science of positive psychology has born this out—people do feel happier when they help others (Otake, Shimai, Tanaka-Matsumi, Otsui, & Fredrickson, 2006). Practicing kindness can enhance a sense of meaningfulness in one's life as well as boost physical and mental health and overall wellbeing (Post, 2005; Schwartz, Meisenhelder, Ma, & Reed, 2003). Altruism, showing concern for the welfare of others, has multiple benefits: "deeper and more positive social integration, distraction from personal problems and the anxiety of self-preoccupation, enhanced meaning and purpose as related to well-being, a more active lifestyle...and the presence of positive emotions such as kindness that displace harmful negative emotions" (Post, 2005, p. 70).

Art therapy provides many opportunities for altruism, kindness, and generosity. To begin with, clients are often spontaneously inspired to give away the creations they've made in art therapy to someone who is important to them. Intentionally making gifts for others can also engage clients in expressing gratitude and achieving a goal. This can include making gifts for others in the group or cards for someone they would like to thank (either dead or alive), or offering objects that provide moral support to others in need, such as the Christmas cards the psychiatric patients made for patients on the medical floors.

Art therapists can also engage clients in *artful* exchanges that create a sense of belonging and being part of something that is bigger than the self (Chilton, Gerity, LaVorgna-Smith, & MacMichael, 2009). This can include art swaps, round robins, practicing random acts of kindness with art, and community projects. These cooperative endeavors might manifest as quilts, murals, altered book collaborations, prayer flags, spirit doll exchanges, art supply swaps and so on.

What Art Therapy Brings to Meaning and Purpose

As positive psychology builds upon the research and theory of meaning and purpose, we now have a more informed view of the benefits and challenges of working with meaning and purpose. Just as with other aspects of wellbeing, we believe that art therapy uniquely contributes to this domain of PERMA. First and foremost, it brings the virtue of creativity, one of the core values of our profession, to the exploration of what is most fundamental and important to our lives. It provides a myriad of innovative ways to examine overarching existential questions such as "Who am I?" and "What am I here for?" that can be illuminating, engaging, and even fun.

For people who need *identity-building* interventions (King et al., 2006, Steger et al., 2013), art therapy is a way of "strengthening selfhood" (Spaniol, 2003, p. 274). It can highlight the strengths, values, beliefs and worldviews that shape who they are. For those who identify a sense of purpose in their lives, art therapy can help refine and deepen that sense of mission. And finally, as we will discuss in the following chapter, for people whose sense of meaning and purpose has been shaken by illness, loss, trauma, or despair, art therapy can highlight their resilience and ways that they have overcome their difficulties.

Discussion Questions

1   What is most important to you and what are your worldviews about those things (people, places, activities, beliefs, spiritual practices, etc.)? How does art fit into those?
2   Looking at the list of values (in Appendix D), pick those that seem important. Do any of your values conflict with others?
3   What are some values that you share with your clients?

CHAPTER 11

Meaning-making and Perception

During a workshop we ran on the theme of "Celebrating Resilience" for people affected by cancer, we engaged in the art process ourselves, as we often do when we work with clients. Gioia had just completed her PhD and returned from a much-needed vacation with her family to celebrate this accomplishment. She was feeling relaxed and inspired. She sketched a woman lost in a pleasant reverie contemplating projects which she was now free to take on (Figure 11.1).

Rebecca, on the other hand, had had a particularly stressful year—her identical twin sister had been near death for months after complicated liver surgery that now Rebecca herself was likely going to have to undergo. She was feeling more optimistic, though, because her sister's health was finally improving, giving Rebecca a sense of hope that, as a natural-born pessimist, she did not usually experience. Rebecca drew a small mandala of a bright sun at the end of a spiral path made of blue for sadness but also healing and gold for prosperity and hope (Figure 11.2).

At the end of the group, we both shared briefly about our images. When Rebecca held up her artwork, several of the group members spontaneously observed that "It looks like a fuse exploding!" She and Gioia chuckled, because, just like our clients, Rebecca had not in any way intended that; however, once it had been pointed out, it did seem inescapable. Seeing the image through their eyes changed Rebecca's perception of it. From that point on, she saw it differently herself.

We were tickled that this encounter so beautifully illustrated that even we—artists for most of our lives and art therapists for the last 25 years—were not even remotely immune to the capacity of imagery to present possibilities of which we might not consciously be aware. This is the beauty of art—it often originates from the conscious realm—e.g., "I'm going to draw a hopeful spiral path ending with a shining sun"—but then it takes on a life of its own.

Once Rebecca became aware that her "bright sun" might also look like an explosion at the end of a fuse, she was able to contemplate meanings that might hold for her. On the one hand, it might suggest that she was "ready to explode"!

With all of the stress she'd been going through, that seemed like a reasonable assumption. On the other hand, although it might not convey the serenity she had initially intended, it seemed to display a level of dynamism that was uncharacteristic for her. In that sense, she thought it might even be *more* hopeful. Maybe it was a spark of celebratory energy!

In this way, Rebecca experienced the same process our clients go through—making something with one intention and then, after receiving input from others and really looking at the visual content, becoming aware of other possibilities. She experienced a *reappraisal* of her assumptions about her artwork and, as a result, a consideration of meanings which might otherwise have escaped her. And finally, as a result of this shift in perception, she saw the image and even her situation differently.

Meaning and Perception

In the last chapter, we delved into *meaning* and *purpose*; we will now discuss *Meaning-making*—the process whereby we construct meaning from our perceptions and how this impacts wellbeing. This chapter is in many ways the apex of this book, the place where all of the elements of PERMA and positive art therapy combine to help us identify and shift how we see and interpret our lives.

Making Sense of "Reality"

Just as we appear to have an essential need to feel that our lives and that life itself has meaning and purpose, we also need to believe life makes sense. In order to establish consistency and stability, we engage in *meaning-making*—the process of taking in, sorting, and interpreting information from our external environment and our internal experience (Baumeiser & Vohs, 2010). We want to know *why* things happen, even if there is no easily discernible cause. If we cannot find a rational answer, our minds naturally *create* one (Terr, 2008). Without some sort of rhyme and reason, life is too chaotic and unpredictable.

Most of us assume that when we are engaging in meaning-making, we are attending to and perceiving an objective *reality*. However, "reality" is always *subjectively* experienced through our own unique and changing perceptions (Lewin, 1943). We "see" the world through a lens of cultural background, worldviews, beliefs, values, feelings, and physiology. These perceptions, in turn, affect our subjective and psychological wellbeing—in short, how happy we are. Positive psychologists have identified that because perception and meaning-making are so critical to wellbeing, we need to develop ways of managing these processes. However, before we look at *changing* our thinking and perceptions, it might be helpful to look at the factors that shape and influence them in the first place.

Factors that Shape Perception

We begin with cognitive influences—beliefs, worldviews, biases, and optimistic and pessimistic explanatory styles—and then consider the role that emotional and physical states play in perception. We explore how cognitive processes, emotions, and physiology influence and are influenced by each other. Finally, we examine the way that stress, trauma, and loss shape our perceptions but also, conversely, how our perceptions shape what we believe about what has happened or is happening to us in our lives.

BELIEFS AND WORLDVIEWS

Beliefs are basic understandings about the world and ourselves that are felt to be true. They begin to form before we can even express ourselves verbally. They are shaped by social and cultural influences—by what we witness and experience through our primary relationships and our immediate environment as our minds are forming and growing. Worldviews are the broader set of beliefs we have about the universe and our place in it. They determine our sense of *what is* and *what ought to be*, what we believe is *good* and *bad*, and where we believe we should direct our energies in life (Koltko-Rivera, 2004).

Aaron Beck (1967), one of the founders of Cognitive Behavioral Therapy (CBT), maintained that we hold core beliefs which shape what we attend to and how we process new information. These serve as shortcuts which allow us to operate automatically without having to devote conscious resources to analyzing and categorizing every piece of incoming data with which we are confronted. Core beliefs tend to be relatively stable despite contradictory information. In other words, we tend to notice things that fit into our schemas. Information that doesn't, we either ignore or write off as exceptions to the rule.

Beck (1967) proposed that *dysfunctional beliefs* cause depression and anxiety. Albert Ellis (1957) similarly suggested that *irrational beliefs* cause people to form negative interpretations of events in their lives and, as a result, to respond in dysfunctional ways that undermine their happiness.

COGNITIVE BIASES

As we alluded to in earlier chapters, there are a range of cognitive mechanisms that we engage in both consciously and unconsciously which affect our perceptions. The *confirmation bias* refers to our tendency to seek out information in the environment which corresponds with our beliefs and expectations (Nickerson, 1998). The *disconfirmation bias* leads us to ignore evidence which does not. The *negativity* bias primes us to perceive cues related to real or imagined threats that might be salient to our survival over more neutral and/or "positive" data.

We are also prone to the *optimism bias*—the illusion that we are immune to risk despite statistical evidence to the contrary (Sharot, Riccardi, Raio, & Phelps, 2007). In addition, we tend to believe that we will be much happier if good things happen than we *actually* are when they do. Conversely, we believe that if bad things happen that we will be much *more unhappy* than we are, and we *underestimate* our capacity to cope when things go wrong (Wilson & Gilbert, 2005).

OPTIMISTIC AND PESSIMISTIC EXPLANATORY STYLES

We are also inclined toward optimistic or pessimistic explanatory styles—ways of "explaining" what we think is happening in and around us. Explanatory styles are characterized by their degree of personalization, permanence, and pervasiveness (Seligman, 2002a):

- Pessimists personalize the bad and depersonalize the good. When bad things happen it is because of who they are, not the situation. Optimists personalize the good and depersonalize the bad.
- Pessimists believe that negative events are permanent, stable, and consistent, and positive events are unstable and transitory. Optimists believe that negative events are isolated incidents and that, generally speaking, things will go well.
- Pessimists see negative events as pervasive, global, and generalized; and positive events as specific. Optimists believe that positive things happen in all domains in their lives and negative events are specific only to a particular situation.

Seligman (2002a) suggests that pessimistic explanatory styles factor significantly in depression, particularly when it undermines motivation and self-efficacy. Conversely, optimistic thinking is associated with positive mood, better health, interpersonal wellbeing, and higher levels of academic and professional performance.

Hope theory examines the role that *agency* and *pathways* play in shaping our expectations (Snyder, 2000). *Agency* refers to our belief in our ability to affect our environment and our motivation to achieve our goals. Optimists tend to believe they can positively influence their circumstances; pessimists are less likely to. *Pathways* refers to the means we perceive that we have at our disposal to do so. Optimists, when they encounter barriers to meeting their goals, are more likely to find alternative pathways to get the job done. Pessimists tend to believe that they can't influence their environment, so they are more likely stop trying.

Growth mindset and *fixed mindset* also figure here (Dweck, 2006). If we have a growth mindset, we are more likely to persist despite setbacks because we see mistakes as part of the learning process, as opportunities to hone our game. If we have a fixed mindset, we are more likely to give up or become risk-averse because we cannot tolerate the possibility of failure.

PHYSICAL STATES

Physical states include not only what we see, feel, hear, touch, smell, and taste, but also level of physiological arousal, stamina, neurological activity, general nutritional health, etc. Although we often think of the body and the mind as two different things, it is increasingly evident they are inseparable. Our physical states impact our perceptions and vice versa. For example, if we are physically depleted, distances/inclines appear more strenuous (Zadra & Clore, 2011). This makes sense—when we are worn down or sick, we know that even the simplest of tasks can seem burdensome. On the other hand, when we feel refreshed, the opposite occurs.

If we are generally hearty and energetic, we may be more naturally resilient and have a corresponding zest for life. If we are struggling with a physical disability, a pain condition, or poor sleep patterns, our attention may be more restricted because our energy is focused on coping and conserving resources. As a result, we may be less attuned to other things (Zadra & Clore, 2011).

EMOTIONS

How we feel affects what we perceive about our experiences, and, conversely, what we perceive affects how we feel. *Emotions* also shape what we attend to and notice. Using the "spotlight" analogy for attention—how we feel determines *where* and *how much* we shine the spotlight. Fear and anxiety narrow attention toward potentially threatening environmental cues (Zadra & Clore, 2011). Positive feelings expand it to perceive possibilities (Fredrickson, 2001).

Emotions also affect how we *appraise* what we notice—they serve as a quick "thumbs up" or "thumbs down" (Kashdan & Biswas-Diener, 2014). For example, when people are afraid, they perceive that a mountain is steeper than when they are calm. If they are sad, distances appear greater (Zadra & Clore, 2011). If they are feeling hopeful, activities that require effort seem easily achievable.

Emotions are also heavily influenced by unconscious beliefs about what we are experiencing. They change rapidly not only as our circumstances change but also as our evaluations of them change (Scherer, 2005). If we've successfully climbed mountains in the past, we are more likely to feel confident when we tackle another one. If we've never climbed a mountain before, we may be anxious about doing so; however, if a mountaineer joins us, we feel reassured. Our brains make quick but complex evaluations that combine and integrate unconscious/implicit information with conscious/explicit thoughts.

Tendencies toward positive or negative emotionality also factor prominently in perception. People with higher positivity ratios like Gioia, because of the broadening effects of positive emotions, tend to see things more optimistically and to perceive more ways to achieve their goals. On the other hand, people who are prone to negative emotionality like Rebecca, because of the narrowing effect of negative emotions, are more likely to perceive things pessimistically. They are less likely to believe that they can change things and see fewer options available to them.

In previous chapters, we looked at the impact that stress can have on our lives and the role that vulnerability to stress can play. Stress has been defined as any environmental, social, biological, or psychological change that requires an adjustment to our usual behaviors (Selye, 1955). Initial approaches to stress suggested that *any* change created stress. Ascertaining our level of stress could be determined by allotting a numerical value to the changes we were experiencing in our lives, both positive and negative (Holmes & Rahe, 1967). Once 300 points accrued, it could be inferred that we were in danger of developing symptoms of stress: gastrointestinal distress, lowered immunity, heart disease, irritability, fatigue, depression, etc.

Folkman and Lazarus (1985) suggested the level of stress depends more on how we *perceive* stressors and our beliefs about our capacity to cope with them. In other words, Rebecca reaching 300 might be quite different from Gioia doing so. This includes perceptions of how given stressors will affect our self-image, health, finances, relationships, and whether they were anticipated or unexpected, desired or not, etc. That is to say, it's not just the objective threat but the *meaning* that it holds for us that determines how stressful we perceive something to be.

We often ask clients to rate their level of stress at a given moment on a scale of 1–10 (1 being extremely agitated and 10 very relaxed). In hospital settings with patients who either are struggling with a life-threatening illness or who are in emotional distress—or the nurses, doctors, and staff helping them—we often hear low numbers followed by exclamations like "I'm in the hospital! Of course my numbers are low!" On the other hand, at the resort, people often report high levels of relaxation and exult "We're in this gorgeous place—who wouldn't be relaxed?!"

We then have them rate their levels of stress *in general*. Many people assume that being in certain environments would naturally be more stressful than others. However, that's not always the case. For example, medical staff often report that they are more relaxed at work, despite the chaos, because the stress is predictable and contained. They know when it will begin and end, exactly what is expected of them, and how to accomplish it. Their personal lives are more complex and unpredictable—whether because of raising teenagers, caring for someone with special needs, managing an illness of their own, paying bills, etc.

In addition, most of us also believe that our level of stress is contingent upon what is happening around us—we're stressed out in a hospital and relaxed at a spa! However, as Jon Kabat-Zinn so aptly put it, "wherever you go, there you are" (1994, p. 11). Those of us who are more prone to anxiety, like Rebecca, often experience stress *regardless* of their circumstances. Those who are generally more relaxed, like Gioia, tend to exhibit that disposition irrespective of how stressful the situation is. As we will explore shortly, knowing our temperament helps us determine how to manage our stress.

TRAUMA AND LOSS

There is no doubt that *loss* and *trauma* impacts our lives. Most of our clients, and we as well, will invariably experience difficulties which may affect us deeply and perhaps change us forever. If that happens at an early age and/or repeatedly, we know it can seriously impede intellectual and emotional development, capacity for attachment and empathy, and ability to regulate emotion (Perry, 2009). In addition, it's not surprising to note most clients and recipients of services in the mental health system are also trauma survivors and many symptoms of mental illness can be seen as remnants of coping strategies which were once adaptive but end up being dysfunctional and/or addictive in the long run (Giller, 1999), such as dissociation, drug addiction, and self-injurious behaviors.

COPING

As mentioned, we tend to *underestimate* our capacity to cope when bad things happen (Wilson & Gilbert, 2005). Even after losses or trauma that are so devastating that we're certain *we will never recover*, we generally bounce back more fully than we could ever have imagined possible. This is partly due to the hedonic treadmill—our tendency to adapt to circumstances *both good and bad*. It is also because, when bad things *actually do happen*, our minds try to make sense of it so that life is still, on some level, understandable and predictable. We construct a narrative that weaves into our overarching schemas and worldviews. This lessens its disorienting impact and allows us to cope. Even if the meaning we arrive at is *negative*, it is often more reassuring than if it has *no meaning at all*.

How we cope with adversity varies from person to person. For example, people who are more buoyant and optimistic tend to face their problems head on and put their efforts toward remediating the situation. When this sort of *problem-focused coping* is not possible, they turn to adaptive, *emotion-focused coping* strategies such as using humor, acceptance, and positive reframing. As a result, they tend to bounce back quicker (Sheier & Carver, 1993). People who are more pessimistic and prone to negative emotionality are more likely to avoid or disengage from problems, regardless of whether or not they could resolve them, which can end up compounding whatever the given stressors might be.

Why Does this Matter?

What we perceive and the meaning that we derive from our perceptions impacts our happiness. People who are generally happier tend to view life's events and their role in them more positively (Seligman, 2002). In turn, perceiving things more positively promotes subjective wellbeing—both by making people feel better and by increasing the likelihood that they experience more satisfaction with important domains of their lives. It also promotes psychological wellbeing by fostering a sense of meaning and purpose, promoting insight and acceptance of oneself, as well as understanding and empathy for others. Life not only makes sense but it seems more hopeful, meaningful, and worthwhile.

In the process of trying to make sense of the world and ourselves in it, perceiving more *positive meaning* from our experiences increases wellbeing and happiness: "A consistent theme throughout meaning-making research is that the people who achieve the greatest benefits are those who transform their perceptions of circumstance from being unfortunate to fortunate" (Baumeiser & Vohs, 2010, p. 614).

Positive Meaning and Benefit-finding

It should be noted that when we are exposed to loss and trauma, we have responses that might be called *negative* but are natural and to be expected. When something bad happens, we suffer and grieve. We may wonder why such a thing happened and if we could have prevented it. That makes us human—it reveals what is important to us. We may also experience symptoms of anxiety, depression, and PTSD. Even if we do not develop any signs of trauma, recovery takes time. It has cycles that may be painful and difficult but are also normal and predictable.

Posttraumatic Growth

Nevertheless, people are actually quite resilient and, as we mentioned earlier, they generally bounce back better than they expect! In fact, often people who have faced some sort of adversity not only return to their previous baseline of functioning, they experience *posttraumatic growth*—positive change that results from struggling with a highly challenging crisis (Tedeschi & Calhoun, 2004). Posttraumatic growth can include an increased sense of meaning and purpose in life, deepened interpersonal relationships, changed priorities, and a greater sense of personal strength. People often identify a particular trauma as a turning point in their lives—the "silver lining" around the cloud of their loss. This might be something about their experience that made them stronger and more resilient or more appreciative of what they have that has endured (Seery, 2011).

Positive psychologists have devoted substantial attention to the role of positive meaning, benefit-finding, and posttraumatic growth in wellbeing (Tennen & Affleck, 1999). They suggest that, although thankfully there is finally much more attention being given the *damaging* effects of trauma—something for which mental health practitioners tirelessly advocated—there is far less focus on the *resilience* that naturally develops when we encounter life-altering adversity.

In fact, we are more likely to experience posttraumatic growth than sympto-matic responses to trauma (Tedeschi & Calhoun, 2004). That is not to say that we won't struggle with grief, anger, guilt, and confusion, as well as periods of disrupted functioning—however, these are "normal" responses to loss. On the other hand, we will also likely experience a broadened perspective of our lives and a richer sense of meaning and purpose.

Unfortunately, as a result of a desire to generate more interest in post-traumatic growth, positive psychologists have been criticized for skating too quickly past loss and trauma (Lazarus, 2003). We also hear this when we train therapists—that rushing to benefit-finding might prevent someone from experiencing vital stages of recovery which, even if painful, are necessary. Without a doubt, this is a valid concern. However, people are naturally resil-ient. More than likely, they will not only survive and recover but also *thrive* from their difficulties. We have dubbed this phenomenon "bouncing back and *bouncing forward.*"

With this in mind, although our role as therapists is always first and foremost to help our clients cope with trauma/loss and to give them a chance to "tell their story," it is also to help them derive positive meaning and opportunities for growth from that which they have experienced. In other words, *when the time is right,* we help them tap into and build on the resources and resilience that got them through their difficulties and to see themselves and their lives in a more purposeful and empowered light.

Positive Art Therapy's Approach to Meaning and Perception

In illustrating how we apply a positive art therapy approach to meaning-making, we outline a progression of steps, with the caveat that they might not always be employed or unfold in precisely the same sequence. Although we describe art therapy processes that are not unique to positive art therapy, we clarify how we utilize these to promote benefit-finding and posttraumatic growth.

We begin with *developing awareness*—of what is occupying our uncon-scious and conscious awareness, where we are putting our attention, and what we are perceiving—and strategies for *increasing awareness*. Then we look at *shifting perceptions*, exploring ways to find positive meaning in the difficulties we have encountered and in life in general, and to experience the increased wellbeing that doing so produces.

Developing Awareness

Before we proceed, it may be useful to review the factors that *generally* shape the way we perceive "reality." As we described above, we filter our experiences through the lens of our beliefs and values, explanatory styles, emotional dis-positions, physiology, developmental history and how we generally cope with change, stress, trauma, and loss. For better or worse, our moods and mindsets are heavily influencing "reality" and shaping the narrative we formulate about what is happening in and around us.

Therapy usually begins with a receptive and supportive inquiry into this "story," into what has led our clients to this moment: what brought them to therapy, what they are hoping for, and how they perceive their situation. As we listen to this account, we are often simultaneously assessing, even if informally, their baseline emotional, physical, and cognitive states as well as their strengths and vulnerabilities in those areas.

Art therapy is ideal for ascertaining this baseline. Because it engages clients in perceptual realms that are not only visual but also tactile and sensorimotor, it provides something unique to the process of developing and increasing awareness right from the start.

Art Engages the Senses and Play

Even before clients actually start manipulating the materials, just seeing art supplies—a rainbow of pastels, markers, paint, clay, found objects, etc.—evokes a sensory response. The creative process initiates a dynamic range of neurobiological activity, what Hass-Cohen calls *creative embodiment* (2016), Rappaport (2016) calls *the felt sense*, and in the Expressive Therapies Continuum, is part of the Kinesthetic and Sensorimotor stage (Hinz, 2009).

The sensorimotor qualities of artmaking serve as a gateway to parts of the brain not usually available to our conscious mind. It allows us to retrieve material—thoughts, feelings, memories—which cannot come to consciousness any other way. The sensory nature of art materials coupled with the reassuring presence of an art therapist is simultaneously stimulating and relaxing at the same time (Hass-Cohen, 2016). It encourages engagement, play, curiosity, and interaction with our environment. This induces a slew of corresponding psychological and psychological processes—e.g., activation of the parasympathetic nervous system, broadened perceptions, and heightened awareness of emotional states.

Expression

Engaging the senses not only facilitates *access to* but also *expression of* both implicit and explicit material. We know that expression is healing and doing so through art can helps clarify thoughts and feelings. As Naumburg (1958) proposed, it serves as *direct communication* of unconscious material. Unlike verbal forms of expression, it circumvents defenses and requires no translation. Nucho (2003) maintained that visual expression served as "a *highly efficient exchange* between various levels of the system and with the external world" (p. 19). Jung (2015) was convinced that art was one of the *most* effective ways of accessing and expressing the unconscious realm.

But what is expression, really? Most simply put, it is how we make our inner experience visible to ourselves and others—through verbalizations, movements, facial expressions, how we make artwork, etc.

Artwork Is Its Own Entity

In art therapy, access and expression of internal processes is taken a step further by the production of artwork which externalizes them *into a form that is separate from its creator*. This may be one of the most extraordinary features that art therapy brings to the meaning-making process—we can literally step away from it, walk around it, approach it from different vantage points, and distance from it. Ulman (1986) believed that because artwork can be observed independently of its maker, therefore allowing them to engage more objectively with what it represents, that it streamlined the therapeutic process.

Art Tells the Story

By giving shape to and revealing the self (Jung, 2015), art says "Look at me, I exist!" It is a testimony to how we see and perceive the world, our version of "reality." Winnicott (1971) suggested that art metaphorically represented the transitional space which connects subjective and objective reality. It gives us a chance to tell our story which, given visual form, becomes more real and takes on a life of its own. It represents both the conscious intention of the artist, but also, as we will explore shortly, many alternative stories which may not, at first, have been evident to its maker but which, through exploration, can come to life.

Increasing Awareness

When sensory impressions, and implicit/explicit feeling, thoughts, and memories take form in artwork, and artists behold these elements of the self, they begin to experience what Joy Schavarien (1999) calls the *dawning of consciousness*. This is the recognition that the artwork and the way it was made mirrors fundamental aspects about the artist and how they operate in the world. There may be times when art therapists might *not* pursue this line of inquiry; e.g., when clients are deeply in flow, or when, because of physical/cognitive challenges, they are not able to voice their associations to their imagery. However, if it makes clinical sense, this is when art therapists and their clients can more consciously engage the making-meaning process, looking at the artwork and considering what it might reveal.

Before we explore this further, we would be remiss if we didn't consider what may be obvious but is nevertheless critical to this discussion—how art therapists approach meaning-making is heavily influenced by *their* beliefs about that process. Rubin (2016) suggests that meanings found in artwork *depend on the theoretical lens through they are perceived*, i.e., the art therapist's worldview.

With this in mind, we categorize that the lens that *we* see through is a composite of psychology, philosophy, anthropology, art and art therapy theories that, for us, combine to form a *positive art therapy* approach.

Like most art therapists, we think that artmaking brings something special to the meaning-making process. Even when we are not formally assessing our clients, we are learning about them through the materials they choose, how they interact with those, and the imagery they make. We also believe that *our clients* fundamentally grasp that their artwork is communicating something (Rubin, 2016). They often look to us to interpret this message—whether grudgingly, because they believe we are "analyzing" their imagery and "know" what it means, or expectantly, for what they think we have magically divined.

Art therapists often attempt to diffuse this power differential by encouraging clients to find their own meanings in the imagery. This is congruent with a client-centered approach that makes *them*, rather than the therapist, the expert of their own experience. However, because art therapy involves not only making art but also *perceiving* it (Betensky, 2001), we suggest that adopting this approach without providing some guidance to our clients on *how to find meaning* in their artwork may downplay the fundamental strength art therapists bring to the meaning-making process: *our expertise in art!*

Not only do we believe that artwork serves as a reflection of the artist's internal world—*the isomorphic mirror* (Cohen & Cox, 1995)—but we also believe that it can be *best* understood by looking at the visual elements in the art. Because art therapists are trained in this domain, we can in turn teach our clients how to observe the visual elements and how the artwork was made in order to explore the meanings these might hold.

Visual Literacy and Mindfulness

We liken examining the formal elements in artwork to a practice of mindfulness. This means bringing our attention more consciously—both client and therapist—to *what is actually in the image.* As we discussed in the chapter on strengths (Chapter 8), although our clients often want to begin talking about their artwork by sharing what they *intended* to communicate in it, before we dive into these associations, we gently steer the process to start *first* with what Betensky (2001) calls *intentional looking.*

We usually begin this process by literally putting distance between the artists and their artwork. We invite them to observe what pops out most to them. What are the dominant visual elements? What patterns emerge? What is the gestalt of the elements when they come together as a whole? What is a surprise? We have them describe their imagery using the language of visual form—texture, value, line quality, direction, style, juxtaposition of shapes, use of space, contrast, balance, depth, focus, etc.

We also explore the process that went into creating it. How did they interact with the art supplies? How engaged were they during its making and did that change as they went along? Carefully attuning to the visual content and the artmaking process allows us to embrace more fully what the image has to say (Betensky, 2001). Then we delve into the content and symbols in the imagery.

Exploring Symbolism

One of the bedrocks of art therapy is *symbolic speech,* the power of artistic imagery and the art process to access and express a range of both conscious and unconscious messages that we might not otherwise be able to convey (Kramer, 1971; Naumburg, 1966). Pioneer art therapist Edith Kramer went so far as to say that the very "aim of art is the making of a symbolic object that contains and communicates an idea" (1971, p. 28). Nucho suggested that images are custom-tailored "information condensers" that come closest to reflecting the immediacy of experience (2003, p. 18). She calls the mind a *metaphor-making machine* that uses symbols to turn abstract and amorphous concepts into concrete anchors that are easier to retrieve and comprehend.

As we described in Chapter 5, on creativity, we often warm up our clients to symbolic thinking by having them call to mind a color, shape, or symbol in response to a particular strength/value, such as spirituality or love. In groups, many people will share the same associations—e.g., for spirituality, purple, white, circles, and infinity signs, or for love, red and pink hearts. We may also get less predictable responses, such as red for spirituality because it signifies passion, or brown for love because it is grounding. The process of visualizing symbols and colors activates imaginative thinking and engages the emotional realm.

Later in the session, we explore the symbolism in their imagery. This includes observing how the visual elements and the process of making the artwork relate to what the artists consciously intended. Invariably they will identify "accidents"—unexpected effects they did *not intend.* We suggest that although these outcomes may be incidental and irrelevant, they might also have metaphorical content. If they *did* have meaning, what might it be? Are there metaphors in the interplay among the formal elements, the process of making the artwork, and the story that have significance and if so what?

SYMBOLISM AND THE COLLECTIVE UNCONSCIOUS

Although we do not often impose interpretations of imagery, we believe that visual symbols derive from a "database" of human knowledge—what Jung (2014) called the *collective unconscious.* As Gantt and Tabone (2011) suggested, when looking at artwork, we decipher visual cues in such a way that we experience an intuitive sense of what it means. For example, color has universal associations. In most cultures, yellow is linked to happiness, enlightenment, energy, and the sun; blue to calm, cool, healing, water and the sky.

In addition, we instantly apprehend and understand the *interrelationship* of visual elements, e.g., smaller objects placed next to larger ones reflect a hierarchy, objects grouped together appear to be related, etc. The same is true of visual elements that have the same color, texture, shape—they are understood to be similar in nature. Differences are interpreted by virtue of their contrast to other elements—e.g., an orange shape in the midst of many blue ones seems significant because it stands out from the latter.

One picture is worth a thousand words. (Barnard, 1927)

In group sessions, we capitalize on this shared knowledge by inviting the artists, if they are comfortable, to hear impressions from other group members. Often they might voice opinions such as "It looks lonely," or "happy," or "It's so beautiful!" When they express diagnostic or aesthetic opinions, we steer them back to the formal elements and ask them to describe what gave them that impression. For *lonely*, they might identify a sky filled with grey clouds made in rapid and dark diagonal lines or a bent and leafless tree. For *happy*, they might refer to creatures playing in a field of colorful flowers. For *beautiful*, they might describe luminous color or a sense of depth and intensity.

Often contradictions between the spoken content and the feel of the image can be explored (Maclagan, 2001), e.g., when a client describes his image as *hopeful* but it has dark ominous clouds and is devoid of life. Another client might say her picture represents her depression but observers point out that, although there *are* clouds in the picture, they are white and fluffy, and behind them is a bright sun and people with smiles on their faces. At times like this, we might step back and talk about universal understandings that people share about imagery and how these may be impacting the way people are seeing it, e.g., how people tend to perceive jagged lines as more dramatic or curvilinear lines as softer and more fluid.

We ask the artists if the discrepancy between what they had intended to depict and what others are perceiving holds any meaning to them and how that relates to the subject matter which the picture was initially meant to portray. If they are properly "warmed up," they often see the implications of identifying parallels and incongruences between the *intended* meaning and the *actual* visual content. They grasp that these serve as metaphors for the situations they reflect and, even more importantly, for their lives in general. The artists experience "a vivid awareness which allows all kinds of things that once seemed inexplicable to make sense" (Rubin, 2016, p. 117)—that *Aha!* moment in which their sense of themselves, their stories, and their place in the world are suddenly visible in a new and surprising way.

When, at the end, the artist was willing to rest his case on what his eyes and hands had arrived at, he had become able to see what he meant. (Arnheim, 1962, p. 135)

Shifting Perception

In articulating ways that we use the art therapy process to develop and increase awareness, it becomes evident that it organically changes how we see things. Artwork reveals our resilience. It showcases strengths, values, and what gives our lives meaning and purpose. It connects us to our humanity. It gives others a glimpse of us that they might not otherwise have seen, and vice versa. Developing and increasing awareness through art therapy naturally shifts perceptions. Art disrupts our assumptions and opens our minds to other possibilities, what Barone and Eisner called "a useful sort of emancipation" from preconceived ideas (2012, p. 16).

Art expresses, documents, contains, and clarifies the condition of the psyche. Placing what is partially known into a shape or form outside of the body not only expands one's awareness, but also frees one from the grips of the complex so that the constructive process of curiosity, reflection, and an eventual shift in viewpoint can occur. (Swan-Foster, 2016, p. 176)

Apart from capitalizing on these inherent attributes, we also strategically employ techniques to *actively shift perception*. We do this in subtle but deliberate ways at the very start of therapy in order to warm up clients to the therapeutic process. This includes, as we have mentioned throughout the book, combining the broadening potential of positive emotions like hope and connection with the simultaneously relaxing/stimulating nature of the artmaking process. This elicits imperceptible changes that may not be consciously recognized but are critical to establishing a strong therapeutic alliance. It helps clients feel safe with us and, in groups, with others which, in turn, makes them more willing to take risks—to experiment with artmaking and self-exploration.

Finding Positive Meaning

In addition to using specific techniques to shift perception early in the therapeutic relationship, we do so at later stages of the process as well to set the stage for *posttraumatic growth* and *benefit-finding*. We move from mindfully observing to actively mining for positive meaning. In other words, we go beyond increasing awareness to *increasing awareness of the good*. As mentioned earlier, posttraumatic growth is facilitated by positive coping, attending to the good, emotional regulation, changing the narrative, and cultivating optimism. We suggest that, because the art therapy process is so effective at shifting perception and amplifying meaning, it enhances the efficacy of these strategies.

Positive Coping

People who engage in *positive coping* appear to devote their resources towards that which they feel can effect change, often called *situational coping*. When they determine that they are not able to change the situation, they switch to *emotional coping* which involves managing their feelings so that they are best able to adapt to the situation. In addition, people who generally experience more positive emotions and optimistic thinking tend to perceive their capacity to cope and the adequacy of their resources more positively. They are also more willing to consider and even welcome challenges to their self-esteem, e.g. negative feedback about themselves, for the sake of personal growth (Aspinwall, 1998).

Mindfully attuning to our physical and emotional needs can help us determine where to channel resources and practice self-care. We also differentiate areas where we can effect change versus those over which we have no control. If we or our clients are more dispositionally anxious, although we might try to manage whatever is causing our anxiety, we may need to focus more on managing the anxiety itself rather "fixing the situation."

Serenity Prayer

God, grant me the serenity
To accept the things I cannot change;
Courage to change the things I can;
And the wisdom to know the difference.
(Adapted from Reinhold Niebuhr, 1892–1971

Artmaking, in and of itself, is a positive coping strategy. As we discussed in previous chapters, it promotes self-expression, it induces the relaxation response, it serves as a productive distraction, it engages states of flow, and it fosters creativity. For example, Puig and colleagues, in their research using creative art therapy with women with breast cancer, found that the participants valued being able to express their feelings, and to relax and devote time to self-care, reflection, and quiet. Perhaps most importantly, it helped shift how they perceived their illness, to "reframe the breast cancer experience and see it as an opportunity for personal transformation and growth" (2006, p. 224).

Art therapy also promotes positive coping by facilitating emotional regulation. Artmaking allows us to vent difficult feelings—*express the stress* as we call it—which in and of itself is satisfying. The art work serves as a container, a place where we can not only channel strong feelings but we can also begin to work through them. Artmaking facilitates emotional arousal in a safe and acceptable way. It reconciles two conflicting demands, the need for emotional release and the need to impose order (Ulman, 1986). At the same time, the art supplies and the art process facilitate the release of neurotransmitters that induce sensory grounding and the relaxation response: "Expressivity and creativity charge the reward circuitry and help maintain a dynamic balance between excitation and tranquility. Such balancing facilitates affect regulation and increases the cognitive capacity to tolerate emotional frustration and to experience joy, satisfaction, and relational security" (Hass-Cohen, 2016).

This is particularly relevant when clients experience *emotional dysregulation*—exaggerated and reactive emotional responses—common for people who struggle with impulse control, addiction, compulsive disorders, borderline personality disorder, anxiety, and bipolar disorder. Because of its capacity to promote emotion regulation, art therapy has been successfully coupled with Dialectical Behavioral Therapy (Heckwolf, Bergland, & Mouratidis, 2014; Huckvale & Learmonth, 2009). It allows people to simultaneously experience and *manage* strong or conflicting feelings; a way to cope with and tolerate emotional distress as well as gain some control over how they are feeling. And then, because the art work provides an object which is literally separate from but generated by the self, it allows for distance and reflection.

An image (Figure 11.3) by Grace, the therapist whose series appeared in Chapter 10, graphically depicts this. She felt overwhelmed by the sense that people easily violated her boundaries—commenting on her appearance and touching her inappropriately—leaving her feeling vulnerable and exposed. When she tried to address it with others, they minimized her reactions, causing her to doubt herself. When she depicted how this made her feel, intensively filling a figure with looping red marks from which arrows shot out, she observed that although it had originated from anger, it actually looked like a stylish spiral "gown." It was not chaotic but instead had beauty and poise. She concluded that expressing her anger and setting boundaries could be powerful, controlled, and even "elegant."

Attending to the Good

Artmaking also allows us to attend to the good, to actively challenge the negativity bias and focus more on what is functional and working in our lives. The interventions that we have explored throughout the book naturally highlight positive aspects of our lives—e.g., visual gratitude journaling, what keeps you strong when times are hard, identifying and developing our strengths and those of others, savoring or visualizing positive emotions, mindful attention to the art and the art process, etc.

These activities spontaneously elicit positive self-image, pleasant memories and experiences, strengths and resilience, what matters to us most, and what gives our lives meaning and purpose. They organically disrupt the negativity bias and bring the positive elements in our lives from the background to the

184 Meaning-making and Perception

foreground. Perception is transformed so that it includes not only the negative and the positive, but all of the in-between. It's not that negative elements
disappear—it's that we see them differently.

Something that might have been perceived as negative or painful, when represented in artwork may seem less disturbing or even visually compelling and/
or aesthetically appealing. When we explore the visual elements that create that
effect, the metaphorical implications are often immediately evident. Rigid and
polarized dichotomies between "good" and "bad" naturally soften to include
more nuanced perception of what is represented in the imagery.

We can also consciously attend to the good. For example, as we have mentioned, we frequently use the "three good things that happened today" exercise
as a warm-up and to shift focus to "the good." We can look at what is going
well in our lives in general, what is going well for others around us, and what
is going well in the world.

A Cherokee fable has an elder telling his grandson that inside of us there
is a battle between two wolves.

One wolf is negativity and one wolf positivity.

"Which wolf wins?" asks the grandson.

The grandfather replies, "The one you feed."

Changing Narratives Through Art Therapy

We can also find positive meaning through "writing our story." Researchers
have discovered that journaling about traumatic experiences can help people put their experiences into a cohesive narrative and find meaning in what
has happened in their lives (Oatley & Djikic, 2008; Park & Blumberg, 2002;
Pennebaker, 1993). Furthermore, writing about trauma appears to help people
generate causal links and foster new understandings and insights, essentially to
move from a negative to a positive understanding of their situation (Tomasulo
& Pawelski, 2012). By telling their story, it allows them to create a *new* narrative
that is more hopeful and life-affirming.

In art therapy, art gives our clients the opportunity to illustrate, paint, or
sculpt their story as they see it and have that witnessed and validated by the
therapist. This is particularly relevant when trauma or loss is dominating their
lives. We don't want to whitewash their struggles in any way. However, as people connect with their creativity, strengths, and humanity, often more positive
and empowering storylines emerge. As they contemplate these alternative
narratives, we can help them be "detectives" searching for "more satisfactory
meanings in the script" (Riley, as cited in Rubin, 2016, p. 4). Again, art does

this naturally. It tells a different story, one that is more personally affirming and empowering.

Art provides opportunities to "reinterpret perceptions that were regarded as immutable" (Riley, as cited in Rubin, 2016, p. 284) and form more coherent and enabling narratives (Hass-Cohen & Carr, 2008). We can also *actively reframe the narrative*—discovering evidence in the artwork of ways that adversity may have made us stronger, more appreciative, more bonded with others, more resolute, etc.—i.e., finding the "silver lining" in the difficulties we have faced.

Dialoguing and Role Reversing with Imagery

We can also dialogue with different elements in art imagery (McNiff, 1992). Doing so can loosen and expand rigid perceptions of elements that they have identified as "negative"—e.g., dysfunctional behaviors or relationships, stressors, trauma, addiction, etc. We might have different parts of an image describe themselves, e.g., Rebecca's path might say "I am a long spiral line made of midnight blue and gold." We might ask what these qualities say about the symbols they depict—"I am dark and intense, but unbroken and winding upward." We might have some parts dialogue with others and see what they have to tell each other—Rebecca's path might say to her sun "Yes, I am blue but I have a thread of hope that ends with you, it lights you up."

We can do this with what initially appears to be contrasting or conflicting elements, or with ones that are similar, or that have subtle differences. We might ask what positive meanings they might hold for each other, what they want and need, what they are trying to accomplish, what purpose they serve, and whether it is acceptable for them to remain as they are or whether something needs to change. We might ask what artistic choices would make that happen, whether they should be made, and how the image should be framed.

Clients can also "role reverse" (Dayton, 1994) with their artwork. For example, Joshua, a client of Gioia's, made a mask of a fox, Mr. Sly, to represent his addiction (Figure 11.4). Mr. Sly wrote to Joshua, "I will not listen to you. It's in my nature to be the trouble I am. Your other half, Mr. Sly". Joshua wrote Mr. Sly back saying "I only want you to show up in my life with good intentions. Any and all appearances should result in positive outcomes. I value your independent strong-willed nature, but your mischievous, sneaky behavior must end." Role reversing with Mr. Sly gave Joshua an opportunity to validate and nurture the self-determination and cleverness that characterized his "other half," but at the same time try to direct that energy more productively.

These exchanges can even lead to performances in which the role of the artist and the artwork are enacted. In a group, other members can be invited to play parts of the image/story. We recommend training in psychodrama to engage in these more complex techniques. And, as always, the clients need to be properly warmed up for role play, which may at first seem uncomfortable.

We can find positive meaning in imagery by encouraging our clients to make response art (making art about another piece of art). This can include amplifying some aspect of an image, free spill-writing, poetry, sound, or movement—the possibilities are endless (Fish 2012; Moon, 2011; McNiff, 2015). Combining the metaphors that emerge in these techniques with visual analysis of the artwork and verbal associations provides opportunities to spotlight the strengths and positive meanings they illustrate. This honors the image and the artist, while also opening the doorway to more positive versions in the story.

These strategies disrupt the negativity bias and open the possibility for more constructive stories to unfold. They work to overcome the general tendency to focus on what's not working and to overlook what is. This can be particularly useful with people who are suffering—with pain, chronic negative affect, loss, or trauma. It helps them to expand the story, which in conscious memory is often incomplete, fragmented, "stuck," or difficult to verbally articulate—so that it includes more detail and breadth. It allows the artist to literally *fill in the picture*, to "finish the story" (Gantt & Greenstone, 2016, p. 359). Negative experiences and feelings are placed in the context of the rest of their lives and then reframed into a more empowering narrative—"a strengths-based view of self" that moves from a victim of misfortune to a "survivor and a thriver" (Steele, Malchiodi, & Kuban, 2008, p. 23).

Cultivating Optimism through Art Therapy

The strategies we use to expand awareness, shift perception, attend to the good, and change the narrative not only show our lives in a more positive light, they also destabilize rigid negative beliefs, particularly those around self-image and our ability to affect change in the world. Because they reframe weaknesses and highlight strengths, they challenge the negative self-talk and helplessness that characterizes pessimistic styles of thinking, and plant seeds of optimism, hope, and self-efficacy.

In addition, because humans generally tend to underestimate their ability to cope—*affective forecasting* as we referred to earlier—these interventions help identify resources and ways to manage challenges. By illustrating who we are and what matters to us most, they also reveal what we are hoping for and how to achieve those aspirations in ways that are congruent with our highest selves.

Art therapy assessments can provide more information about resources, goals, explanatory styles, pathways, and agency. For example, Darewych's (2013) "Bridge Drawing with Path" highlights what clients aspire to and how they imagine they will get there. In addition, because *any* artwork invariably reflects something about the artists' worldviews and beliefs, whether related to a specific art therapy assessment or organically in the art therapy process, it provides clues about what the artists value and what they are trying to accomplish. It shows us their internal landscape and the inhabitants therein.

From there we can determine where to devote our resources which, as we will explore in greater detail in the next chapter on Accomplishment, then becomes the "treatment plan." It outlines the roadmap with the ends toward which we are striving and the means we have to get there.

Art Therapy Transforms Perceptions

As Rebecca's drawing of a path to the sun eloquently shows, art can be a fascinating way to shift our perceptions. Regardless of what we are trying to represent and our level of artistic skill, interesting "accidents" happen—visual effects of which we are not aware. Even Rebecca, a seasoned artist and art therapist, is not immune to this magic.

When others pointed out to her that her spiral path might be a fuse, Rebecca's initial reaction—being that she is naturally anxious and "stressed out"—was to question whether or not she was "ready to explode"! But then she put on her "positive art therapy cap" and considered other meanings. First, she checked in with herself about feeling "explosive." She noted that she didn't really feel that distraught, but she flagged that as something to revisit if it showed up again in her artwork. When she really looked at the image, she noticed that it reflected dynamic energy and upward movement. There was also a richness and depth to the colors which underscored a sense that it might be more about generativity than destruction. Perhaps instead of an explosion, it was a firecracker!

This just scratches the surface of insights Rebecca's image might contain. She could further uncover meaning by using strategies we listed above—analyzing the visual content, reflecting on the process of making it, comparing that to her intentions, dialoguing further with the imagery, writing letters to/from her image, embodying the image through movement, and so forth.

These techniques naturally deepen and expand the meaning-making process. They are certainly helpful for someone like Rebecca, who, like so many of our clients, was struggling with both internal and external challenges. It revealed more hopeful and galvanizing possibilities. These meaning-making strategies can be just as powerful for someone like Gioia, who was at a good place in her life, but who might also enjoy contemplating the layers of meaning her imagery might hold.

For example, although Gioia was feeling inspired and her artwork reflected that, there were many visual elements that lent themselves to deeper exploration—e.g., the page with the woman's face is brighter than the other side; the face is more dimensional whereas the owl on the tree limb is a silhouette, etc. We could also explore the words that she included; is the figure in the image asking for inspiration, or is Gioia asking to be inspired by her? Or perhaps, because the letters are also stenciled like the owl, the figure is dialoguing with that animal spirit. The dreamy nature of the image also seems to literally "inspire" a story—like a fairytale begging to be told.

In this chapter, we've reviewed how art is a way that we not only find but we also *make* meaning. Making artwork helps us get to know ourselves better—both through our own and the eyes of others. It does this through multiple channels. It engages our senses; it provides us with gateways to parts of the brain and consciousness otherwise not accessible; it facilitates externalization/expression of thoughts and feelings; it evokes positive emotions and it contains and transforms negative emotions; it enables symbolic communication; it is inherently social in nature; it promotes feelings of empathy and connection; it offers opportunities to visualize strengths and attend to the good; it helps identify assumptions and beliefs; it shifts narratives; it challenges negative and pessimistic modes of thinking, and it fosters benefit-finding and posttraumatic growth.

We are excited about sharing these strengths with the world of positive psychology. In turn, we suggest that we, as art therapists, can help our clients mine not just for insight, but also for *positive meaning* in the art therapy process. We propose that one of the greatest tools for doing so lies in mindful observation of the formal elements and the process whereby the art was made. This metaphorical content serves as the terrain which we navigate, in tandem, with our clients. We combine the other elements of PERMA and the positive art therapy approach to steer that process towards finding the most enabling and empowering narratives.

Regardless of whether we or our clients have experienced trauma or loss, whether we are stressed out or feeling stuck, or even if we are content and just want to keep growing, this can help us experience more happiness and wellbeing. It shifts our perceptions so that we are more appreciative of ourselves and others, we are more optimistic and hopeful, we are more aware of our capacity to cope, we are more willing to take on risk, we bounce back quicker from adversity, and we notice what's working in our lives and in the world around us. It gives us a chance to rewrite our stories and shows us not only the silver lining in the clouds—but also the sun behind them, the garden below, the creatures that live there, and maybe even a pot of gold at the end of the rainbow!

Discussion Questions

1   How have your heritage and cultural background, gender, sexual orientation, class, and physical attributes influenced your worldviews?
2   Are you more of a pessimist or an optimist? Your clients?
3   Do you experience a shift in your perceptions when others give you feedback about what they notice in your artwork?
4   How do your clients respond when getting input from others?

CHAPTER 12

Accomplishment

Many of the workshops we run, whether in corporate settings, substance abuse treatment, or psychiatric units, are attended by people who did not realize that they would be making artwork. We get varying responses when folks see the art supplies laid out—excitement, wariness, irritation. We use techniques such as "three good things" or strengths lists and introductions to get them warmed up to each other and the art process. We provide mandalas and stencils along with a brief demonstration of how to use the materials to help ease their anxiety about not being able to draw. Within about five minutes, everyone is completely absorbed in their artwork. After another 20–30 minutes, as attendees show signs that they are finishing up, we begin processing the artwork. They are usually surprised at how quickly time flew and how much they "got into it."

They are even more astounded when they realize that, despite their conviction that they could only make "stick figures," they completed an unexpectedly well-developed drawing. In addition, when they see similarities and differences in each other's visual imagery, they grasp that each piece bears both the unique signature of the artist and common visual themes—abstract, figurative, flowing, structured, cool, warm, etc. There is a new appreciation for the expressive capacity of art and some satisfaction that their drawing turned out much better than they had expected. Rarely do they discard it. Instead, they usually place it carefully in the folders we provide, commenting that their family, friends, or co-workers will get a kick out of seeing it.

This happens frequently in art therapy: People are often surprisingly proud of what they've made, particularly because they did not believe they had it in them. It gives them a sense of accomplishment and a little boost of pride.

The "A" in PERMA

Accomplishment, aka achievement, was added to Seligman's formula for well-being (2011) after one of his students challenged him that "people pursue success, accomplishment, winning, achievement, and mastery for their own sake" (p. 8). There might be some irony that Seligman needed to have this pointed out to him, considering that he, himself, has been ranked among the top one hundred eminent psychologists of the twentieth century (Haggbloom et al., 2002). Although his own life has been full of achievement, he didn't initially recognize its relevance to wellbeing!

Achievement is often used synonymously with accomplishment, and is defined as the completion of goals which a person highly values. Perhaps the term "achievement" represents the realization of a goal which society values and "accomplishment" the realization of goals that are more mundane. Both can be used as verbs or nouns—you can accomplish achievements and achieve accomplishments. Accomplishment is also associated with mastery. Humans have a basic need to feel a sense of competence and to be able to exert some control over their environment (Maslow, 1943; Seligman, 2011).

As it does with the other domains of PERMA, art therapy brings something unique to accomplishment. This goes back to the roots of art therapy (Hill, 1945; Kramer, 1971), to the notion that art provides opportunities for building skills, enhancing self-esteem, and promoting feelings of mastery and pride. Even people who insist that they are not artists, for whom we have to pull out all of the stops to warm them up to doing art, are amazed when, lo and behold, they've actually made a piece of art! They are even more surprised if they share their artwork in a group, when others instantly "get it"! They see that however humble their artwork might be, it has eloquently communicated who they are and what matters to them most. It may not be "fine art" but it is expressive and often even aesthetically pleasing.

When Seligman (2011) introduced accomplishment into the PERMA model, he was referring mostly to the inherent gratification we get from the sheer pleasure of accomplishing something. This suggests that we might first need to establish what someone is *trying to accomplish*. What are their goals and what are they hoping to achieve?

Accomplishment in the Therapy Process

Before considering what *our clients* might be trying to accomplish, we realized that we had to examine first what *we* were trying to accomplish. What are *our* goals and aspirations in undertaking the art therapy venture with our clients? This suggests that we step back even further to the purpose of therapy in general.

If we are operating from a positive psychology perspective, we can assume that unlike a psychology-as-usual approach which focuses more on identifying problems, treating mental illness, reducing symptoms, and decreasing pain and suffering, *our* primary purpose is promoting mental health, wellbeing, and flourishing. This might include adopting Diener's model of subjective wellbeing—increasing positive emotions, decreasing negative emotions, and experiencing greater satisfaction with the important domains in one's life. It might mean using Ryff's model of psychological wellbeing, which includes promoting autonomy, personal growth, strengths, connecting meaningfully with others, mastering the complexities of life, and knowing and accepting oneself. As we have made clear throughout the book, because it fit well with the practice of art therapy, we adopted PERMA, Seligman's model, which identifies positive emotions, engagement, relationships, meaning, and achievement as the core elements of wellbeing.

We had to step back again to consider what *positive art therapy* is trying accomplish by *combining* positive psychology with art therapy. What art therapy approaches were most instrumental in the positive art therapy model? Obviously, as Rubin (2016) suggests, the approach that guides an art therapist—art psychotherapy, art-as-therapy, gestalt, cognitive-behavioral, or what-have-you—is instrumental in shaping what they perceive is the focus of art therapy. Adopting an overarching theory would presumably include developing goals that incorporate what art therapy uniquely brings to that paradigm—e.g., accessing and externalizing parts of consciousness that we cannot articulate verbally, expressing that content in visual form, channeling overwhelming emotions, etc.

Regardless of their orientation, we can safely say that most art therapists are usually trying to help people suffer less and improve the quality of their lives. However, as we have mentioned, because of the subtle and yet pervasive dominance of the medical model and the fact that most art therapy training takes place in clinical settings (Vick, 2003), art therapy is often applied in the service of ameliorating, reducing, or managing symptoms related to a so-called "presenting problem" or a DSM diagnosis—depression, anxiety, PTSD, ADHD, etc.

We would be hypocritical if we did not admit that even as "positive" art therapists, we do the same. In fact, a significant number of our clients come to us through "clinical" channels—be it through our work in substance abuse treatment, in psychiatric settings, with people affected by cancer, or in our private practice with people struggling with anxiety and depression. Even the clients Rebecca meets with at the resort are usually referred to her because they are stuck or somehow dissatisfied with their lives—what Keyes would call *languishing* and our corporate clients are trying to address challenges such as low employee morale, burnout, or communication problems among their team members.

In addition, because we usually begin our work with some variation of "what brought you here today?" this often elicits some difficulty or concern with which the person/dyad/group is struggling. As we will talk about shortly, that is the "pain" that is motivating them to seek our help. However, even as we are determining what "the issue" is, we are wearing our *positive art therapy* hats and this is shaping what we consider to be the objectives of our work together. In other words, regardless of who our clients are, our "treatment plan" is going to be modeled on a positive art therapy approach.

Saying "*regardless* of who our clients are" might seem inconsistent with a person-centered point of view. After all, in order to be culturally relevant and empower our clients, therapy should be based upon *what our clients want and need*. However, as we explored in the previous chapter, if we presume that we are all biased in our perceptions, when we as therapists are discerning what our clients want and need, we are doing so through all sorts of conscious and unconscious filters. Therefore, rather than attempting to maintain some form of neutral stance, we emphatically acknowledge our biases.

What Is Positive Art Therapy Trying to Accomplish?

We are positive art therapists. We have a clear and unambiguous agenda. It is driven by our desire to help people live the highest quality of life given their strengths and limitations—the latter which might not only be difficult, but life-threatening—and what we believe is the best way to go about doing so. It is also undeniably influenced by the challenges (and successes!) that we have encountered with trying to increase *our own* wellbeing and happiness.

Many of these objectives are ones that most therapists would value; providing support, managing difficult feelings, developing insight, etc. And certainly those that are inherent to the art process are ones to which most art therapists ascribe, e.g., promoting expression, engagement, self-esteem, and mastery. This should really be no surprise if we consider that the practice of positive psychology and art therapy are both rooted in similar traditions—psychodynamic theory, humanism, cognitive behavioral therapy, education, even behaviorism—and therefore include activities which derive from these models. However, in contrast to other psychology and art therapy approaches, we are proposing an *unabashedly* "positive" agenda that harnesses and magnifies the healing potential of the art process to that end. Again, although it may at times seem like a subtle shift, it is significant in that it presumes that "building what is strong" may be the most effective way of "fixing what is wrong," not the other way around.

Not only do we resolutely believe this, but we share this bias with our clients from the very beginning. We specify that this is the lens through which we approach our work so that if/when they begin working with us, they grasp that other art therapists might adopt very different strategies. We also suggest that our approach might at times contradict those approaches and even what they themselves believe would be most helpful. As a result, we suggest that if we do work together, we will collaborate to determine the best path for managing their concerns and improving their overall wellbeing.

What Is the Client Trying to Accomplish?

Having acknowledged that we are approaching our work from a positive art therapy viewpoint, with our own underlying agenda, we do need to find out what our clients are hoping to get out of therapy. Even if *they* are not the ones who instigated the work—e.g., children with behavioral problems, involuntarily hospitalized psychiatric patients, people in prison or court-ordered to substance abuse treatment, those with severe developmental delays, etc.—we can explore what motivates them and how we can help. Since we now find ourselves working together, like it or not, how might we make the best use of that time?

Motivation

In order to identify what our clients' goals are, we want to ask what's motivating them to change, if anything at all. What do *they* want in their lives? *Motivation* can be defined as a willingness do something, a desire to move forward toward goals, to be, as Seligman says, *pulled by the future*. Our clients may be driven by goals that are very different than we, as positive art therapists, perceive to be the purpose of our work together. Without reconciling the two and figuring out goals that we *both* want to accomplish, the therapeutic "alliance" won't "ally"—that is, we won't have the common ground needed to move forward.

For most of us, motivations are complex. We have *intrinsic* motivation for activities which we find rewarding in their own right. They engage us, are fun, provide challenge, and are flow-inducing. We also have *extrinsic* motivation— we do things because we expect external rewards. For example, we might be motivated to go to work because we enjoy it and it gives us a sense of purpose and meaning (intrinsic), but we might also be motivated by our paycheck and the prospect of a promotion (extrinsic). Gioia's substance-abuse clients may be internally motivated to participate in art therapy because it is relaxing, but they might also be externally motivated to report to their probation officer that they are participating in treatment.

Although there is nothing inherently "bad" or "good" about either kind of motivation, internal motivation is likely to be more sustainable because it is inherently rewarding and tied to core interests, strengths, and values. External motivation may be less reliable because it depends on factors outside the person and over which they may have little control. With respect to the therapy process, it appears that people who are primarily externally motivated are less likely to complete treatment. People who are *both* internally and externally motivated are most likely to continue in treatment, and those who are *predominantly* internally motivated have been shown to have the most positive treatment outcomes (Brown, 2007). External motivation might help us for a while, but to achieve long-term goals, we need to feel that they align with who we truly are.

Goals We Care About

Working toward our goals provides focus, opportunities for learning, skill-building, a sense of purpose, and, frequently, social connections. Pursuing goals provides structure to our days, organizing our experiences and reinforcing a sense of coherence and meaning in life (Lyubomirsky, 2008). Putting effort toward these goals leads not only to everyday rewards, but also to an overall sense of accomplishment which, over time, fosters increasingly greater well-being.

Sheldon and Elliot (1999) found that goals which are *self-concordant*—personally valued and associated with growth, connection, and autonomy—promote sustained effort. Self-concordant goals link us back to purpose and meaning, identity, to who we think we are and who we want to be. This provides the perseverance and passion necessary to achieve long-term goals, what positive psychologist Angela Duckworth and colleagues have characterized as *grit* (Duckworth, Peterson, Matthews, & Kelly, 2007). Grit and resilience give us strength to overcome barriers we encounter when trying to meet our goals.

MOTIVATIONAL INTERVIEWING

So, how do we determine what goals will be self-concordant? How do we find out what intrinsically motivates our clients, what fuels their passion to succeed and activates their grit when they run into obstacles? How do we find what they are trying to accomplish in therapy—*their* goals? We ask them!

Miller and Rollnick (2002) developed a technique called Motivational Interviewing (MI), which can help us to discover what is driving our clients and what they are trying to achieve. MI is a person-centered inquiry designed to ally with clients by asking them questions which highlight their intrinsic values and goals. It is meant to promote autonomy and engender motivation for change by asking questions such as, "What makes you think you need to change?" "If you make changes, how would your life be different from what it is today?" Or, "If you were to decide to change, what would you have to do to make this happen?"

MI resists attempts to convince our clients to make changes which, in *our* opinion, would be "good for them." Instead, it opens doors for both client and therapist to embrace the natural ambivalence that arises when contemplating the pros and cons of change. We want to find out *why* they think they need to change, or if they think they need change *at all*.

We might approach this inquiry as a practice in mindful observation. Open-minded curiosity on *our* part kindles interest in *theirs*. Creating the psychological space for non-judgmental contemplation of the benefits of *not changing* can provide a springboard for mobilizing their underlying motivation *to change*. We, both therapist and client, want to simply notice what comes up when ambivalence to change arises, i.e., to *roll with resistance* (Miller & Rollnick, 2002). That means refraining from arguing, educating, debating, or "experting," none of which actually work to boost motivation. Maintaining an attitude of non-judgmental awareness and rolling with resistance supports the therapeutic alliance and keeps the ball where it should be, squarely in the clients' court. After all, *they* need to invest in their own success in order to sustain the perseverance and passion—the grit—they'll need to accomplish long-term, self-concordant goals.

Motivational interviewing has been found to be effective with a broad range of populations (Rubak, Sandbæk, Lauritzen, & Christensen, 2005). Traditionally MI involves asking open-ended questions, however art therapist Horay (2006) recommends that we incorporate non-verbal interviewing to help our clients explore their goals and motivations. This might include encouraging them to illustrate their ideas about how change happens (Duncan & Miller, 2000). What do they believe? What is their worldview? Is change something that derives from their own perseverance or divine intervention? All of these questions can be asked and answered through art.

For example, Gioia suggested creating "a machine which makes change" to young male clients struggling with addiction. One jokester with the strength of humor quipped that he would draw an ATM machine! Another young man, Darrel, made a game board on paper for his "machine," placing small clay objects like "landmines" that blocked his way to the finish line—sobriety. He explained that they represented friends who still used drugs. When the clay figures dried, he discovered that these "obstacles" did not stick to the paper. They could easily be removed. This allowed for a clear path toward his goal—becoming drug-free! Together, Darrell and Gioia laughed at the metaphor that these barriers could both literally and figuratively be "swept away"!

When Darrell actually did so, however, because he had made the "landmines" with great detail and care, removing them left a void. They had been one of the most interesting parts of the game board! For a moment, he and Gioia reflected that altering his artwork, which initially seemed unambiguously positive, had also symbolically represented the loss of his friends. This helped Darrell identify that grieving the loss of his using buddies might temporarily take precedence over other goals such as developing new positive friendships.

APPROACH AND AVOIDANT GOALS

Darrell's "change machine" essentially illustrates *approach* goals, that is, what he wanted, his desire to get sober. Although as positive art therapists, we intentionally attune to and develop *positive* motivations, when we are setting goals we also need to include *avoidant goals*. As Bannink (2014) describes, approach and avoidant goals include not just what we want to achieve and the rewards that holds (the "carrot"), but also what we are trying to leave behind or the pain (the "stick"). When people are motivated by both the fear of failure and the hope for success, they will work harder than when they are driven by a desire for achievement alone (Wong, 2011).

As we discussed in the chapter on positive emotions (Chapter 5), we'll often start our work by paradoxically exploring "the negative"—what we are avoiding—because it provides the context for articulating the positive. For example, for someone who is experiencing anxiety, they are usually clear that they'd like to be "less agitated." Then, by exploring the anxiety more deeply, we can "flesh out" what, in contrast, they would like to experience—more serenity, more peace, being more present, etc. By articulating their avoidance goal, we discover their approach goal.

Often, people will say that their goal is to "just be happy." We respond by narrowing this down—after all, "happiness" covers a lot of territory! Not surprisingly, people want to *feel* better! They want to feel less anger, resentment, and fear and more love, joy, peace, and hope. The Subjective Wellbeing model accounts for the profound impact having a higher ratio of positive to negative emotions has on happiness. Positive emotions and interpersonal connections are huge motivators *in and of themselves.*

Art directives such as using a folded page to illustrate both avoidant and approach goals can be instructive. If people want to feel more connected and less lonely, more loved and less isolated, more "happy" and less miserable, what does this look like to them? We could create a variation of *scaling*, a technique from MI, by using visual diagrams to measure their confidence and readiness to move in one direction or the other. Other directives might include drawing "what I want in my life and what I don't" or tracing one's hands and filling them in with "what I want to hold on to and what I'd like to let go of" (Nobis, 2010). These artful possibilities literally draw out conflicting impulses, as well help to clarify goals and boost motivation.

GOALS AND STRENGTHS

In order for goals to be motivating and sustainable, they also need to stem from strengths. Research by positive psychologists found that "given that strengths are, by definition, associated with personal values and the expression of an integrated psychological core, they are likely to suggest a self-concordant approach to goals and, therefore, to maximize the chances for greater wellbeing and goal attainment" (Linley, Nielsen, Gillett, & Biswas-Diener, 2010, p. 13). Using one's strengths helps us tap into the grit and resilience needed to achieve goals, and art therapy is an avenue for doing just that.

Because art therapy can provide such a personal glimpse of our clients' motivations it gives us the "language" from which to develop highly personalized treatment goals. Strengths that are revealed, especially those that are most engaging, become *the means to realize these goals.* In other words, the artwork illustrates not only the *what,* i.e. the "goals" of treatment, but also the *how* to make it happen, i.e., the strategies to achieve them. Artwork illustrates the destination and the means to get there.

Specific directives like the "Bridge Drawing with Path" (BDP) (Darewych, 2014) elicit meaningful goals and future-orientation. The path illustrates how we conceive of the journey as well as barriers/obstacles/impasses (or lack thereof) we might encounter on the way. Strengths and resources that have helped us thus far and will sustain us on the rest of the journey often appear in the imagery.

Whether or not the specific focus of the artwork is to delineate goals and determine strategies to meet them, artwork reveals these naturally. Generally speaking, what is most rewarding, meaningful, hopeful, will look different— brighter, closer, larger, more detailed, made with more care and deliberation, emphasized, etc. In addition, because even the simplest of images are more layered and metaphorically rich than the concepts they are illustrating, and the formal elements clearly reflect the unique signature of the artist, the latter's perceptions of the content shift. Combining that with the metaphors that are revealed in the way the artwork was made also highlights particular strengths such as organizational skill, spontaneity, simplicity, industry, independence, interdependence. It reveals ways to pursue what we care about that will be most energizing and congruent.

PROBLEM-SOLVING AND DECISION-MAKING

Because this kind of review so often reveals dynamics of which the artists had not previously been aware, it can also engender a reset of goals and provide information needed to make them more self-concordant. By illustrating the core of who we are and the strengths that empower us most, the art process continuously guides us to paths that are more meaningful and congruent with our true selves. This is another one of art therapy's inherent assets; it provides opportunities to explore options and experiment with solutions.

Rebecca harnesses this dynamic at the resort in "Transforming Awareness" workshops and consults. She is referred clients who want to explore barriers to their creativity or who feel that they are somehow "stuck" at a crossroads in their jobs, relationships, or their lives in general. In essence, they are trying to answer questions like "Should I stay or should I go?" or "Now or later?"

She usually begins with prompts such as: use symbols to represent "what keeps you strong?"; "what would it look like if this situation were the best it could be?" or, "if you had more work–life balance?"; or, with couples, "you were on the same page and your relationship was more gratifying?" Even in these brief encounters, she always introduces the notion that useful information can be gleaned from the congruencies and discrepancies that emerge when reflecting on the artwork, the process of making it, and their associations to it.

For example, Jason, who was from Oregon but was contemplating taking a job in New Jersey, drew a map showing the things he wanted in his life. Upon reflection, he was struck that his map was "all Oregon." He had not even included NJ! In addition, it wasn't just that Oregon was so large, but it was more colorful, richly detailed, and full of the things that he loved. It literally "dominated the map." He realized that, although he had thought he was resolved about moving east, both his artwork and verbal associations revealed something else altogether and he decided not to take the job in New Jersey.

In another session, a mother who had been ill was conflicted about resuming work. She thought that because her kids were now in preschool and she seemed to be recovering, she should be more productive. When she filled her mandala, including symbols for her children, exercise, and nutrition, her work was outside of the circle's boundary. She concluded that, although working was there, it wasn't part of the "inner circle." Based on her image, she determined that, for now, she needed to focus on her kids and her health.

Czamanski-Cohen and colleagues (2012, 2014), in their research with cancer patients who were experiencing *decisional conflict*—anxiety, ambivalence, and doubt that arises over choices that might lead to undesirable or even fatal outcomes—also observed that art therapy facilitated decision-making. It helped them externalize, get some distance from, and sort through chaotic thoughts and feelings provoked by having to make potentially terminal treatment choices. Their imagery gave them confidence and certainty about how to proceed. In addition, it helped them identify coping strategies to deal with the symptoms of their illness. Czamanski-Cohen also discovered that it helped patients manage ambivalence and uncertainty about *past* decisions that they had doubted or regretted.

When our clients are feeling overwhelmed, we can have them do artwork about ways they are coping. It reveals their resilience and gives them more of a sense of control. They can also explore *past successes*—ways they have managed in the past—to find additional tools for dealing with current stressors.

TRANSFORMING AWARENESS: IS THERE REALLY A PROBLEM?

As we stated above, even as positive art therapists, we usually begin treatment with "the problem." Because of the dominance of the negativity bias, whether or not we are more optimistic or have higher ratios of positivity, we often unconsciously perceive our challenges through a negative lens. By providing a means to more fully express the thoughts and feelings associated with those difficulties, art therapy can often paradoxically provide some distance and relief from "the problem." In fact, when we engage visual analysis of the formal elements, and we compare and contrast that to the metaphors in the art process and verbal associations, often what was initially perceived as a problem is transformed. As we explored in the previous chapter, the art therapy process induces a *positive reappraisal*.

For example, Martha had been divorced from her husband for a couple of years but they had an amicable relationship and were still very united in raising their son. Her ex was pressuring her to remarry him, as were her family members. Given that she had not met anyone else, a part of her agreed. She was conflicted about what to do and felt guilty that she was not embracing him more wholeheartedly. However, when she drew symbols for what her life would look like if it were more satisfying, she did not include an image for her ex. At first, she thought it might have been an oversight, but when Rebecca asked her if she wanted to add him, Martha said, "there isn't room." It did not take much for her to grasp the metaphor that was revealed by his absence from the picture and her decision not to add him. It empowered her to pursue a relationship that would be more fulfilling, despite pressure from others.

The opposite might also occur. For example, many times clients say they are ending a relationship either because of misunderstandings, incompatibilities, buried anger, or resentments. However, in their artwork, they include symbols for those significant others, perhaps even close to or at the center of their image. They might also be drawn in the same colors as others elements, such as pets or loved ones, that have positive associations. The client realizes that, despite their hurt or anger, the other person is an important part of their lives.

The art therapy process gives us unexpected and clear answers to complex questions. It reveals the way to proceed in situations about which we are ambivalent and conflicted. It provides a different perception of what the conscious mind perceives to be "the problem." We connect with parts of ourselves that may even have "resolved" the problem. And, although the challenge may not completely disappear, it is experienced differently. Positive aspects are perceived such that the situation may not only seem less daunting, but it may also feel manageable or even hopeful.

Moving into Action

As we have suggested above, the art therapy process clarifies goals as well as providing us with the pathways and resources to go about making them happen. It also gives us strategies for moving into action. Recall from the chapters on creativity and flow (Chapters 6 and 7) that we need to warm up to taking action—the art therapy process also reveals the way our clients are most likely to make that shift.

For example, a woman who was feeling isolated made a mandala with symbols for what would be in her life if she felt more connected. She drew a symbol of her husband in the center as a bright yellow sun whose rays were extending beyond the mandala's circumference to the edge of the page. She had drawn him this way because he "lightens my spirits when I'm down." She mused that the way the sun's rays extended beyond the circle reflected his ability to help her "get out of herself."

She noticed that she had drawn a couple of small white circles near the part of the rays that were at the edge of the paper. At first, she didn't know what they represented, but then she chuckled and thought that maybe they symbolized his love of baseball. She remembered that he played on a summer league with co-workers. He had often invited her to join but she had always turned him down. She decided that she would start to go when the season began so that she could meet some of his colleagues and their mates. At the end of the session, she not only felt less isolated, but she felt like she had a clear strategy to "get out more." It also became clear to her that her husband was not only a source of support for her, but that his energy and warmth provided a safe and congruent path to "extend" herself out into the world. Her artwork even gave her the exact route through which to do so—his love of baseball!

Changing the imagery in artwork becomes a metaphor for taking action and making changes in life. If something is awry or disorganized, we can alter it to make it more congruent and organized. If something is missing, we can add it. Modifying the image "metaphorically suggests new resolutions to old scripts" (Riley, 1999, p. 285).

The art imagery and the creative process provides a virtual realm within which we can enact a range of alternative possibilities—we can imagine various outcomes, project ourselves into those scenarios, and experiment with different conclusions. We can discern from our options, reflect upon the consequence of these possibilities, and determine which one(s) might serve us and others best.

Art Illustrates Accomplishment and the Process of Getting There

As these examples illustrate, artwork provides us with a great deal of infor-mation. It not only illustrates accomplishments of which we are aware, but it reveals previously unnoticed progress. Even if improvement and change is not seen, the art can indicate that a therapeutic process has happened and time was invested. Art therapist Shirley Riley (1999) stated, "art therapy makes the evolution of the therapeutic process a visible event shared and respected by the creators and the therapist-observer" (p. 284). Artmaking can be used to review the course of therapy, identify changes, determine if any goals have been met, and illustrate what has been accomplished.

As Seligman's student rightly identified, accomplishment is rewarding in and of itself. This includes not only the product of our efforts, but also *the process* of trying to accomplish something—i.e., the reward is often just in "the doing." Art therapy, because it involves making art, is a "doing" therapy. As a result, it brings something completely unique to the "A" in PERMA. It involves both the process of creation and formation of a tangible object, something that has its own autonomous presence in the world. Art therapy is not only *rooted* in accomplishment, we could even say art therapy *is* accom-plishment therapy.

Ironically, art therapy is often trivialized as an "activity" therapy; however, that may be one of its greatest assets. For example, one of the most eminent positive psychologists, Ed Diener, noted that many of the more effective well-being interventions mix "positive thinking with activity theories" (Diener & Ryan, 2009, p. 400). He referred to Csíkszentmihályi's (1991) theory of flow, stressing the importance of *paratelic* endeavors—activities whereby the process is as rewarding as meeting the objective it serves. This includes activities that inspire interest, spontaneity, curiosity, play, exploration, engagement in the-here-and-now, and flow. Positive psychologist Frisch (2006), in his Quality of Life Therapy, strongly advocates for activities which promote "the type of crea-tivity aimed at *losing the self* in flow experiences" (p. 282; original emphasis).

Art therapy naturally meets these criteria. It is an inherently rewarding activity that galvanizes all of the above—play, curiosity, exploration, etc. In addition, as we explored in the chapters on creativity and flow, even people who are initially resistant to engaging in art, once they are properly warmed up, frequently enter into flow. This is the "process" part of art therapy, the fact that just doing artwork is not only healing, but it is also enjoyable and engaging.

It is often implicitly understood that the "art" made in art therapy is more for self-expression and less for aesthetic purposes. Art therapists underscore this by reiterating that it is not a classroom, and no one will be graded. They don't even have to show their artwork if they don't want to. This also encourages adopting a *growth mindset*. Recall from the chapter on creativity that this includes the willingness to take risks and make mistakes. It is interesting to note that Frisch (2006) recognized this, stressing that creative endeavors are not only fun but they reduce "perfectionism" and "self-criticism" (p. 282). He even suggests that therapists participate in the activity in order to model successfully overcoming the risk of failure.

Art therapists are particularly well equipped to simultaneously inspire and mitigate the risk of engaging in creative endeavors. They have the expertise to match their clients with activities that maximize the skill/challenge balance. In addition, they have the technical knowledge to provide support when their clients encounter difficulties. This helps ensure that their clients achieve some degree of success—that they are able to create something that helps express what they were trying to communicate.

Kramer identified this as sublimation—suggesting that making art allows for a "synthesis of emotional freedom and structured expression" (1975, p. 33). Kramer suggested that artmaking empowered people to discharge feelings but also to bring order to their experience:

> It is a process wherein drive energy is deflected from its original goal and displaced onto achievement, which is highly valued by the ego, and is, in most instances, socially productive ... An essential feature of sublimation is the great amount of genuine pleasure the substitute activity affords. (1971, pp. 68–9)

Kramer found that art therapy, because it encouraged autonomy, self-control, and goal attainment, was particularly useful with children who struggle with impulse control or who could not express themselves verbally. As Wadeson (1980/2010) wrote, "The pleasure they may derive from expressing themselves in visual form can be not only satisfying in and of itself but it can also enhance a sense of mastery and self-esteem" (p. 14). Making something, however simple, provides opportunities to master challenges and induce corresponding feelings of competence, optimism, and pride. Landgarten (1981) described the art in art therapy as evidence of an assertive self-directed act, inherently empowering. As artists living with cancer taught us, sometimes art simply marks our presence in the world, providing evidence that we are still alive: "I make, therefore I am."

Pride

Pride is a positive emotion we experience when we've accomplished something in which we believe that we had a pivotal role (Tracy, Weidman, Cheng, & Martens, 2014). We feel that our hard work has paid off. We get a boost of energy and confidence. Nucho (2003) explored ways that art can be used to highlight accomplishments. For example, with adults, adolescents, and even with children, artwork can illustrate moments in which they felt very proud of themselves. It can also depict challenges they encountered and how they overcame them, bolstering pride in their resilience and capacity to survive.

In addition, artmaking itself, because if it is both a tangible accomplishment and a living testimony to *our efforts*, evokes experiences of *authentic* pride ("I *did* great!"). In contrast to its darker side, *hubris*, authentic pride boosts self-esteem in a positive way. Hubris—boastfulness or arrogance that signals an underlying narcissism and low self-esteem—is more likely associated with a fixed mindset ("I *am* great!"). While both kinds of pride indicate triumph about success, authentic pride facilitates feelings of social empowerment and genuine self-confidence (Tracy et al., 2014). It strengthens a sense of identity and positive self-appraisal.

Pride is physiologically activating (Kreibig, 2014). In cultures around the world, when we feel proud, we jump up, expand our chest, and raise our arms and fists high above our heads, exclaiming to everyone that we won! Woohoo! In artmaking, although that sense of achievement may not be quite as dramatic as crossing the finish line or hitting a home run, the resulting feeling of accomplishment is no less rewarding. As Hass-Cohen and Carr (2008) identified, sensory pleasure and pride in the art product stimulate the secretion of oxytocin, the brain's natural reward hormone.

Pride and exuberance naturally inspire us to share our accomplishments with others. In art therapy, pride is enhanced by the therapist's acknowledgment both of the artwork and the effort that went into making it, what Rubin (2011) described as the confirming gleam in the therapist's eye. The artwork produced is understood to be an extension of the person, something that has value and deserves care and respect.

As we identified in Chapter 9 on relationships, celebrating accomplishments is key to building positive relationships. It is a critical component in strengthening the therapeutic alliance. In art therapy, the art therapist *capitalizes* on their clients' accomplishment by active constructive responding—"Wow! Look at that, can you tell me about it?" The joint pride which the client and therapist and/or group voice about the imagery helps to further expand positive feelings of validation and universality. This fuels motivation in future artmaking ventures. The art is then a visible reminder of mastery. It reflects the ability to manifest change in the world.

In art therapy, we often reassure participants that they do not need to be trained artists. The goal is to express and explore feelings and enjoy the process, not necessarily to create a highly finished product. But clients do want to make aesthetically successful artwork. We know this because they tell us so! They are invested in "the product" and want the sense of pride and achievement that making visually pleasing art can bring—art that can be valued as much for its aesthetic appeal as its expressive power (Spaniol, 1998).

This is confirmed by research that Hartz and Thick (2005) conducted with female juvenile offenders; focusing on both *process and product* in art therapy was most effective for increasing feelings of mastery and self-worth. Therefore, in order to help our clients build the skills they need to achieve something that *looks good to them*, we advise that art therapists not shy away from the role of "art teacher." We want to model artistic techniques that increase our clients' ability to successfully express themselves with art media. We can teach them how to change the pressure on pencils or oil pastels to create softer lines or bolder marks, blend chalk pastels for shading, or score clay and apply slip to create a secure bond between clay coils. These skills give them better dexterity and control over what they are trying to create and greater satisfaction in the resulting product.

For example, Bruce Moon (2012) wrote about teaching adolescents to stretch their own canvases, a process which entails time and effort. It's not an easy task—pulling the fabric over the stretchers, stapling it down evenly! But after this hard work, when his clients finally got to paint, it was more much meaningful to them than if they'd used pre-stretched canvases. We understand that such labor-intensive preparations may not be practical for all art therapy studios, but it illustrates the point. Real effort and determination heighten the sense of pride and achievement that comes when we have successfully accomplished something!

Displaying artwork has also been used to boost pride. "Art exhibits" can range from hanging client artwork inside or outside the studio, to local gallery exhibits, community-sponsored displays, or even national events that raise awareness about art therapy, such as AATA's exhibition at the US Senate in 2001 or the annual National Veterans' Creative Arts Festival. This can be heightened by involving the artists in framing or staging their piece and, if appropriate, having them attend the exhibit.

In summary, art therapy contributes to accomplishment in multiple ways. It helps us articulate not only what we are moving away from, but also what we are moving toward. It reveals what matters to us most and it show us the means to go about achieving what we want in our lives in ways that are congruent with our highest selves. In addition, because art therapy involves focused and engaged "doing," it offers the benefits that come from activities that promote creativity, play, and flow.

We also literally make something in art therapy which often induces feelings of mastery, accomplishment, and authentic pride. Having the therapist facilitate self-expression provides a sense of being acknowledged. We can heighten this experience by teaching our clients skills to hone their ability to express themselves and, when appropriate, by giving them opportunities to display their artwork to a larger audience.

Having explored Accomplishment, the last domain in PERMA, we now move to applications in training and professional development and future directions that positive art therapy might take.

Discussion Questions

1 What achievement are you most proud of? Is it also valued by others around you?
2 What values underlie your goals?
3 What motivates your clients? Are there differences between their goals and what you are trying to accomplish with them?

CHAPTER 13

Professional Applications and Future Directions

When we first entered the realm of positive psychology, we resonated most with the observation that *psychology-as-usual* appeared to focus most on pathology—on what was wrong with a person. It seemed like both a revelation and yet a confirmation of something that we had sensed throughout our careers. We noticed that *art therapy-as-usual* appeared to have a similar imbalance. Art therapy, to our newly opened eyes, seemed to have evolved around its capacity to help troubled spirits express themselves and find some relief from their suffering through the healing practice of making art, as well as its ability to reveal their struggles in a way that circumvented verbal defenses. These were certainly outstanding attributes, but they seemed to be predominantly *problem-focused*. Although there was some merit to this observation, at the same time we recognized that our critique of art therapy-as-usual, in and of itself, was "problem-focused." This irony did not escape us. The negativity bias was at play even as we were attempting to bring to the field a more positive paradigm!

With this in mind, we now try to be much more appreciative of the diverse viewpoints that shape our field. Like positive psychologists whose work derives from theoretical foundations laid down by their predecessors, most of what we know as positive art therapists grows from seeds planted by the pioneers of art therapy and our contemporary colleagues. Positive art therapy emerges through comparison and contrast to the wealth of research, theory, and anecdotal wisdom they have contributed.

We employed PERMA, Seligman's model of wellbeing, as the framework to merge the principles of positive psychology with the field of art therapy because it seemed to fit most logically with *the way it had unfolded for us*. However, as we have hopefully conveyed, there are different models that might be used—psychological wellbeing, subjective wellbeing, flourishing, etc. In addition, although we have divided the content into domains and subtopics of PERMA, they are all so intricately interwoven and interdependent that separating them creates artificial division which, *in vivo*, instantly dissolve.

Exploring the intersection between positive psychology and art therapy over the last 10+ years has had profound impact on our professional practice. Perhaps, even more importantly, it has completely transformed our lives. As a result of this work, Rebecca, who is naturally depressive, pessimistic, anxious, and low-energy, is much more hopeful, resilient, hearty, and serene. And Gioia, who is naturally buoyant, optimistic, and energetic, is even more engaged than before. In addition, our relationships have greatly improved and we are much more appreciative of the strengths that others bring to our lives.

On top of the many personal gifts we've gotten from learning about positive psychology, we feel an even deeper appreciation for our own field. We have always known, as all art therapists do, that we are different than other mental health professions. Even when we have succumbed to apologetic defensiveness for doing something that isn't traditional therapy, we've always felt proud of art therapy's capacity to facilitate expression, meaningfully engage our clients, and reveal something new and different. After diving into positive psychology—discovering strategies that improve wellbeing and happiness despite hardship and trauma—we were beside ourselves with excitement at what art therapy could bring to those efforts. And now, having written this book, we might go even further to say that we think art therapy may be *one of the best ways* to implement a positive psychology paradigm.

This has inspired us to train other art therapists, students, and mental health practitioners so they, too, could apply these techniques to their work. It also sparked a passion to bring these practices to a broader audience—other health providers, educators, corporate teams, guests at resorts, the general public—really *anyone* who is hoping to improve the quality of their lives.

Workshops and Trainings

We provide here a brief review of how we facilitate trainings with "non-client" populations. This includes "frontline" providers—people who work in high-intensity environments as servants to the public, i.e., hospital personnel, police officers, schoolteachers, or government employees. We also do corporate trainings in organizational settings—in technology, the fashion industry, public relations, hospitality, and management—an area of art therapy practice that has yet to be fully tapped but that holds a great deal of promise. The few art therapists who have ventured down this path suggest that it can be particularly useful because it provides unique ways to explore staff dynamics and facilitate creative problem-solving (Babyak, 2015; Ault, 1986; Huet, 2011; Huss & Sarid, 2014; Italia, Favara-Scacco, Di Cataldo, & Russo, 2008; Salzano, Lindemann, & Trostky, 2013; Turner & Clark-Schock, 1990; Winkel & Junge, 2012).

As many of these authors caution, professional boundaries need to be maintained in organizational trainings, particularly because they often include not only peers but also the supervisors who will be evaluating them. We orchestrate discussions so that sharing is genuine and personal and yet less revealing and emotional than it might be in a therapy group. Even when it is structured this way, it is often quite authentic and meaningful. Winkel and Junge (2012) maintain that art therapists, because of their training in group therapy skills, are well equipped to contain the depth of sharing so that it ensures the psychological safety necessary for professional settings.

We start most of our workshops with introductions and the "three good things" warm-up. We then provide psycho-education on whichever element of PERMA the workshop addresses. It might be promoting positivity—shifting cognitive and emotional dynamics in ourselves, our relationships and/or the workplace so that we are experiencing less conflict and more wellbeing in our lives. It might speak more generally to managing stress, e.g., coping with challenges, developing resilience, increasing positivity and optimism, etc.

In all of these groups, we always focus on the aspirations they are working toward, strengths and values they share, and aspects of their work that reflect those qualities. Seeing these illustrated through art imagery gives them an appreciation for their individual contributions and the culture they have collectively created. They access a sense of being relevant, useful, and supported. It helps them feel better not only about their work, but that of their co-workers and the organizations that employ them. This provides context for what they are doing in the bigger picture of their lives, even if they may not stay in their job or in that particular field.

Team Building

When we are running longer workshops in healthcare and corporate settings, we have the luxury of doing group activities such as the "Island Exercise," a classic directive with murky origins. Before the workshop, we draw kidney-shaped "islands" on large butcher paper. Based on the purpose of the group, we divide the audience into teams of 4–6 people and tell them they have found themselves together on an island that they can equip with anything that they might want or need. We playfully add that they have been given a magical set of drawing materials that can materialize anything that they can imagine!

We suggest that everyone participate in the drawing process, even those who insist they are not artists and that they'll just sit and watch, or supervisors who maintain they are there to observe. We explain that doing artwork activates parts of the mind that can be useful in problem-solving and creative thinking. If they are anxious about their drawing skills, we recommend a simple task like coloring in or around the island.

When the islands are complete, the teams name them and, if possible, display them. We then provide colored paper, scissors, tape, and glue and tell them that they can create pathways to other islands or construct the means for other teams to visit them. The teams then share what they notice about their island compared to the other teams. There is usually lighthearted joking as they playfully boast about or apologize for their resolution to the task. We explore metaphors and insights that are revealed in their islands and the process of making them. In particular, we ask how their personal strengths and values support the larger mission of the group, and how they worked together using those strengths.

We close with sharing our own observations about the unique qualities we noticed among the individuals, the teams, and the group as a whole. We also list specific strategies they can use that build on what they discovered in the workshop to enhance communication, support, and efficacy in the team. At the end of the session, we provide the point of contact with additional observations about their teams' dynamics.

PERMA in Workshops

The workshops and trainings that we run, regardless of who they are with and what particular focus they are highlighting, generally address multiple aspects of PERMA. They generate *positive emotions* through artmaking, laughter, playfulness, enjoyment, and sense of connection with others. They promote *engagement* through creativity, strengths, and flow. They fortify *relationships* through team-building, collaborative problem-solving, and appreciative exchanges. They provide a sense of *accomplishment* by producing a tangible record of their unexpected success as artists and through the successful completion of a collaborative venture.

By providing a glimpse of themselves and their peers through visual imagery and group dynamics, the art process also shifts *meaning and perception* as well as boosting insight. It illustrates personal strengths and values and demonstrates how many of these resonate with others in the workshop, their profession, and/or the organizations that brought them together. This aligns their personal and professional sense of *meaning and purpose.*

At the end of all of our trainings, we distribute anonymous evaluations which ask attendees when they were most/least engaged, an important takeaway, something that was new and different, and what was most surprising. Usually, they are *least* engaged during the psycho-educational portion; however, they always report that the information was nevertheless very useful. Invariably, they are *most* engaged during the artmaking and processing of the artwork. They usually comment that they hadn't realized how important wellbeing was in their lives. They are most surprised that they were not only able to do artwork, but that they actually enjoyed it and learned something from it.

When we are working in organizational settings and running workshops, we are always linking art therapy with positivity in the minds of the people with whom we interact. We do this in order to increase the likelihood they will advocate for art therapy in the future—for themselves, their loved ones, the people with whom they work, and the institutions with whom they are affiliated.

Professional Development

When we train art therapists and clinicians in positive art therapy, we employ similar strategies as those we listed above. However, we also explore topics that are particularly relevant to the mental health professions, e.g., compassion satisfaction, self-care, and positive ethics. Below we will describe some of the continuing education trainings that we run and then we will discuss how we apply positive art therapy to supervision and consultation.

Training and Continuing Education

Transforming Burnout and Compassion Fatigue into Compassion Satisfaction

Compassion satisfaction refers to the gratification we experience when we enjoy our work, we find it engaging, we feel that we are able to successfully help our patients, and we are supported by our peers and supervisors (Stamm, 2002). Compassion satisfaction also emerges when we are connected to the values that bring us to our profession and we see our work as a calling. It's what keeps us committed to our work, even when it is difficult and stressful.

Psychology-as-usual has focused more on *burnout* and *compassion fatigue*— understandable when one considers their prevalence among healthcare and human service providers. Burnout results from excessive and prolonged stress on the job. It is described as a gradual "loss of enthusiasm, excitement, and a sense of mission in one's work" (Cherniss, 1980, p. 16). It is characterized by emotional exhaustion, depersonalization, perceived unfairness, lack of control, and high turnover (Maslach, 1982).

Compassion fatigue is a condition in which healthcare workers experience vicarious trauma as a result of caring for people who have witnessed or experienced trauma (Stamm, 1997). Unlike burnout, which is usually progressive, compassion fatigue can occur after just one incident of secondary exposure to trauma; however, it most frequently develops as a result of chronic encounters with situations which leave healthcare workers feeling helpless and overwhelmed (Niemiec, 2013). Compassion fatigue produces symptoms similar to PTSD—anxiety, disconnection, depersonalization, somatization, and depression.

When we run workshops with healthcare professionals, we often measure their level of burnout, compassion fatigue, and compassion satisfaction using the "Professional Quality of Life" tool (Stamm, 2010). We invite them to talk about challenges people in their profession encounter. For example, in inpatient hospitals, it's usually aggressive patients, poorly trained support staff, long hours, burdensome paperwork, and institutional politics. Giving them a chance to "express the stress" is a great entrée to query, "With all of these stressors, what sustains you and brings you back to this work?" There is a palpable shift in energy as they begin to report things such as seeing their patients improve, solving complex problems, support from co-workers, etc.

We provide attendees with strengths cards (Booth, 2007) or a list of strengths, such as the ones we offer in Appendix C. We have them pick a strength they identify with and one they admire in a colleague and then discuss those in dyads. We might do the same with a list of values and ask them which ones they personally identify with and which represent their profession.

At any point in this process, we offer an art directive—related to strengths, values, or the support they feel in their team. Invariably, when they reflect on their imagery, they are struck by common strengths that emerges—humor, resilience, kindness, patience, flexibility, compassion, and advocating for their patients. They are energized by reconnecting to their passion to make a difference in people's lives. When they are given opportunities to reflect on their values and what drew them to mental health, many of them realize that despite the arduous nature of their work, they have a deep sense of purpose and an enduring belief that their lives are mission-driven.

Self-care

Although self-care—finding ways to balance and nurture our personal and professional needs—can apply to any demographic, it is particularly relevant to healthcare providers. It is positively correlated with increasing compassion satisfaction and reducing burnout and compassion fatigue (Alkema, Linton, & Davies, 2008). Determining whether a person is experiencing either or both of the latter is important because they may require different interventions. We provide a handout (adapted from the ACA's Self-Care Assessment, 2002) which outlines five domains of self-care—physical, emotional, psychological, professional, and spiritual—and provides activities designed to address each.

We suggest that they put a symbol for themselves in the middle of a mandala and add symbols which represent the things that are most important to their self-care. During the processing, we use the artwork to highlight what it reveals about their needs and priorities, ways they are taking care of themselves, and areas upon which they might need to address in order to make their work more gratifying and sustainable.

Positive Ethics

Handelsman, Knapp, and Gottlieb (2009) coined the term *Positive Ethics* after identifying that ethics trainings generally operate from a risk-management paradigm in which practitioners are deterred from ethical violations out of fear of reprisal. Handelsman and colleagues suggest that rather than being preoccupied with avoiding ethical *dilemmas*, we can proactively explore the ethical *dimensions* inherent to our work—e.g., ethical nuances, grey areas, and competing ethical demands. This is particularly important because Ethics Boards, when investigating ethical violations, consider whether a clinician used supervision to address the ethical complexities of the case under review.

Gottlieb, Handelsman, and Knapp (2008) recommend that ethics trainings be more aspirational—that they explore the values that ground ethical standards and inspire people to practice in alignment with those ideals. Gottlieb and colleagues liken the transition from personal to professional values to an acculturation process—i.e., new practitioners are like immigrants coming to a new land. They must learn to identify which of their values are congruent and which conflict with those of their profession—their "new country."

Lisa Hinz (2011) was the first to introduce positive ethics to the art therapy profession. Her suggestions were added to the latest revision of AATA's Code of Ethics. AATA also added *creativity* to their list of values, a virtue that might not be relevant to other professions but is fundamental to ours: "Art therapists cultivate imagination for furthering understanding of self, others and the world. Art therapists support creative processes for decision-making and problem-solving, as well as, meaning-making and healing" (AATA, 2013).

The positive ethics workshops we run combine an exploration of strengths and values with a "Vision/Mission Map" exercise adapted from the work of Robert Biswas-Diener (personal communication, May 5, 2014) (see Appendix A, "Positive Art Therapy Directives"). These workshops help professionals connect with ethics in a new and different way. Participants often report that they had never perceived ethics as anything other than sanctions that might be imposed on them by credentialing or licensing bodies. They tell us that they are no longer as fearful of inadvertently violating ethical codes because they feel more personally connected to the values and principles from which those codes derive. They are also more motivated to seek consultation when ethical complexities arise.

Positive Art Therapy in Supervision and Consultation

When we train art therapists and students in the strategies we use to adopt a positive art therapy approach, they are usually surprised at how this challenges their view of themselves and their clients; especially if they have been immersed in institutions which emphasize the medical model—identifying problems, trauma, and pathology. This is even more so if, in their own lives their attention has focused on compensating for areas they perceive to be weaknesses, rather than building on their strengths and competencies. We invite them into the same process we engage in with our clients.

STRENGTHS AND VALUES IN RELATIONSHIPS

Not surprisingly, most art therapists we work with share *appreciation of beauty and excellence*. Ironically, they are often embarrassed by this attribute, which at first blush might seem superficial. However, when they realize that their visual intelligence and aesthetic sensibilities are *the very things* that distinguish them from other mental health professionals, they own that strength with pride.

Sometimes looking at their strengths can be uncomfortable, particularly if they score high in *modesty* and *humility*. However, as they become more proficient at strengths spotting in others, they grasp that collectively our strengths complement and enhance what we are *all* bringing to the table. This can be heightened by exercises such as doing artwork about *strengths in a client/a colleague/someone in their community* which help them see their strengths functioning in relationship to others. This applies to values as well. Identifying what is important and what motivates them, their clients, co-workers, managers, and even the institutions for whom they work helps them to collaborate more effectively.

As we mentioned in Chapter 9 on relationships, we also use *Appreciative Inquiry (AI)* to help supervisees expand on the best in what they do (Fialkov & Haddad, 2012). When they are struggling with challenges, be it with clients, colleagues, supervisors, or organizations, it can help them perceive these situations differently. AI stimulates curiosity and interest in what it would look like if things were the best they could be and builds on existing resources to make that happen.

FEELINGS AND BELIEFS ABOUT THERAPY

We use response art and replicating client artwork to explore their perceptions of and learn more about their clients (Fish, 2012; Deaver & McAuliffe, 2009). We identify how they *feel* about their clients and their work—what energizes them and gives them joy, peace, and gratitude. We also mindfully explore the negative emotions they encounter, aiming to discern what purpose they are serving and what needs they might be identifying. In supervision, as in therapy, we want to increase the ratio of positive to negative emotions, and to induce the attendant broadening of perceptions and building of physical, social, and emotional resources that help them cope more effectively and manage those challenges. This keeps the flame of hope burning, something that is vital not only for our clients but also for us if we are to persist with the kind of work that we do.

We use art to explore their beliefs about therapy in general and art therapy in particular, as well as how they see themselves in the therapy process—are they a mirror, a container, a safe place, etc.? What do they think their role is with respect to their clients—teacher, guide, witness, advocate, collaborator, fellow artist?

We have occasionally used the directive "Draw yourself as a source of light" in supervision. Art therapist Eileen M.'s "Light in a Brick Room" illustrates this beautifully (Figure 13.1). She identified that it often felt difficult to stay "lit" when she was confronted with the wall of darkness and emptiness she saw in her clients (in personal communication). However, rather than trying to tear the wall down, she wanted to help illuminate the bricks and examine how the wall was built. She determined that, although the light was not "grounded," the fact that it was shining nevertheless meant that sometimes her presence in a client's life was enough.

We sometimes have art therapists dialogue with their light source, asking it where it gets its energy and telling it how much they appreciate its glow.

THERAPIST IDENTITY

We also look at discouraging myths that pervade the healing professions and common culture about therapists/art therapists. For example, in their article, "Choosing psychotherapy as a career: Why did we cross that road?", Farber and colleagues (Farber, Manevich, Metzger, & Saypol, 2005) confront assumptions such as that therapists work with others in order to fulfill unmet needs for attention or intimacy. This includes stigmatizing beliefs that therapists are motivated "'knowingly or unknowingly, by position of authority, by the dependence of others, by the image of benevolence, by the promise of adulation, or by a hope of vicariously helping themselves through helping others'" (Maeder, in Farber et al., 2005, p. 1014).

Research confirms that, although many therapists *do* come to their careers as a way to explore and resolve their problems and that, indeed, personal history *does* play a role in their choice of careers, it is not always because the latter was dysfunctional (Farber et al., 2005). In addition, although many therapists appear to have served as mediators and confidantes in their family of origin, we suggest this may derive as much from strengths—e.g., social intelligence and diplomacy—as from vestiges of unresolved family dynamics. Becoming therapists may not be as much to fill an emotional void as to gain mastery over their lives in ways that are congruent with their strengths.

We even challenge more elevated impressions of therapists, e.g., the archetype of *Wounded Healers* who empathize with their clients because they have suffered and overcome their *own* challenges. Farber and colleagues point out that "all those wounded in childhood do not become healers; and all those who become healers have not been profoundly wounded" (2005, p. 1015). They suggest that therapists are no different from the general population—everybody has emotional problems. We would say that just as our clients are works in progress, so too are we. Therefore, there is very little chance that we will overcome *all* of our challenges. Rebecca, the pessimist, jokingly suggests that there may be doubt that we overcome *any* of them.

Therapists are human. At any given moment, they might be struggling with losses, trauma, and physiological, emotional, and psychological conditions over which they have little or no control. Some of those "wounds" might still be open and not yet "healed." However, this does not render them incapable of assisting others.

What seems to make therapists different from others is a desire not just to *help* people but also to *understand* them. Therapists appear to be curious, psychologically minded, and introspective. They are intrinsically motivated and proactive in the service of others (Farber et al., 2005). They also seem to be "at home in the darkness of suffering" (Stone, 2008, p. 48). Their compassion may derive as much from their strengths of humanity and their ability to handle seeing others in pain as from having overcome difficulties.

With this in mind, we suggest embracing more empowering archetypes for our work: perhaps the *Explorer* who ventures into uncharted territories to discover hidden treasures, or the *Rebel* who disrupts the status quo and fights against oppression, or even the *Jester*, who uses humor to call attention to painful truths and take life less seriously (Pearson, 1991). Art therapists might resonate with the Creator, who finds novel solutions to challenging situations or with the Magician whose "wand"—art—magically changes perceptions and opens our eyes to beauty that is already there.

We often wonder what draws art therapists to this line of work and not to related fields like counseling or social work. Especially when we consider the challenges that art therapists face with establishing their validity in the workplace. Riddle and riddle [*sic*] (2007), in their research with male art therapists, discovered that they scored very high in appreciation of beauty and excellence and creativity. We suspect that these characteristics likely differentiate most art therapists from practitioners in other mental health fields.

GOALS AND ACCOMPLISHMENTS

Seeing the transformation art therapy brings about in our clients often heightens the pride our work can inspire. There are very few art therapists who don't love what they do. They love it because it is so unbelievably effective! Not only are our clients surprised by how much they enjoy art therapy, how relaxing it is, and how much it reveals, we ourselves are always struck that no amount of insight or divination could help us learn as much about our clients and ourselves as we do from the art therapy process.

Naturally, art therapists, like all other professionals, are grappling with varying levels of competency in their work. Depending on the number of years we've been in the field, in the helping professions in general, and what life experience we had before becoming therapists, we are somewhere on a continuum of *novice* to *seasoned*. That marker can change depending on the setting and the populations with whom we're working. Nevertheless, regardless of our level of expertise, we try to adopt a growth mindset toward our work—to maintain an attitude of curiosity and interest, to assume that we are continuously learning about our clients and they about us. We are always navigating this journey in tandem and teaching each other how to do so most effectively given what, together, we have set out to accomplish. We take pride in our efforts, celebrate our successes, and mine for positive meaning in our mistakes.

In addition, because we can rarely *fully* understand what is happening in our work with our clients, we use art and consultation with others to help us see what our minds cannot always consciously comprehend. This also helps us identify and manage the complexities and ethical dimensions of our work. When we run into challenges, we examine our motivations and see if they are congruent with what our clients are trying to achieve or what they can reasonably be expected to do. We try to maintain our optimism and hope but also to set expectations so that they are not impossible to meet.

For example, when working with people with schizophrenia, we do not attempt to rid them of their delusional ideation, but rather to help them be more mindful and aware of their environment and to connect safely with others. Art helps them do both. With clients who abuse substances, we help them identify what purpose their drug of choice served, as well as the reasons, if any, that it stopped being effective, and ways they might meet those needs more productively. Art helps them do that too.

We do the same for the institutions where we work. For example, on psychiatric units, even though we would like to run art therapy groups without interruption, we recognize that we are in settings that prioritize medical interventions over clinical ones. We accommodate the needs of other professionals while keeping our focus on the clients. We might even note to the group members that therapy, just like life, can experience inconvenient interruptions and we can model staying on track despite these distractions.

We use all of these strategies to make *us* better equipped to help our clients and to model them for others—clients, other art therapists, other clinicians, and others in general. In addition, and perhaps most importantly, because doing so on a professional level cannot help but affect us on a personal level, it is likely to improve *our overall wellbeing*. It will make our work much more enjoyable and sustainable in the long run.

Limitations

As we bring this book to a close, we hope that we have described the theory and research upon which a positive art therapy approach is founded and provided context for its emergence in art therapy. We have also attempted to provide a broad range of interventions for applying this approach in both our professional practice and our personal lives. In doing so, we have tried to consider feedback we received from art therapy educator Michael Franklin—that we risked losing novice art therapists if we didn't tailor our delivery of this content to all levels of professional development. We kept this in mind by trying to present the material in ways we hoped would be accessible for beginning, intermediate, and advanced practitioners.

However, we recognize that some of the material we have covered is complex and at times it may require a level of clinical finesse that comes only through experience. There is also an implicit assumption that readers of this book are trained in basic counseling skills. In addition, a background in studio art—the fluidity of paint, the difference between chalk and oil pastels, the properties of clay, safety issues around different media, etc.—would naturally aid in understanding the complexities we refer to in the artmaking process.

The Physical Domain

We only briefly covered the vital role that physical health plays in mental health. This critique that has also been leveled against the field of positive psychology. Although our workshops often address the physical components of self-care—sleep, diet, exercise, etc.—we did not explore in depth the links between physiology, art therapy, and wellbeing. We see exciting possibilities in this realm.

For example, research is revealing the complex neurophysiology of engaging in the art therapy process. Several art therapists are venturing further into this terrain, e.g., Hass-Cohen (2016) in *Art Therapy Relational Neuroscience* and Czamanski-Cohen (2016) in the *Bodymind Model*. Kaimal, Ray and Muniz's (2016) recent pilot study showed using open artmaking with an art therapist resulted in statistically significant lowering of cortisol levels (a biological marker of stress response). We look forward to further developments in this area.

Community-based Applications

We also would have liked to have brought more attention to applications of this content through community and arts-based agencies. For example, we are fans of the work of Dr. Janis Timm-Bottos, who has been promoting social inclusion through "Art Hives" (http://www.arthives.org/), small publicly accessible arts studios throughout Canada and the world. In the US, PSA Art Awakenings in Arizona has opened 15 state-funded art studios, as well as mobile art services, providing expressive art therapies to over 2,500 adults and children with behavioral health problems. We know this only touches on some of the inventive ways that art is being used to build more social inclusion, justice, and healing. We imagine that continuing to broaden the scope of our work beyond clinical settings might help repair some of the deep social fractures we are struggling with in the world. We look forward to collaborating with others already active in such endeavors!

Aesthetics and Environment

Although we briefly discussed the role of culture in wellbeing, we did not delve as deeply into its impact on aesthetics and the role of aesthetics in perception. For example, Cathy Moon's exploration (2016) of relational aesthetics, which includes using our aesthetic sensibilities to facilitate empathy and encourage aesthetic satisfaction in our clients toward their artwork, is congruent with a positive art therapy approach. The interplay between aesthetics and the environment, and how these combine to improve wellbeing, also deserves more attention. We imagine that *environmental art therapy* (Davis, 1999; Farrelly-Hansen, 2001), which emphasizes engaging with community and connecting with nature through sustainable art practices, will figure more prominently in the evolution of positive art therapy.

Future Directions

Reframing Misconceptions about Art Therapy

Although we identify ourselves as operating from a positive psychology paradigm, at our core we are first and foremost art therapists. We always capitalize on opportunities to advocate for the field and embrace any associations that people have to art therapy, correct or incorrect. For example, increasingly when we share that we are art therapists, we are asked if art therapy is akin to the adult coloring books that have become so popular. We used to bristle at this association until we realized our reaction might reflect an internalization of negative stereotypes—the assumption that ties to coloring further marginalized art therapy as a form of recreational activity or as "childish." Now we see it differently. We perceive that the global attention coloring has brought to art therapy has substantially increased our visibility and garnered well-deserved appreciation, even if it includes some misconceptions about what we do.

We determined that, rather than presuming that ties to coloring devalue art therapy, we could instead see these connections as elevating the healing nature of doing art. In addition, the fact that coloring books now cater to adults suggests that doing everyday art is no longer relegated only to children. So now, when people ask if art therapy is coloring, we say "Yes! Absolutely!" However, we clarify that coloring is more of a "self-help" tool, similar to anxiety workbooks or gratitude lists.

This gives us a platform from which to differentiate between *therapeutic art* and *art therapy*. We explain that like other therapies, we work with people who are struggling with a problem or want to improve the quality of their lives and that art provides unique ways to express ourselves, it gives us information we couldn't have discovered in any other way, it provides us with a way to channel difficult feelings, it relaxes us, etc. This starts a conversation about when and why someone might take that a step further and actually employ an art therapist.

Research Opportunities

As Robert Biswas-Diener noted in his foreword to this book, positive psychology has gained prominence in the last two decades because it has employed sophisticated research techniques to build a substantial psychological science. We know that art therapy needs to do the same. Despite the recent gains we have made in establishing our relevance and efficacy, both in general and in areas germane to positive psychology, we must substantiate claims we make about the benefits clients receive from our services.

This includes fundamental assumptions about our work, e.g., that artmaking is healing, that it helps people express themselves differently and better than other forms of communication, that it reveals aspects of memory and experience that cannot be accessed in other ways, that it induces flow, the relaxation response, and positive emotions, etc. Art therapy experts state "the most important area of research [should be] quantitative experimental designs that test the effectiveness of art therapy interventions compared to other forms of treatment...[such as] outcome studies using control groups, randomization, and measures with good psychometric properties" (Kaiser & Deaver, 2013, pp. 119–20). Unfortunately, the skills and financial resources needed for such research endeavors are challenging to access and develop.

Currently the only *quantitative* experimental study using positive art therapy we know of was conducted by art therapist Donna Radel and funded in part by the National Endowment for the Arts. Her dissertation described a randomized, controlled trial with female cancer patients which incorporated a positive psychology-informed, standardized art therapy protocol developed by art therapist Mary Donald (2013). Radel found that Donald's approach helped "decrease emotional distress and enhance spiritual well-being" (Radel, 2015, p. xi).

Using Our Strengths in Research

Part of what has kept most art therapists from engaging in more traditional research is that it is too costly and ambitious to those of us who, at our hearts, are clinicians/artists/teachers. Grant-writing, social science, and statistics are not usually our most energizing strengths! In addition, experimental research methods often seem too complex and mathematical, too distant from the soulful art studio.

More than twenty years ago, art therapists Junge and Linesch (1993) urged art therapists to use their strengths when doing research. When Gioia decided to get a PhD in Creative Art Therapies, she vividly recalled those words. They particularly resonated when she faced the thought of engaging in research methods which did little to activate and engage her highest strengths.

ARTS-BASED RESEARCH

Reading McNiff's (1998) book, *Art-Based Research*, Gioia had an epiphany—she could be a researcher *and* use her strengths! If art is a way of knowing, of learning, of asking questions that can reveal new and compelling answers, artmaking could be research! This is the basis for art-based research (ABR), which uses visual, literary, and/or performing arts to explore social, emotional, spiritual, and artistic questions.

In many ways, ABR is similar to art therapy, because, as creative art therapist Kossak (2012) wrote, *it's what we do!* In both, we are using art to explore and learn, to create meaning and new knowledge, and to express the otherwise ineffable. In ABR, art made *by the researcher(s)* becomes the primary investigative method. It becomes the vehicle for the artists/researchers to be systematically curious (McNiff, 1998; Kapitan, 2010; Leavy, 2015)

ABR provides a way for art therapists to do research that congruently uses our character strengths such as creativity, delight in and appreciation of beauty and excellence, curiosity, love of learning, authenticity, and passion for social justice. At the same time, it employs our unique skills in the visual arts and in making art with collaborative teams of artists-researchers.

While positive psychologists would heartily endorse art therapists using their strengths, arts-based research may be unfamiliar to them. It's not the kind of quantitative statistical analysis that most positive psychologists have used to research happiness and wellbeing. For so long those topics themselves were thought to be "fluffy" enough on their own. As a result, hard numbers were needed, not just to build a reliable body of knowledge, but to combat the underlying prejudice the subject of happiness seemed to engender.

This kind of stigma is familiar to art therapists, who are used to having their work trivialized because it involves art supplies and can look, on the surface, like a leisure activity. Ironically, it often brushed off as "just for fun" when that very quality is one of its greatest strengths. It engages clients more than other therapies and keeps them coming back! The impression that it is *fun* is no accident. When people are doing artwork, it evokes positive emotions. However, that does not mean that complex therapeutic processes are not occurring at the same time.

Oddly enough, art therapists often exhibit a kind of "internalized oppression," wherein they also believe that only quantitative outcome studies qualify as research. In order to move forward, art therapists will need to educate themselves about diverse kinds of research and the importance of finding the right fit between research questions and methods. For example, randomized controlled trials are best for determining *if* a specific intervention has an effect—and we desperately need these studies to help us move forward the science of art therapy!—but research methods such as ABR are best for determining *in what way* or *how* an intervention has an effect.

For example, we might use quantitative research to examine *differences* between *art therapy-as-usual* and *positive art therapy*, and *therapeutic art activities* versus *art therapy with a therapist*; or to determine the effectiveness of positive art therapy directives such as loving-kindness meditation followed by artmaking, or drawing a favorite positive emotion. We might use qualitative and arts-based methods to explore positive art therapy communities and discover new insights into how art can connect us to our greater humanity.

ALLYING WITH RESEARCHERS IN OTHER FIELDS

Art therapists can also use their social intelligence to collaborate with positive psychologists and others versed in research. For example, recently Gioia reached out to Steven Robbins at Arcadia University in Pennsylvania to discuss a quantitative study showing that drawing mandalas boosts mood (Babouchkina & Robbins, 2015). She congratulated him on his work with his students who are investigating questions fascinating to art therapists. He was surprised and delighted to hear from her and they discussed potential collaborations. Hooray! If we can create more trans-disciplinary alliances like these, we can advance the science of art therapy and its applications—be it in positive psychology, body/mind connection, trauma and posttraumatic growth, etc. We can empower art therapists to use their unique strengths in research and create opportunities for positive psychologists and others to advocate for the benefits of the arts in healthcare, social welfare, and global wellbeing as a whole.

Let's connect with positive psychologists like Frederickson on positive emotions, Csíkszentmihályi on flow, Emmons on gratitude, Simonton on creativity, Linley and Biswas-Diener on energizing and engaging strengths, Wong and Steger on meaning, Davidson on mindfulness, Gable and Gottman on relationships, Kashdan on curiosity and psychological flexibility, and so forth. We can also ally with positive psychologists and others who are taking this work into education, such as Charles Walker at St. Bonaventure University in New York. We can collaborate with other creative arts therapists, like Dan Tomasulo who has incorporated positive psychology into psychodrama or Sabine Koch, who researched joy in dance-movement therapy (Koch, Morlinghaus, & Fuchs, 2007).

Defining Ourselves

Potash and colleagues (Potash, Mann, Martinez, Roach, & Wallace, 2016) recently reviewed the archives of *Art Therapy, the Journal of the American Art Therapy Association* in order to determine how art therapists actually practice art therapy, rather than how we have traditionally defined our work. They discovered that keywords that appeared most often were prevention, lifestyle management, wellness, therapy, rehabilitation, as well as assessment and social action. The authors proposed a new and expanded definition of the field art therapy:

> Art therapy is an integrative mental health profession that combines knowledge and understanding of human development and psychological theories with training in visual arts to provide a unique approach for improving physical, mental, and community health. Art therapists use art media, creative processes, imagination, and verbal reflections of produced imagery, to help people resolve problems, foster expression, increase self-awareness, manage behavior, reduce stress, restore health, promote creativity, support resiliency, enhance well-being, achieve insight, develop interpersonal skills, and build community. (Potash et al., 2016, p. 124)

Their definition is *proactive* rather than *problem-focused*. Not only does it include *wellbeing*, but it also includes a wide range of factors that contribute to wellbeing. We imagine that as we continue to discover the factors that make art therapy so effective and expand how we practice in the world, we will continue to refine who we are and what we do best.

The Positive Art Therapy Agenda

As we suggested in the introduction, we believe that an alliance between art therapy and positive psychology will not only be mutually rewarding but that the synergy of our combined efforts can make the pursuit of wellbeing more accessible, enjoyable, and beautiful. Although we assume that most people reading this book will be art therapists, we also hope it reaches the world of positive psychology and beyond.

This book provides a systematic method for combining positive psychology and art therapy, what we have called positive art therapy, by applying the PERMA model of wellbeing to the principles of art therapy. In addition, as promised, we have included a list of directives at the end of the book that can be adapted to the needs of different clients. These strategies use the art therapy process to induce positive emotions, transform negativity, inspire creativity, promote engagement, heighten connection to others, and explore meaning, purpose, and perception.

In the end, however, we suggest that at its core, positive art therapy is more a philosophy than a set of techniques. Positive art therapy applies positive psychology's commitment to identifying and developing the factors that promote mental health, happiness, and wellbeing to the field of art therapy. It incorporates the notion that *building what's strong* not only improves wellbeing, fosters resilience, and buffers against stressors, but that it may be as effective, if not more so, at reducing suffering than focusing on problems and *fixing what's wrong*. Positive art therapy also derives from the belief that, because art therapy has unique benefits, it contributes something distinctive to improving wellbeing. It is intrinsically enjoyable and engaging, it promotes feelings of mastery and accomplishment, it connects us to each other and to meaning and purpose, and it naturally shifts the way we see things and helps us attend to the good. Positive art therapy holds that combining art therapy and positive psychology can enhance wellbeing *above and beyond what either can do alone*.

To go back to the analogy of a reservoir, we think of this synergy as a refreshing infusion of positivity that can offset the drain caused by compassion fatigue, burnout, and despair. To mix metaphors, we also think of it as a fire that lights our energy, compassion, and hope, and as fuel that powers our mission to bring more love and beauty into the world. Of course, because we are art therapists, other metaphors come to mind, e.g., a renewable resource, water that hydrates the roots of a growing tree, seeds to plant in an already fertile field, or rays of sunshine that reveal the silver lining around the clouds of difficulty we have faced and that transform what before was murky and dark.

These metaphors, and this book for that matter, represent how *we* conceptualize the crossover between art therapy and positive psychology. However, we realize that there are countless ways that these two fields could impact each other, some which we alluded to above and others that we might not even have considered. Let's hear how *you* envision this friendship. We hope you write, illustrate, blog, post, share, present, research, create, and sing and dance about how positive art therapy works for you!

Before we close, we suggest you go back to your image of "a happy and fulfilled life." What does it reveal to you now, based on what you have learned? You might create another piece that captures newfound impressions you have of wellbeing. What, if anything, is different? Moving forward, how will this inform your practice? Your perceptions of your clients and your work? Your life? We hope that, just as it has for us, it will sustain you in your passion and mission and make *you* happier!

Positive Art Therapy Directives

These directives can be modified to most media and art forms. We often use stencils, mandalas, hand and/or body outlines (small or life-size), found-object "shrines" from boxes, altered books, wire/cloth dolls, artists trading cards, and masks. In groups, we modify directives to be collaborative, such as murals, round-robins, quilts (paper/cloth), to increase group cohesion and team building. Depending on the clients/setting, we often include writing, visual journaling, letter writing, poetry, dialoguing, and role-reversing either before as warm-up, during as a part of the process, or after as reflection.

Accomplishment Inventory: Write things you accomplished—at the end of the day, the year, at work, on a project, in therapy, toward life goals, etc. Note little things you did regularly, major achievements, what you took care of, places you traveled, people you spent time with, etc. Sketch little images with each. Having accomplished those things, sketch what you would like to do next.

Achievement/Authentic Pride Scrapbook: Create a scrapbook to celebrate and honor your accomplishments and the things for which you are proud. You can do this with families, teams, and your community.

Affirmation Touchstones: Use clear jumbo decorative glass fillers (from craft stores). On same-size bits of paper, design affirmations following the "three Ps" rule: *present* tense as if already happening, *personally* meaningful, and associated with *positive* feelings like safety, comfort, achievement and connection. Modge-podge the affirmations to the back of glass fillers.

Appreciating Small Things: Notice small things throughout the day that positively impact the quality of your daily life.

Attending to the Good/Negativity Bias: Do art about something that is bothering you. See if the visual elements reveal positive aspects of the situation that you might not have noticed before.

Awe: Remember a place, experience, or person that inspired awe in you.

Beautiful Day: Your vision of a beautiful day.

Best Possible Life: Pretend you are looking back on your whole life. Makes symbols of things that would be in your life if it turned out to be the best that you could have imagined? (Can be modified to look back from any point in time—six months; one, two, five years, etc.).

Body Scan: Respond to a body scan (self-initiated, from a recording, or conducted by the art therapist) focused on observing what is happening in the body, the emotions, the mind, and the environment.

Bracelets: Using regular beads and alphabet beads, make bracelets spelling out strengths, values, affirmations, names of comforting others, positive emotions you want to feel, etc.

The Carrot and the Stick: What is the carrot (the reward) and what is the stick (the pain) that motivates you to change?

Coloring Mandala: Make an ink drawing of pleasing imagery or designs. Xerox the image onto heavier paper (as many copies as you want). Color them for relaxation. Have others make coloring images and compare how you colored them similarly/differently.

Community of Service: Make a list of groups you belong to—work, church, family, recreational, neighborhood. Focus on one that serves the greater good in some way.

Congruent Goals: What are you trying to achieve? What internal and external strengths and resources will help you accomplish these. What barriers do you foresee? How will you overcome these?

Coping Tools: Make a toolbox with symbols for the "tools" that keep you well.

Dark Night of the Soul/ What Keeps You Strong?   When times have been tough and you have encountered difficulties, what has kept you going? Using a folded page, create shapes and symbols for internal and external qualities or things that have kept you strong.

Downward Comparison Card: Make a card for someone who, because they are struggling, made you aware of blessings in your life.

Environmental Art: Take a moment to appreciate the natural world around you. Make artwork using natural materials: rocks, sticks, snow, leaves, sand, etc. Make a design using living plants (also known as gardening).

Exceptions: Think about moments you felt better or when you had felt in control of a situation that has been difficult for you. What was different? What made it better?

Golden Moments: Depict key/cherished memories. Celebrate what is pleasant and rewarding in your life.

Good in the Bad: Think about a behavior that you are trying to stop because it has somehow become dysfunctional. What purpose has it served you? How has it helped? What benefits has it given you? Why would you stop doing it? What could help you in the same way?

Good Wolf/Bad Wolf: A grandfather tells his grandson that inside of us there is a battle between two wolves—negativity and positivity. "Which wolf wins?" asks the grandson. Grandfather replies, "The one you feed." Do artwork about the good/bad wolves.

Gratitude: List what makes you feel grateful. Think about what is going well at this moment; today; in general; in a particular situation (at work, home, with another person); for others in your life; in the world. Do this regularly in a visual gratitude journal.

Gratitude Gift: Make an art gift for a person/team/organization toward whom you feel grateful.

Group Appreciations: Groups members pass around art that is identifiably theirs (a card, mandala, basket, with their names on them) and others contribute appreciations (drawing or writing on small slips of paper, magazine images, affirmation pebbles, etc.).

Happy and Fulfilled Life: What does a happy and fulfilled life include for you? What would you be doing and where would you be? Who would be there with you? How would you be feeling?

Hope Journey: What path has your hope taken? What threatens it, what sustains it? When is it strongest? Who makes you feel most hopeful?

Illuminated Path: Make a path leading from where you've been to where you're going that is lit by a source of light. Visualize a path from where you were to where you are going that is illuminated. What is the source of light?

Inner Critic/Inner Muse: Make artwork of these two characters. What strengths do they represent? Have them dialogue with each other about what they are hoping to accomplish and how they can work together.

Intrinsic/Extrinsic Goals: What do you want to accomplish in specific areas of your life? What part of them is inherently rewarding and intrinsically motivated (to feel better, stronger, more energetic) and what parts derive from external consequences (to get a raise, get more recognition, etc.)?

Island Exercise: Draw kidney-shaped "islands" on mural paper. Teams of 4–6 people find themselves on an island which they can equip with anything that they might want/need. Their "magical" art supplies can materialize anything they can imagine! Have teams name and display islands. Using paper, scissors, tape, and glue, teams then create pathways to other islands or construct the means for other teams to visit their island.

Interests/Passions: What interests you? What you are passionate about? How is this connected to your life story? Do your interests give your life deeper purpose and meaning?

Kindness in the Midst of Struggle: Think about a time when you were struggling, yet still found a way to help someone else and it made you feel better.

Love-Kindness Meditation Art: Bring your attention to the area of your heart. See if you can feel your breath and your heart together as if you could breathe into the heart and out from the heart. Then bring to mind a person/creature in your life who you absolutely love, who, the second that you think about them, you start to smile, this could be someone in your family, a close friend, it might be a child, or a pet. Focus on sending them loving thoughts. May they be well, may they be happy, may they be protected from harm. Take a few more breaths and try and stay connected with that feeling, sending it to all of humanity. Respond artistically.

Love Map: With your significant other, each do artwork about what you think is important to you: worries, hopes, hobbies, dreams, friends, favorite foods, etc. Combine your love maps into a single image or a three-dimensional sculpture. Reflect on challenges and successes along the way.

Machine Which Makes Change: What makes change happen?

Making Mistakes: Draw an object you like—an apple, a stapler, a coffee cup. After holding the image at arm's length, deliberately exaggerate any "mistakes." Repeat this for several days.

Meaning and Purpose: What gives your life meaning and purpose?

Meaningful People and/or Creature: Who has been/is meaningful to you?

- Friend/family member/ancestor
- Teacher or mentor
- Pet
- Celebrity, historical/religious figure, fictional character
- Admired politician/activist
- Community member

Mission and Vision Map: Draw a small mandala with symbols for three core strengths (see Appendix C). Write down three core values (see Appendix D)—that make you think, "This is me!" Write three sentences about "What I want to do with my life?" Look to the core values you wrote earlier as a guide. This is the aspiration: "Why (do) I get up in the morning!?" Write three sentences about "How do I want to achieve that?' Make an imaginary map using collage materials (old maps) that represents the way to move toward your life mission using the strengths mandala as the guide. Include any personal ephemera (business cards, photographs). Frame in a visible place to inspire motivation.

Noticing Positive Emotions: Make a piece of artwork simply showing how you are feeling today. Then, ask yourself, does this artwork express any positive emotions? Make a second picture to further explore those feelings. Write a few thoughts about the experience.

One Door Closes, Another One Opens: Make artwork with two doors—one that closed due to a challenge and one that then opened as a result.

Optimism/Pessimism: Fold paper in half. On one side, represent something that you feel proud of or good about having changed in your life and on the other, a challenge you are facing. On the back, write about the images.

Personalize the good thing by identifying your contribution to that event, what role you had in making it happen. Then see if you can find something surprising or visually pleasing on the challenge side even though it's about something unpleasant.

Positive Emotions You Would Like to Experience More: Remember or imagine a positive emotion you'd like to feel more.

Positive Meaning: Think about an experience you struggled with in your life. What did it teach you? How did it make you stronger? What did it make you appreciate more?

Positive Poems/Art: Write on a PERMA topic for 5–10 minutes. Circle words/phrases that stand out. Compose a short poem from those. It does not have to rhyme. Respond with art. (Altered Books variation, have people circle words in the book's text relevant to PERMA topics and do same as above).

Relationship House: What is the foundation, what protects it (the roof), what different floors/levels does it have?

Relationship Preferences/Needs: Identify what you would want/prefer and what you need in your relationships (with family, friends, co-workers, clients, therapist, etc.). If other relevant parties are there, compare images.

Renewable Source of Energy: Remember a time when you felt energized, engaged, and invigorated. Create a symbol for that sensation as if it were a source of renewable energy. If it's a river, what keeps it flowing; a light, what keeps it illuminated; battery, what keeps it charged?

Safe Place: Create a visual reminder of a place of comfort and security.

Savor Beauty: Mindfully attend to a pleasant visual/sensory experience.

Self-care Mandala: Divide a mandala by the domains of self-care that are most important to you—physical, emotional, psychological, professional, and spiritual—with symbols for the activities that will support your health in those areas.

Self-symbols: Create a self-symbol as an animal, tree, house, monster, sandwich, toy, city, weather pattern, etc. Notice values, strengths, worldviews, beliefs, emotional, and physical qualities that might reflect core identity.

Social Action Art: Make art for others, give art gifts to people you appreciate, to people or a group in need, leave small pieces of art in public places for people to find.

Social Atoms/Support Network: Draw an image or make a 3-D sculpture of your social support network, placing yourself in the center and mapping out the network of people around you in order of closeness/intimacy. Variations can be used to explore current, past, or future relationships. Perhaps using different colors to locate different people or different kinds of support (emotional, practical, financial, informational, companionship, etc.).

Strength Sanctuary: Create a shelter from any size/shape of box for your strengths as represented by found objects.

Strengths Family Tree: Create a family tree of strengths.

Strengths Mobile: Make a mobile of your strengths working together.

Strengths Partner/Couples: Create art work about the strengths of your relationship or about the strengths you each bring to the relationship.

Strengths Realized and Unrealized: Make artwork about strengths you use, ways could use them differently, and ones you would like to use more.

Strengths spotting: Make a metaphor which represent tools for spotting strengths—glasses, microscopes, telescopes, binoculars, etc. Illustrate what you appreciate about someone close to you, a colleague, a public figure, or an organization you admire.

Strengths Stretching: Make art using your strengths in a new and challenging way.

Strengths Symbols: Using lists of strengths (see Appendix C), make symbols for your signature strengths. Make a set of cards for the strengths you see in yourself and others. Create a cartoon about using these in new ways.

Strengths That Deplete vs. Energize You: Divide a page in four and represent your energizing realized and unrealized strengths, learned behaviors (depleting strengths), and your weaknesses. Use images that represent people, places, or activities that remind you of each domain.

Strengths in Your Community: Create a triptych that features the strengths of three individuals in your life such as a close friend or family member, a mentor or colleague, and a client or customer.

Super-strengths Superhero: If you were a superhero, what would be your super strengths? Who are the other superheroes in your life?

Therapist Role and Archetypes: Do artwork of how you see yourself as a therapist—teacher, guide, co-traveler, co-pilot, etc.? What archetypes resonate for you—Magician, Explorer, Creator, etc.?

Three Good Things: Write about and make symbols for three good things that happened that day (or during a specific event). You can write on the back what about you or the situation made you appreciate it.

Three Things I Love About You: Make symbols for characteristics you appreciate in a loved one.

Values Mandala: Put a symbol of yourself at the center of a mandala. Place symbols for your values in proximity to the self-symbol, based upon how essential they are to you. Recreate the mandala, placing the symbols of the values relative to how much you *act* on those values. Include marks or symbols for barriers to enacting the values as well as motivations to enact them more.

Values Wall Hanging/Mobile: Identify and celebrate your values in relationship to each other.

Warm-ups to Creative Flow:

- Keep art supplies in places you inhabit most—the kitchen, your purse/backpack, at your office, in your car, etc.
- Spill write about anything that's on your mind for three minutes without pausing. Write to visualize about anything with a positive focus—positive emotions, attending to the good, hopes, purpose, and meaning—or to "express the stress."

- Play with your art supplies—mess around with them, scribble, use a handful of markers at the same time, play with a ball of clay, squeeze some paint out of the tube, rip paper.
- Flip through magazines, find images that inspire you, cut them out and arrange them in different ways.
- Make something silly and "ugly" that you're not attached to.
- Dialogue with your art supplies—ask them what they need.

What's Most Important to You?   Make symbols for the people, creatures, places, activities, beliefs, religious/spiritual practices, that are most important to you.

When It's Bad/When It's Good/What Makes It Better?   List and make artwork about those categories.

Who Is in Charge?   Who is running the show? Who/what is your higher power? What connects to your higher power?

You at Your Best: Make a picture of you/your family/your team/your community at their best.

Your People: Who are your people culturally, ethnically, professionally, personally? What strengths do you share with these groups?

Glossary

Accomplishment/Achievement: the completion of goals which a person highly values.

Appraisal: quick cognitive evaluations of what's relevant/important.

Appreciative inquiry: the process of discovering effective practices through a collaborative search for the best of a person/group/organization.

Attending to the good: countering the negativity bias and consciously noticing what is positive and functional in our lives.

Attention: a cognitive process in the brain which enables focusing awareness.

Beliefs: basic understandings that are felt to be true; fundamental ideas and assumptions about how things are related to each other.

Benefit-finding: positive meaning found in difficulties and challenges.

Broaden-and-build theory: the theory that positive emotions serve the evolutionary function to broaden our thinking and to build enduring psychological, social, and physical resources.

Character strengths: core traits that are relatively stable and inherently valuable.

Compassion fatigue: a condition affecting healthcare workers which leads to anxiety, disconnection, somatization, and depression, sometimes termed vicarious trauma or secondary trauma.

Compassion satisfaction: the gratification healthcare workers experience when they feel supported in what they do, empowered, and they perceive their work as a calling.

Creative process: the progressive stages of innovation—preparation, incubation, illumination, and verification.

Creativity: using cognitive flexibility to imagine, produce, or design original thoughts/objects that are adaptive and appropriate to cultural conditions.

Decisional-conflict: anxiety, ambivalence, and doubt that arises over choices that might lead to undesirable or even fatal outcomes.

Emotional regulation: awareness of and control over our affective experience; learning to tolerate emotions.

Explanatory styles: ways we make sense of our experiences, we account for what we perceive is happening around us, to us, and in us.

Explicit information processing system: higher order cognitive processes that are accessible to conscious awareness which acquire, represent, and implement knowledge.

Fixed mindset: believing intelligence is heritable, that failure is bad and should be avoided.

Flourishing: optimal functioning which includes high levels of emotional, psychological, and social wellbeing.

Flow: effortless state of attention wherein concentration is focused and activities are inherently rewarding and challenging but achievable.

Growth mindset: believing intelligence is malleable and can be increased through perseverance, that failure provides learning opportunities.

Identity: an individual's sense of self/personhood, unique from others.

Implicit information processing system: cognitive processes which hold experience-based, non-verbal knowledge and are generally inaccessible to conscious awareness.

Inner Critic: disparaging internal conscious and/or unconscious self-talk which censors idea-generating thinking critical to creativity.

Inner Muse: the inspired, intuitive, and imaginative parts of our creativity.

Languishing: lack of vitality, emptiness; although no signs of psychiatric illness are evident, the person is not happy or satisfied.

Learned behaviors: behaviors one performs competently, but at a cost to personal energy or zest.

Meaning in life: what is most important to us and gives our lives meaning and purpose.

Meaning-making: the active process of sorting and interpreting information from our external environment and our internal experience.

Mindfulness: attuning to mental, emotional, and physical experience and the *here and now* while attempting to suspend judgment.

Mission: a simple, clear, and global statement that reflects core values and purpose.

Motivational interviewing: a method of increasing motivation for change by exploring ambivalence to change.

Negativity bias: an evolutionary mechanism that drives us to notice negative internal and external information that might be salient to our survival.

Optimism: an explanatory style whereby individuals personalize positive events and believe they will persist and that negative events are specific, isolated occurrences which could happen to anyone.

Passions: self-defining activities which are sources of joy and meaning.

Perception: the process of interpreting information we receive through our senses.

Pessimism: an explanatory style whereby individual believe negative events are personal and they will persist and that positive events are specific, isolated occurrences which are not genuinely related to them.

Positive emotions: feelings that are considered desirable and feel good.

Positive ethics: basing ethics in the aspirational values that ground ethical standards rather than approaching ethics from a risk-management perspective.

Positivity ratio: the proposition that a higher ratio of positive/negative emotions contributes to flourishing and a lower ratio leads to languishing.

Positive relationships: relationships in which we feel safe, cared for, supported, and connected.

Posttraumatic growth: positive change that occurs as a result of a highly challenging life crisis.

Psychological wellbeing: also called eudemonic wellbeing, the psychological factors, such as meaning and purpose, autonomy, connection, personal growth, mastery, self-acceptance, and engaging our strengths, that contribute to reaching our fullest potential.

Purpose: an intention to accomplish something beyond self-interest, a belief that one is alive for a reason, a sense of having a mission or calling.

Reappraisal: a shift in one's initial cognitive evaluation.

Self-compassion: accepting and understanding oneself as imperfect yet worthy of esteem.

Self-concordant goals: goals that are personally valued and intrinsically rewarding, usually related to autonomy and strengths.

Strengths-based approach: approach to psychotherapy/counseling which emphasizes a person's unique resources, talents, strengths, skills, and abilities.

Strengths blindness: a tendency to overlook one's strengths.

Strengths spotting: noticing strengths in oneself and others.

Stress: environmental, social, biological, or psychological demands that require a person to adjust their usual behaviors.

Subjective wellbeing: also called hedonic wellbeing, the ratio of positive to negative emotions that we experience and how satisfied we are with important domains in our life.

Symbol: an idea/association which may or may not be conscious, e.g., visual images, that represent multiple ideas.

Values: guiding principles or enduring standards about what is most important and worthwhile.

Vision: a clear statement of the desired impact of one's mission.

Visual literacy: the ability to discern and articulate visual content and relationships in imagery such as line, shape, form, color, texture, proportion, perspective, etc.

Warm up: priming the creative process by inspiring receptivity to new ideas; activities designed to build trust and increase willingness to take interpersonal risks.

List of Strengths

Able to change one's mind
Accept others' shortcomings
Accept own shortcomings
Achiever
Act on convictions
Activator
Adaptive
Adventurous
Altruistic
Appreciate beauty and excellence
Appreciate everyday experience
Artistic
Authentic
Aware of others
Believe that life has meaning
Brave
Caring
Citizenship
Commitment
Compassion
Competitive
Connector
Consistent
Courageous
Creative
Critical thinker
Curious
Deliberate
Disciplined
Discoverer

Do good deeds
Do one's share
Elevate others
Emotionally intelligent
Energetic
Enthusiastic
Excited
Expect the best
Explorer
Fair
Faith
Flexible
Forgiveness
Future orientation
Generosity
Gratitude
Grit
Help others
Honest
Hopeful
Humanity
Humble
Humility
Humor
Industriousness
Ingenious
Inspirational
Integrity
Intellectual
Interest

Intimacy
Judgment
Justice
Kindness
Knowledge
Leadership
Love of learning
Loving
Loyalty
Mastering new skills
Musical
Nice
Not jumping to conclusions
Not taking undue risks
Noticing nature
Novelty-seeking
Nurturing
Open to experience
Open-minded
Optimistic
Organizer
Originality
Passion
Perseverance
Persistent
Personally intelligent
Perspective
Playful
Provide wise counsel
Prudence

Purpose
Resilient
Seeing the lighter side
Self-control
Self-Regulation
Sense of purpose and meaning
Serenity
Smiling
Social responsibility
Socially intelligent
Speaking the truth
Speaking up for what is right
Spirituality
Taking care of others
Taking responsibility
Teamwork
Temperance
Tender and befriender
Thankful
Transcendence
Valor
Vigor
Vitality
Weigh all evidence
Will to accomplish goals
Willingness
Wisdom
Wonder
Zestful

List of Values

Accountability	Curiosity
Accuracy	Decisiveness
Achievement	Dependability
Adventurousness	Determination
Altruism	Devotion
Ambition	Diligence
Assertiveness	Diplomacy
Authenticity	Discipline
Awesomeness	Discretion
Balance	Diversity
Belonging	Economy
Benevolence	Effectiveness
Boldness	Efficiency
Calmness	Elegance
Carefulness	Eloquence
Challenge	Embodied
Cheerfulness	Empathy
Clarity	Enjoyment
Commitment	Enthusiasm
Community	Equality
Compassion	Ethical
Competitiveness	Excellence
Consistency	Excitement
Contentment	Expertise
Contribution	Exploration
Control	Expressiveness
Cooperation	Fairness
Correctness	Faith
Courtesy	Family
Creativity	Feminism

Fitness
Flexibility
Fluency
Focus
Freedom
Fun
Generosity
Goodness
Grace
Growth
Hand-crafted
Happiness
Hard work
Health
Helping
Holiness
Honesty
Honor
Humanity
Humility
Improvement
Inclusion
Independence
Individuality
Ingenuity
Inner harmony
Innovation
Inquisitiveness
Insightfulness
Integrity
Intelligence
Intuition
Irreverence
Joy
Justice
Laughter
Leadership
Legacy
Love
Loyalty
Making a difference
Mastery
Merit

Moral
Motivation
Musical
Natural
Nurturance
Obedience
Openness
Order
Originality
Patriotism
Perfection
Philanthropy
Playfulness
Positivity
Power
Practicality
Preparedness
Privacy
Professionalism
Prudence
Reliability
Resourcefulness
Respect
Restraint
Results-oriented
Rigor
Sacrifice
Safety
Satisfaction
Security
Self-actualization
Self-control
Selflessness
Self-reflection
Self-regulation
Self-reliance
Sensitivity
Sensuality
Serenity
Service
Shrewdness
Silence
Simplicity

Sobriety
Society
Sophistication
Soundness
Speed
Spirituality
Spontaneity
Stability
Strategic
Strength
Structure
Success
Support
Surprise
Teamwork
Temperance
Thankfulness
Thoroughness
Thoughtfulness
Thriftiness

Tidiness
Timeliness
Tolerance
Traditionalism
Tranquility
Trustworthiness
Truth-seeking
Understanding
Vision
Vitality
Wealth
Willingness
Winning
Wisdom
Wittiness
Wonder
Youthfulness
Zeal
Zest

Bibliography

Abuhamdeh, S., & Csíkszentmihályi, M. (2014). The artistic personality: A systems perspective. *The systems model of creativity* (pp. 227–237). Netherlands: Springer.

Adler, A. (1979). *Superiority and social interest: A collection of later writings.* H. L. Ansbacher & R. R. Ansbacher (Eds.). New York: Norton.

Adler, J. M., & Hershfield, H. E. (2012). Mixed emotional experience is associated with and precedes improvements in psychological well-being. *PloS one, 7*(4), 1. doi:http://dx.doi.org/10.1371/journal.pone.0035633

Algoe, S. B., & Stanton, A. L. (2012). Gratitude when it is needed most: Social functions of gratitude in women with metastatic breast cancer. *Emotion, 12*(1), 163–168.

Alkema, K., Linton, J. M., & Davies, R. (2008). A study of the relationship between self-care, compassion satisfaction, compassion fatigue, and burnout among hospice professionals. *Journal of Social Work in End-of-Life & Palliative Care, 4*(2), 101–119.

Allen, P. B. (1992). Artist in residence: An alternative to "clinification" for art therapists. *Art Therapy: Journal of the American Art Therapy Association, 9*(1), 22–29.

Allen, P. B. (1995). *Art is a way of knowing.* Boston, MA: Shambhala.

Allen, P. B. (2012). Art as enquiry: Towards a research method that holds soul truth. *Journal of Applied Arts & Health, 3*(1), 13–20. doi:10.1386/jaah.3.1.13_1

Alter-Muri, S. B. (2002). Viktor Lowenfeld revisited: A review of Lowenfeld's preschematic, schematic, and gang age stages. *American Journal of Art Therapy, 40*(3), 170–192.

AATA (American Art Therapy Association) (2013). Ethical principles for art therapists. www.americanarttherapyassociation.org/upload/ethicalprinciples.pdf

ACA (American Counseling Association) (2002). Self-care assessment. Adapted from K.W. Saakvitne, L.A. Pearlman, & Staff of TSI/CAAP (1996). *Transforming the pain: A workbook on vicarious traumatization.* New York: W.W. Norton.

APA (American Psychiatric Association) (1952). *Diagnostic and statistical manual of mental disorders*, 1st ed. Washington, DC: Author.

APA (American Psychiatric Association) (2013). *Diagnostic and statistical manual of mental disorders*, 5th ed. Washington, DC: Author.

Andersen, S. M., & Berk, M. S. (1998). Transference in everyday experience: Implications of experimental research for relevant clinical phenomena. *Review of General Psychology, 2*(1), 81.

Anderson, J. R. (2004). *Cognitive psychology and its implications*. New York: Worth Publications.

Antonacopoulou, E. P., & Gabriel, Y. (2001). Emotion, learning and organizational change: towards an integration of psychoanalytic and other perspectives. *Journal of Organizational Change Management, 14*(5), 435–451.

Arieti, S. (1976). *Creativity: The magic synthesis*. New York: Basic Books.

Arnheim, R. (1962). *Picasso's Guernica: The genesis of a painting*. Berkeley: University of California Press.

Arnheim, R. (1974). *Art and visual perception: A psychology of the creative eye*. Berkeley: University of California Press.

Art Therapy Credentials Board. (2016). Code of ethics, conduct, and disciplinary procedures. https://www.atcb.org/resource/pdf/2016-ATCB-Code-of-Ethics-Cond uct-DisciplinaryProcedures.pdf

Aspinwall, L. G. (1998). Rethinking the role of positive affect in self-regulation. *Motivation and Emotion, 22*(1), 1–32.

Assagioli, R. (1942). Spiritual joy. *The Beacon* (June), p. 168. www.psykosyntese.dk/

Assagioli, R. (1959). *Dynamic psychology and psychosynthesis*. New York: Psychosynthesis Research Foundation.

Ault, R. E. (1986). Draw on new lines of communication. *Personnel Journal, 72*–77.

Baas, M., De Dreu, C. K. W., & Nijstad, B. A. (2008). A meta-analysis of 25 years of mood-creativity research: Hedonic tone, activation, or regulatory focus? *Psychological Bulletin, 134*(6), 779–806.

Babouchkina, A., & Robbins, S. J. (2015). Reducing negative mood through mandala creation: A randomized controlled trial. *Art Therapy, 32*(1), 34–39.

Babyak, K. L. (2015). Art therapy informed organizational consulting: An international survey study (Doctoral dissertation), Drexel University, Philadephia, PA.

Bandura, A. (1977). *Social learning theory*. New York: General Learning Press.

Bannink, F. (2014). *Post traumatic success: Positive psychology and solution-focused strategies to help clients survive and thrive*. New York: Norton.

Barnard, F.R. (1927). One picture is worth a thousand words, *Printer's Ink*, March 10.

Barone, T., & Eisner, E. W. (2012). *Arts based research*. Thousand Oaks, CA: Sage.

Bartlett, M. Y., & DeSteno, D. (2006). Gratitude and prosocial behavior: Helping when it costs you. *Psychological Science, 17*(4), 319–325. doi: 10.1111/j.1467-9280.2006.01705.x

Baumeiser, R. F. (1991). *Meanings of life*. New York: Guilford Press.

Baumeiser, R., & Vohs, K. (2010). The pursuit of meaningfulness in life. In C. Snyder & S. Lopez (Eds.), *Handbook of positive psychology* (pp. 608–617). New York: Oxford University Press.

Baumeister, R., Bratslavsky, E., Finkenauer, C., & Vohs, K. (2001). Bad is stronger than good. *Review of General Psychology, 5*(4), 323–370.

Beck, A. T. (1993). Cognitive therapy: Past, present, and future. *Journal of Consulting and Clinical Psychology, 61*(2), 194–198. doi:10.1037/0022-006X.61.2.194

Beck, A.T. (1967). *The diagnosis and management of depression*. Philadelphia, PA: University of Pennsylvania Press.

Belkofer, C. M., & Konopka, L. M. (2008). Conducting art therapy research using quantitative EEG measures. *Art Therapy: Journal of the American Art Therapy Association Association, 25*(2), 8.

Bell, C., & Robbins, S. (2007). Effect of art production on negative mood: A randomized, controlled trial. *Art Therapy: Journal of the American Art Therapy Association, 24*(2), 5.

Bell, S. (2011). Art Therapy and Spirituality. *Journal for the Study of Spirituality, 1*(2), 215–230. doi:10.1558/jss.v1i2.215

Benson, H. (2009). *Timeless healing*. New York: Simon and Schuster.

Benson, H., Greenwood, M. M., & Klemchuk, H. (1975). The relaxation response: Psychophysiologic aspects and clinical applications. *The International Journal of Psychiatry in Medicine, 6*(1–2), 87–98.

Bentzen, M. (2015). Dances of connection: Neuroaffective development in clinical work with attachment, *Body, Movement and Dance in Psychotherapy, 10*(4), 211–226, doi:10.1080/17432979.2015.1064479

Betensky, M. (2001). Phenomenological art therapy. In J. A. Rubin (Ed.), *Approaches to Art Therapy: Theory and Technique*, 2nd ed. (pp. 121–133). New York: Routledge.

Betts, D. J. (2011). Positive art therapy assessment: Looking towards positive psychology for new directions in the art therapy evaluation process. In A. Gilroy, R. Tipple, & C. Brown (Eds.), *Assessment in art therapy* (pp. 203–218). London: Routledge.

Biswas-Diener, R. (2010). *Positive psychology as social change*: New York: Springer.

Biswas-Diener, R. (2011). *Practicing positive psychology in coaching: Assessment, activities, and strategies for success*. Hoboken, NJ: Wiley & Sons.

Biswas-Diener, R. (2013). *Invitation to positive psychology: Research and tools for the professional*. London: Saffron.

Biswas-Diener, R., & Kashdan, T. B. (2013). What happy people do differently. *Psychology Today Blog*, July 2. https://www.psychologytoday.com/articles/201307/what-happy-people-do-differently

Biswas-Diener, R., Kashdan, T., & Minhas, G. (2011). A dynamic approach to psychological strength development and intervention. *Journal of Positive Psychology, 6*(2), 106–118. doi:10.1080/17439760.2010.545429

Booth, M., & Sleeman, J. (2007). *Strengths in a Box*. Northmead, Australia: Holllyhox Positive Resources.

Bowlby, J. (1988). *A secure base: Clinical applications of attachment theory*. New York: Basic Books.

Braiker, H. B., & Kelley, H. H. (1979). Conflict in the development of close relationships. In R. Burgess & T. Huston (Eds.), *Social exchange in developing relationships* (pp. 135–168). New York: Academic Press.

Bramesfeld, K. D., & Gasper, K. (2008). Happily putting the pieces together: A test of two explanations for the effects of mood on group-level information processing. *British Journal of Social Psychology, 47*, 285–309.

Brassaï. (1999). *Conversations with Picasso*. Chicago, IL: University of Chicago Press.

Brown, L. V. (2007). *Psychology of motivation*. New York: Nova Publishers.

Brown, N. J. L., Sokal, A. D., & Friedman, H. L. (2013). The complex dynamics of wishful thinking: The critical positivity ratio. *American Psychologist*, no pagination specified. doi:10.1037/a0032850

Bucciarelli, A. (2011). A normative study of the Person Picking an Apple From a Tree (PPAT) assessment. *Art Therapy: Journal of the American Art Therapy Association*, *28*(1), 31–36. doi:10.1080/07421656.2011.557349

Buckingham, M., & Clifton, D. O. (2001). *Now, discover your strengths*. New York: Simon and Schuster.

Burdette, H. L., & Whitaker, R. C. (2005). Resurrecting free play in young children: Looking beyond fitness and fatness to attention, affiliation, and affect. *Archives of Pediatrics and Adolescent Medicine*, *159*(1), 46.

Burkewitz, J. N. (2014). *Coming to the studio, going with the flow: A study on artmaking to enhance flourishing* (MA thesis), Florida State Univesity. http://diginole.lib.fsu.edu/cgi/viewcontent.cgi?article=8168&context=etd (Electronic Theses, Treatises and Dissertations, Paper 8947).

Burnes, B., & Cooke, B. (2013). Kurt Lewin's field theory: A review and re-evaluation. *International Journal of Management Reviews*, *15*(4), 408–425. doi:10.1111/j.1468-2370.2012.00348.x

Burton, J. (1990). *Conflict resolution and prevention*. New York: St. Martin's Press.

Busfield, J. (2010). "A pill for every ill": Explaining the expansion in medicine use. *Social Science & Medicine*, *70*(6), 934–941. doi:http://dx.doi.org/10.1016/j.socscimed.2009.10.068

Butler, T. (2010). *Getting unstuck: A guide to discovering your next career path*. Boston, MA: Harvard Business Press.

Calish, A. (1994). The metatherapy of supervision using art with transference/counter transference phenomena. *Clinical Supervisor*, *12*(2), 119–127.

Cane, F. (1951). *The artist in each of us*. London: Thames and Hudson.

Carnes, J. J. (1979). Toward a cognitive theory of art therapy. *Art Psychotherapy*, *6*(2), 69–75.

Carr, D. (2014). *Worried sick: How stress hurts and how to bounce back*. New Brunswick, NJ: Rutgers University Press.

Carter E. (2006). Pre-packaged guided imagery for stress reduction: Initial results. *Counselling, Psychotherapy, and Health*, *2*(2), 27–39, July 2006.

Chaplin, L. N. (2009). Please may I have a bike? Better yet, may I have a hug? An examination of children's and adolescents' happiness. *Journal of Happiness Studies*, *10*(5), 541–562.

Chapman, L., Morabito, D., Ladakakos, C., Schreier, H., & Knudson, M. (2001). The effectiveness of art therapy interventions in reducing post traumatic stress disorder (PTSD) symptoms in pediatric trauma patients. *Art Therapy: Journal of the American Art Therapy Association*, *19*(2), 100–104.

Chávez-Eakle, R. A., Graff-Guerrero, A., García-Reyna, J. C., Vaugier, V., & Cruz-Fuentes, C. (2007). Cerebral blood flow associated with creative performance: A comparative study. *Neuroimage*, *38*(3), 519–528.

Cheavens, J. S., Strunk, D. R., Lazarus, S. A., & Goldstein, L. A. (2012). The compensation and capitalization models: A test of two approaches to individualizing the treatment of depression. *Behaviour Research and Therapy*, *50*(11), 699–706.

Cherniss, C. (1980). *Staff burnout: Job stress in the human services*. New York: Praeger.

Chilton, G. (2013). Flow in art therapy: A review of the literature and applications. *Art Therapy: Journal of the American Art Therapy Association*, *30*(2), 64–70. doi:10.1080/07421656.2013.787211

Chilton, G. (2014). *An arts-based study of the dynamics of expressing positive emotions within the intersubjective art making process* (Doctoral dissertation), Drexel University, Philadelphia, PA.

Chilton, G., Gerber, N., Bechtel, A., Councill, T., Dreyer, M., & Yingling, E. (2015). The art of positive emotions: Expressing positive emotions within the intersubjective art making process (L'art des émotions positives : exprimer des émotions positives à travers le processus artistique intersubjectif). *Canadian Art Therapy Association Journal, 28*(1–2), 12–25. doi:10.1080/08322473.2015.1100580

Chilton, G., Gerber, N., Councill, T., & Dreyer, M. (2015). I followed the butterflies: Poetry of positive emotions in art therapy research. *Cogent Arts and Humanities, 2*(1), 1026019. doi:10.1080/23311983.2015.1026019

Chilton, G., Gerity, L., LaVorgna-Smith, M., & MacMichael, H. N. (2009). An online art exchange group: 14 secrets for a happy artist. *Art Therapy: Journal of the American Art Therapy Association, 26*(2), 66–72.

Chilton, G., & Leavy, P. (2014). Arts-based research practice: Merging social research and the creative arts. In P. Leavy (Ed.), *Oxford handbook of qualitative research* (pp. 403–422). New York: Oxford University Press.

Chilton, G., & Wilkinson, R. A. (2009). Positive art therapy: Envisioning the intersection of art therapy and positive psychology. *Australia and New Zealand Journal of Art Therapy, 4*(1), 27–35.

Chilton, G., & Wilkinson, R. A. (2016). Positive art therapy. In J. A. Rubin (Ed.), *Approaches to art therapy: Theory and technique*, 3rd ed. (pp. 249–268). London: Routledge.

Chomsky, N. (1965). *Aspects of the theory of syntax*. Boston, MA: MIT Press.

Christopher, J. C. (1999). Situating psychological well-being: Exploring the cultural roots of its theory and research. *Journal of Counseling and Development, 77*(2), 141–152.

Clover, D. (2011). Successes and challenges of feminist arts-based participatory methodologies with homeless/street-involved women in Victoria. *Action Research, 9*(1), 12.

Cobb, R. A., & Negash, S. (2010). Altered book making as a form of art therapy: A narrative approach. *Journal of Family Psychotherapy, 21*(1), 54–69.

Cohen, B. M., Barnes, M.-M., & Rankin, A. B. (1995). *Managing traumatic stress through art: Drawing from the center*. Baltimore, MD: Sidran Press.

Cohen, B. M., Mills, A., & Kijak, A. K. (1994). An introduction to the Diagnostic Drawing Series: A standardized tool for diagnostic and clinical use. *Art Therapy: Journal of the American Art Therapy Association, 11*(2), 105–110. doi: 10.1080/07421656.1994.10759060

Cohen, B., & Cox, C. (1995). *Telling without talking: Art as a window into the world of multiple personality*. New York: W. W. Norton.

Cohen, S., Kamarck, T., & Mermelstein R (1983). A global measure of perceived stress. *Journal of Health and Social Behavior, 24*(4): 385–396. doi:10.2307/2136404

Collie, K., Bottorff, J. L., & Long, B. C. (2006). A narrative view of art therapy and art making by women with breast cancer. *Journal of Health Psychology, 11*(5), 761–775.

Collier, A. F. (2011). The well-being of women who create with textiles: Implications for art therapy. *Art Therapy: Journal of the American Art Therapy Association, 28*(3), 104–112.

Collins, A. L., Sarkisian, N., & Winner, E. (2009). Flow and happiness in later life: An investigation into the role of daily and weekly flow experiences. *Journal of Happiness Studies, 10*(6), 703–719.

Congdon, K. G. (1990). Normalizing art therapy. *Art Education, 43*(3), 19–43.

Conoley, C. W., Padula, M. A., Payton, D. S., & Daniels, J. A. (1994). Predictors of client implementation of counselor recommendations: Match with problem, difficulty level, and building on client strengths. *Journal of Counseling Psychology, 41*(1), 3–7. doi:10.1037/0022-0167.41.1.3

Coombs, M. M., Coleman, D., & Jones, E. E. (2002). Working with feelings: The importance of emotion in both cognitive-behavioral and interpersonal therapy in the NIMH Treatment of Depression Collaborative Research Program. *Psychotherapy: Theory, Research, Practice, Training, 39*(3), 233.

Cooperrider, D. L., & Srivastva, S. (1987). Appreciative inquiry in organizational life. *Research in Organizational Change and Development, 1*(1), 129–169.

Cosgrove, L., Krimsky, S., Vijayaraghavan, M., & Schneider, L. (2006). Financial ties between DSM-IV panel members and the pharmaceutical industry. *Psychotherapy and Psychosomatics, 75*(3), 154–160.

Cozolino, L. (2014). *The neuroscience of human relationships: Attachment and the developing social brain* (Norton Series on Interpersonal Neurobiology). New York: Norton.

Crocetti, E., Avanzi, L., Hawk, S. T., Fraccaroli, F., & Meeus, W. (2013). Personal and social facets of job identity: A person-centered approach. *Journal of Business and Psychology, 29*(2), 281–300. doi:10.1007/s10869-013-9313-x

Croghan, C. (2013). Knitting is the new yoga? Comparing techniques; physiological and psychological indicators of the relaxation response. http://esource.dbs.ie/han dle/10788/1586

Crooks, T. (2013). *Spirituality, Creativity, Identity, and Art Therapy* (Master's thesis). LMU/LLS Theses and Dissertations. Paper 61. http://digitalcommons.lmu.edu/etd/61

Csíkszentmihályi, M. (1991). *Flow: The psychology of optimal experience.* New York: HarperPerennial.

Csíkszentmihályi, M. (1996). *Creativity: Flow and the psychology of discovery and invention.* New York: HarperCollins.

Csíkszentmihályi, M. (1997a). *Finding flow: The psychology of engagement with everyday life*: New York: Basic Books.

Csíkszentmihályi, M. (1997b). Happiness and creativity: Going with the flow. *The Futurist, 31*(5), 8–12.

Csíkszentmihályi, M. (2014). Toward a psychology of optimal experience. In *Flow and the foundations of positive psychology: The collected works of Mihaly Csíkszentmihályi* (pp. 209–226). Dordrecht: Springer Netherlands.

Curl, K. (2008). Assessing stress reduction as a function of artistic creation and cognitive focus. *Art Therapy: Journal of the American Art Therapy Association Association, 25*(4), 164–169.

Czamanski-Cohen, J. (2012). The use of art in the medical decision–making process of oncology patients. *Art Therapy: Journal of the American Art Therapy Association, 29*(2), 60–67.

Czamanski-Cohen, J. (2016). The bodymind model: A platform for studying the mechanisms of change induced by art therapy. *The Arts in Psychotherapy, 51,* 63–71. doi:10.1016/j.aip.2016.08.006

Czamanski-Cohen, J., Sarid, O., Huss, E., Ifergane, A., Niego, L., & Cwikel, J. (2014). CB-ART—The use of a hybrid cognitive behavioral and art based protocol for treating pain and symptoms accompanying coping with chronic illness. *The Arts in Psychotherapy, 41*(4), 320–328. doi:https://doi.org/10.1016/j.aip.2014.05.002

Czamanski-Cohen, J., & Weihs, K. L. (2016). The bodymind model: A platform for studying the mechanisms of change induced by art therapy. *The Arts in Psychotherapy, 51*, 63–71. doi:https://doi.org/10.1016/j.aip.2016.08.006

Dalebroux, A., Goldstein, T., & Winner, E. (2008). Short-term mood repair through art-making: Positive emotion is more effective than venting. *Motivation and Emotion, 32*(4), 288–295.

Damon, W., Menon, J., & Cotton Bronk, K. (2003). The development of purpose during adolescence. *Applied Developmental Science, 7*(3), 119–128.

Darewych, O. (2013). Building bridges with institutionalized orphans in Ukraine: An art therapy pilot study. *The Arts in Psychotherapy, 40*(1), 85–93.

Darewych, O. (2014). *The bridge drawing with path art-based assessment: Measuring meaningful life pathways in higher education students* (Doctoral dissertation). Lesley University, Cambridge, MA.

Davidson, K. W., Mostofsky, E., & Whang, W. (2010). Don't worry, be happy: Positive affect and reduced 10-year incident coronary heart disease: The Canadian Nova Scotia Health Survey. *European Heart Journal, 31*(9), 1065–1070. doi:10.1093/eurheartj/ehp603

Davidson, R. (2010). Mindfulness training and emotion regulation: clinical and neuroscience perspectives. *Emotion, 10*(1), pp. 8–11.

Davis, B. (2010). Hermeneutic methods in art therapy research with international students. *The Arts in Psychotherapy, 37*(3), 179–189.

Davis, C. G., Nolen-Hoeksema, S., & Larson, J. (1998). Making sense of loss and benefiting from the experience: Two construals of meaning. *Journal of Personality and Social Psychology, 75*(2), 561.

Davis, J. (1999). Report: environmental art therapy: Metaphors in the field. *The Arts in Psychotherapy, 26*(1), 45–50.

Dayton, T. (1994). *The drama within: Psychodrama and experiential therapy.* Deerfield Beach, FL: Health Communications.

De Petrillo, L., & Winner, E. (2005). Does art improve mood? A test of a key assumption underlying art therapy. *Art Therapy: Journal of the American Art Therapy Association, 22*(4), 8.

De Shazer, S. (1985). *Keys to solution in brief therapy.* New York: Norton.

De Shazer, S., & Dolan, Y. (2012). *More than miracles: The state of the art of solution-focused brief therapy.* New York: Routledge.

Deaver, S. P. (2009). A normative study of children's drawings: Preliminary research findings. *Art Therapy, 26*(1), 4–11. doi:10.1080/07421656.2009.10129309

Deaver, S. P. (2012). Art-based learning strategies in art therapy graduate education. *Art Therapy: Journal of the American Art Therapy Association, 29*(4), 158–165. doi: 10.1080/07421656.2012.730029

Deaver, S. P., & McAuliffe, G. (2009). Reflective visual journaling during art therapy and counselling internships: A qualitative study. *Reflective Practice, 10*(5), 615–632.

Deaver, S. P., & Shiflett, C. (2011). Art-based supervision techniques. *The Clinical Supervisor, 30*(2), 257–276. doi:10.1080/07325223.2011.619456

Decety, J., & Meyer, M. (2008). From emotion resonance to empathic understanding: A social developmental neuroscience account. *Development and Psychopathology, 20*(Special Issue 04), 1053–1080. doi:10.1017/S0954579408000503

Deci, E. L., & Ryan, R. M. (1985). *Intrinsic motivation and self-determination in human behavior.* New York: Springer.

DeLue, C. H. (1999). Physiological effects of creating mandalas. In C. Malchiodi (Ed.), *Medical art therapy with children* (pp. 33–49). Philadelphia, PA: Jessica Kingsley.

Demir, M., & Özdemir, M. (2010). Friendship, need satisfaction and happiness. *Journal of Happiness Studies, 11*(2), 243–259.

Demir, M., Özdemir, M., & Weitekamp, L. (2007). Looking to happy tomorrows with friends: Best and close friendships as they predict happiness. *Journal of Happiness Studies, 8*(2), 243–271.

Demir, M., Özen, A., Doğan, A., Bilyk, N.A., & Tyrell, F.A. (2010). I matter to my friend, therefore I am happy: Friendship, mattering, and happiness. *Journal of Happiness Studies, 12*(6), 1–23.

Derryberry, D., Reed, M.A., Pilkenton-Taylor, (2003). Temperament and coping: Advantages of an individual differences perspective. *Development and Psychopathology, 15*, 1049–1066.

Diener, E. (1994). Assessing subjective well-being: Progress and opportunities. *Social Indicators Research, 31*(2), 103–157.

Diener, E. (2003). What is positive about positive psychology: The curmudgeon and Pollyanna. *Psychological Inquiry, 14*(2), 115–120.

Diener, E. (2012). New findings and future directions for subjective well-being research. *American Psychologist, 67*(8), 590–597. doi:10.1037/a0029541

Diener, E., & Biswas-Diener, R. (2008). *Happiness: Unlocking the mysteries of psychological wealth*. New York: Wiley-Blackwell.

Diener, E., & Chan, M. (2011). Happy people live longer: Subjective well-being contributes to health and longevity. *Applied Psychology: Health and Well-being, 3*, 1–43.

Diener, E., Lucas, R.E., Scollon, C. N. (2006). Beyond the hedonic treadmill. *American Psychologist, 61*(4), p. 305–314.

Diener, E., Oishi, S., & Lucas, R. E. (2003). Personality, culture, and subjective well-being: Emotional and cognitive evaluations of life. *Annual Review of Psychology, 54*(1), 403–425.

Diener, E., & Ryan, K. (2009). Subjective well-being: A general overview. *South African Journal of Psychology, 39*(4), 391–406.

Diener, E., Suh, E., Lucas, R., & Smith, H. (1999). Subjective well-being: three decades of progress. *Psychological Bulletin, 125*, 276–302.

Dietrich, A. & Stoll, O. (2010). Effortless attention, hypofrontality and perfectionism. In B. Bruya (Ed.), *Effortless attention: A new perspective in the cognitive science of attention and action*. Cambridge, MA: MIT Press.

Dietrich, A. (2003). Functional neuroanatomy of altered states of consciousness: The transient hypofrontality hypothesis. *Consciousness and Cognition, 12*(2), 231–256.

Dietrich, A. (2004a). Neurocognitive mechanisms underlying the experience of flow. *Consciousness and Cognition, 13*(4), 746–761.

Dietrich, A. (2004b). The cognitive neuroscience of creativity. *Psychonomic Bulletin and Review, 11*(6), 1011.

Digman, J. M. (1990). Personality structure: Emergence of the five-factor model. *Annual Review of Psychology, 41*(1), 417–440.

Dissanayake, E. (1999). "Making special": An undescribed human universal and the core of a behavior of art. In B. Cooke & F. Turner (Eds.), *Biopoetics: Evolutionary explorations in the arts* (pp. 27–46). Lexington, KY: ICUS.

Donald, M. (2008). Art therapy and quality-of-life with newly diagnosed breast cancer patients: A quantitative pilot study (Unpublished pilot study). The Cancer Center at Paoli Memorial Hospital, Paoli, PA.

Donald, M. (2013). *The Self-Book© Art Therapy Intervention 6-Session Curriculum.* www.selfbookarttherapy.com/curriculum.html

Dondis, D. A. (1974). *A primer of visual literacy.* Cambridge, MA: MIT Press.

Doran, G. T. (1981). "There's a S.M.A.R.T. way to write management's goals and objectives." Management review. *AMA FORUM, 70*(11): 35–36.

Drake, J. E., & Hodge, A. (2015). Drawing versus writing: The role of preference in regulating short-term affect. *Art Therapy: Journal of the American Art Therapy Association, 32*(1), 27–33.

Drake, J., & Winner, E. (2012). Confronting sadness through art-making: Distraction is more beneficial than venting. *Psychology of Aesthetics, Creativity, and the Arts, 6*(2), No pagination specified. doi:doi: 10.1037/a0026909

Drake, J., Coleman, K., & Winner, E. (2011). Short-term mood repair through art: Effects of medium and strategy. *Art Therapy: Journal of the American Art Therapy Association, 28*(1), 26–30.

Drass, J. M. (2015). Art therapy for individuals with borderline personality: Using a dialectical behavior therapy framework. *Art Therapy: Journal of the American Art Therapy Association, 32*(4), 168–176. doi:10.1080/07421656.2015.1092716

Duckworth, A. L., Peterson, C., Matthews, M. D., & Kelly, D. R. (2007). Grit: Perseverance and passion for long-term goals. *Journal of Personality and Social Psychology, 92*(6), 1087.

Duckworth, A., Steen, T. A., & Seligman, M. E. P. (2005). Positive psychology in clinical practice. *Annual Review of Clinical Psychology, 1*(1), 629–651. doi:10.1146/annurev. clinpsy.1.102803.144154

Duncan, B. L. & Miller, S. D. (2000). The client's theory of change: Consulting the client in the integrative process. *Journal of Psychotherapy Integration, 10*(2), 169–187. http:// dx.doi.org/10.1023/A:1009448200244

Dunn, E. W., Gilbert, D. T., & Wilson, T. D. (2011). If money doesn't make you happy, then you probably aren't spending it right. *Journal of Consumer Psychology, 21*(2), 115–125.

Dweck, C. (2006). *Mindset: The new psychology of success.* New York: Random House.

Elkins, D. N. (2009). The medical model in psychotherapy: Its limitations and failures. *Journal of Humanistic Psychology, 49*(1), 66–84. doi:10.1177/0022167807307901

Elliot, A. J., Sheldon, K. M., & Church, M. A. (1997). Avoidance personal goals and subjective well-being. *Personality and Social Psychology Bulletin, 23*(9), 915–927. doi:10.1177/0146167297239001

Elliott, R., Bohart, A. C., Watson, J. C., & Greenberg, L. S. (2011). Empathy. *Psychotherapy, 48*(1), 43–49. doi:10.1037/a0022187

Ellis, A. (1957). Rational psychotherapy and individual psychology. *Journal of Individual Psychology, 13*, 38–44.

Ellis, A. (1977). Rational-emotive therapy: Research data that supports the clinical and personality hypotheses of RET and other modes of Cognitive-Behavior Therapy. *The Counseling Psychologist, 7*(1), 2–42. doi:10.1177/001100007700700102

Epstein, M. H., & Sharma, J. (1998). *Behavioral and emotional rating scale: A strength-based approach to assessment.* Austin, TX: PRO-ED.

Everly, G. S., McCormack, D. K., & Strouse, D. A. (2012). Seven characteristics of highly resilient people: Insights from Navy SEALs to the "Greatest Generation." *International Journal of Emergency Mental Health, 14*(2), 137–143.

Farber, B. A., Manevich, I., Metzger, J., & Saypol, E. (2005). Choosing psychotherapy as a career: Why did we cross that road? *Journal of Clinical Psychology, 61*(8), 1009–1031.

Farran, C. J., Wilken, C. & Popovich, J. M (1992). Clinical assessment of hope. *Issues in Mental Health Nursing, 13*(2), 129–138.

Farrelly-Hansen, M. (Ed.) (2001). *Spirituality and art therapy: Living the connection.* London: Jessica Kingsley.

Feen-Callgan, H. (1995). The use of art therapy in treatment programs to promote spiritual recovery from addiction. *Art Therapy: Journal of the American Art Therapy Association, 12*(1), 46–50.

Festinger, L. (1954). A theory of social comparison process. *Human Relations, 7,* 117–140. doi:10.1177/001872675400700202

Fialkov, C., & Haddad, D. (2012). Appreciative clinical training. *Training and Education in Professional Psychology, 6*(4), 204–210. doi:10.1037/a0030832

Fish, B. J. (2012). Response art: The art of the art therapist. *Art Therapy: Journal of the American Art Therapy Association, 29*(3), 138–143.

Fitzpatrick, M. R., & Stalikas, A. (2008). Positive emotions as generators of therapeutic change. *Journal of Psychotherapy Integration, 18*(2), 137–154. doi:10.1037/1053-0479.18.2.137

Flückiger, C., & Grosse Holtforth, M. (2008). Focusing the therapist's attention on the patient's strengths: A preliminary study to foster a mechanism of change in outpatient psychotherapy. *Journal of Clinical Psychology, 64*(7), 876–890.

Folkman, S., & Lazarus, R. S. (1985). If it changes it must be a process: Study of emotion and coping during three stages of a college examination. *Journal of Personality and Social Psychology, 48*(1), 150.

Folkman, S., & Moskowitz, J. T. (2000). Positive affect and the other side of coping. *American Psychologist, 55*(6), 647.

Forgeard, M. J. C., & Seligman, M. E. P. (2012). Seeing the glass half full: A review of the causes and consequences of optimism. *Pratiques Psychologiques, 18*(2), 107–120. doi:http://dx.doi.org/10.1016/j.prps.2012.02.002

Frances, A. (2012). DSM-5 is a guide, not a Bible: Simply ignore its 10 worst changes. *Huffington Post Science.* www.huffingtonpost.com/allen-frances/dsm-5_b_2227626.html

Frank, G., (1984). The Boulder model: History, rationale, and critique. *Professional Psychology: Research and Practice, 15*(3), 417–435. doi:10.1037/0735-7028.15.3.417

Frankl, V. E. (1959). *From death-camp to existentialism: A psychiatrist's path to a new therapy.* Boston, MA: Beacon Press.

Frankl, V. E. (1985). *Man's search for meaning.* New York: Pocket.

Franklin, M. (2010). Affect regulation, mirror neurons, and the Third Hand: Formulating mindful empathic art interventions. *Art Therapy: Journal of the American Art Therapy Association, 27*(4), 160–167.

Franklin, M. (2016). Contemplative wisdom traditions in art therapy. In J. A. Rubin (Ed.), *Approaches to art therapy,* 3rd Ed. New York: Routledge.

Franklin, M., Farrelly-Hansen, M., Marek, B., Swan-Foster, N., & Wallingford, S. (2000). Transpersonal art therapy education. *Art Therapy, 17*(2), 101–110. doi:10.1080/07421656.2000.10129507

Franzini, L. R. (2001). Humor in therapy: The case for training therapists in its uses and risks. *Journal of General Psychology, 128*(2), 170–193.

Fredrickson, B. L. (1998). What good are positive emotions? *Review of General Psychology, 2*(3), 300.

Fredrickson, B. L. (2001). The role of positive emotions in positive psychology: The broaden-and-build theory of positive emotions. *The American Psychologist, 56*(3), 218–226.

Fredrickson, B. L. (2004). The broaden-and-build theory of positive emotions. *Philosophical Transactions of the Royal Society B: Biological Sciences, 359*(1449), 1367.

Fredrickson, B. L. (2009). *Positivity: Groundbreaking research reveals how to embrace the hidden strength of positive emotions, overcome negativity, and thrive.* New York: Crown.

Fredrickson, B. L. (2013). *Love 2.0: How our supreme emotion affects everything we feel, think, do, and become.* New York: Hudson Street Press.

Fredrickson, B. L., & Joiner, T. (2002). Positive emotions trigger upward spirals toward emotional well-being. *Psychological Science, 13*(2), 172.

Fredrickson, B. L., & Kurtz, L. E. (2011). Cultivating positive emotions to enhance human flourishing. In S. I. Donaldson, M. Csíkszentmihályi, & J. Nakamura (Eds.), *Applied positive psychology: Improving everyday life, health, schools, work, and society* (pp. 35–47). Hove: Routledge.

Fredrickson, B. L., Tugade, M. M., Waugh, C. E., & Larkin, G. R. (2003). What good are positive emotions in crisis? A prospective study of resilience and emotions following the terrorist attacks on the United States on September 11th, 2001. *Journal of Personality and Social Psychology, 84*(2), 365.

Freud, S. (1930). Civilization and Its Discontents. London: Penguin.

Freud, S. (1955). Two case histories ("Little Hans" and the "Rat Man"). Standard Edition, Vol. 10. London: Hogarth Press (original work published 1909).

Freud, S. (1957a). Creative writers and day-dreaming. Standard Edition, Vol. 9, pp. 141–153. London: Hogarth Press (original work published 1908).

Freud, S. (1957b). The unconscious. Standard Edition, Vol. 14, pp. 159–215. London: Hogarth Press (original work published 1915).

Freud, S. (1958). The dynamics of transference. Standard Edition, Vol. 12: 99–108. London: Hogarth (original work published 1912).

Frisch, M. (2006). *Quality of life therapy: Applying a life satisfaction approach to positive psychology and cognitive therapy.* Hoboken, NJ: Wiley & Sons.

Fulmer, C. A., Gelfand, M. J., Knuglanski, A. W., Kim-Prieto, C., Diener, E., Pierro, A., & Higgines, E. T. (2010). On "feeling right" in cultural contexts: How person-culture match affects self-esteem and subjective wellbeing. *Psychological Science, 21*(11), 1563–1569.

Gable, S. L., Gonzaga, G. C., & Strachman, A. (2006). Will you be there for me when things go right? Supportive responses to positive event disclosures. *Journal of Personality and Social Psychology, 91*(5), 904–917.

Gable, S. L., & Haidt, J. (2005). What (and why) is positive psychology? *Review of General Psychology, 9*(2), 103.

Gallese, V., Eagle, M. N., & Migone, P. (2007). Intentional attunement: Mirror neurons and the neural underpinnings of interpersonal relations. *Journal of the American Psychoanaytic Association, 55*, 131–175.

Gantt, L. (1990). *A validity study of the Formal Elements Art Therapy Scale (FEATS) for diagnostic information in patients' drawings* (Doctoral dissertation), University of Pittsburgh, Pittsburgh, PA.

Gantt, L. (2009). The Formal Elements Art Therapy Scale: A measurement system for global variables in art. *Art Therapy: Journal of the American Art Therapy Association, 26*(3), 6.

Gantt, L. & Tabone, C. (2011). The Formal Elements Art Therapy Scale and "Draw a person picking an apple from a tree." In Malchiodi, Cathy A. (Ed.), *Handbook of art therapy* (pp. 420–427). New York: Guilford Press.

Gantt, L., & Greenstone, L. (2016). Narrative art therapy in trauma treatment. In J. A. Rubin (Ed.), *Approaches to art therapy*, 3rd Ed. New York: Routledge.

Gantt, L. & Tinnin, L. W. (2007). Intensive trauma therapy of PTSD and dissociation: An outcome study. *The Arts in Psychotherapy, 34*(1), 69–80.

Gantt, L. & Tinnin, L. W. (2009). Support for a neurobiological view of trauma with implications for art therapy. *The Arts in Psychotherapy, 36*(3), 148–153. doi:http://dx.doi.org/10.1016/j.aip.2008.12.005

Gardner, H. (2011). *Frames of mind: The theory of multiple intelligences.* New York: Basic Books.

Garland, E. L., Fredrickson, B., Kring, A. M., Johnson, D. P., Meyer, P. S., & Penn, D. L. (2010). Upward spirals of positive emotions counter downward spirals of negativity: Insights from the broaden-and-build theory and affective neuroscience on the treatment of emotion dysfunctions and deficits in psychopathology. *Clinical Psychology Review, 30*(7), 849–864.

Gelso, C. J. (2002). Real relationship: The "something more" of psychotherapy. *Journal of Contemporary Psychotherapy, 32*(1), 35–40.

George, J. M., & Zhou, J. (2001). When openness to experience and conscientiousness are related to creative behavior: An interactional approach. *Journal of Applied Psychology, 86*(3), 513.

Gerity, L. (Producer). (2009). The Artist Happiness Challenge eWorkshop. www.artellaland.com/shop/index.php?main_page=product_info&products_id=626

Getzels, J. W., & Csíkszentmihályi, M. (1976). *The creative vision: A longitudinal study of problem finding in art.* New York: Wiley.

Gilbert, D. (2009). *Stumbling on happiness.* Toronto: Vintage Canada.

Giller, E. (1999). What is psychological trauma? www.soberrecovery.com/forums/friends-family-alcoholics/214177-what-psychological-trauma.html

Gipson, L. R. (2015). Is cultural competence enough? Deepening social justice pedagogy in art therapy. *Art Therapy: Journal of the American Art Therapy Association, 32*(3), 142–145. doi:10.1080/07421656.2015.1060835

Goleman, D. P. (1995). *Emotional intelligence: Why it can matter more than IQ for character, health and lifelong achievement.* New York: Bantam Books.

Goleman, D. (1998). *Working with emotional intelligence.* New York. Bantam Books.

Gorelick, K. (1989). Rappochement between the arts and psychotherapies: Metaphor the mediator. *The Arts in Psychotherapy, 16*, 149–155.

Gottlieb, M. C., Handelsman, M. M., & Knapp, S. (2008). Some principles for ethics education: Implementing the acculturation model. *Training and Education in Professional Psychology, 2*(3), 123–128. doi:10.1037/1931-3918.2.3.123

Gottman, J. M. (1999). *The marriage clinic: A scientifically-based marital therapy.* New York: W.W. Norton.

Gottman, J.M., & Silver, N. (2000). *Seven principles for making marriage work: A practical guide from the country's foremost relationship expert.* New York: Three Rivers Press.

Graham, S. M., Huang, J. Y., Clark, M. S., & Helgeson, V. S. (2008). The positives of negative emotions: Willingness to express negative emotions promotes relationships. *Personality and Social Psychology Bulletin, 34*(3), 394–406.

Graham, J. E., Lobel, M., Glass, P., & Lokshina, I. (2008). Effects of written anger expression in chronic pain patients: Making meaning from pain. *Journal of Behavioral Medicine*, *31*(3), 201–212. doi:10.1007/s10865-008-9149-4

Gross, J. J., & Levenson, R. W. (1993). Emotional suppression: Physiology, self-report, and expressive behavior. *Journal of Personality and Social Psychology*, 64, 970–998.

Gross, J. J., & Thompson, R. A. (2007). Emotion regulation: Conceptual foundations. In J. J. Gross (Ed.), *Handbook of emotion regulation* (pp. 3–24). New York: Guilford Press.

Gruber, J. (2011). A review and synthesis of positive emotion and reward disturbance in bipolar disorder. *Clinical Psychology and Psychotherapy*, *18*(5), 356–365. doi:10.1002/cpp.776

Gruber, J., Mauss, I. B., & Tamir, M. (2011). A dark side of happiness? How, when, and why happiness is not always good. *Perspectives on Psychological Science*, *6*(3), 222–233.

Guttmann, J., & Regev, D. (2004). The phenomenological approach to art therapy. *Journal of Contemporary Psychotherapy*, *34*(2), 153–162.

Haggbloom, S. J., Warnick, R., Warnick, J. E., Jones, V. K., Yarbrough, G. L., Russell, T. M., . . . & Monte, E. (2002). The 100 most eminent psychologists of the 20th century. *Review of General Psychology*, *6*(2), 139–152. doi:10.1037/1089-2680.6.2.139

Handelsman, M. M., Knapp, S., & Gottlieb, M. C. (2009). Positive ethics: Themes and variations. In C. R. Snyder, & S. J. Lopez (Eds.), *Oxford handbook of positive psychology* (pp. 105–113). Oxford: Oxford University Press.

Hanes, M. J. (1995). Utilizing road drawings as a therapeutic metaphor in art therapy. *Art Therapy: Journal of the American Art Therapy Association*, *34*(1), 19–23.

Hanson, R. (2009). *Buddha's brain: The practical neuroscience of happiness, love, and wisdom*. Oakland, CA: New Harbinger Publications

Harker, L., & Keltner, D. (2001). Expressions of positive emotion in women's college yearbook pictures and their relationship to personality and life outcomes across adulthood. *Journal of Personality and Social Psychology*, *80*(1), 112.

Hart, S. L., Vella, L., & Mohr, D. C. (2008). Relationships among depressive symptoms, benefit-finding, optimism, and positive affect in multiple sclerosis patients after psychotherapy for depression. *Health Psychology*, *27*(2), 230.

Hartz, L., & Thick, L. (2005). Art therapy strategies to raise self-esteem in female juvenile offenders: A comparison of art psychotherapy and art as therapy approaches. *Art Therapy: Journal of the American Art Therapy Association*, *22*(2), 70–80.

Hasan, H., & Hasan, T. F. (2009). Laugh yourself into a healthier person: A cross cultural analysis of the effects of varying levels of laughter on health. *International Journal of Medical Sciences*, *6*(4), 200–211.

Hass-Cohen, N. (2016). Review of the neuroscience of chronic trauma and adaptive resilient responding. In J. King. (Ed.), *Art therapy, trauma and neuroscience: Theoretical and practical perspectives*. London and New York: Routledge Publishers.

Hass-Cohen, N., & Carr, R. (2008). *Art therapy and clinical neuroscience*. London: Jessica Kingsley.

Hayes, S. C., Strosahl, K. D., & Wilson, K. G. (1999). *Acceptance and commitment therapy*. New York: Guilford Press.

Hays, R. E., & Lyons, S. J. (1981). The bridge drawing: A projective technique for assessment in art therapy. *The Arts in Psychotherapy*, *8*(3–4), 207–217. doi:http://dx.doi.org/10.1016/0197-4556(81)90033-2

Heckwolf, J. I., Bergland, M. C., & Mouratidis, M. (2014). Coordinating principles of art therapy and DBT. *The Arts in Psychotherapy, 41*(4), 329–335. doi:http://dx.doi.org/10.1016/j.aip.2014.03.006

Heintzelman, S. J., & King, L. A. (2014). Life is pretty meaningful. *American Psychologist, 69*(6), 561–574. doi:10.1037/a0035049

Helgeson, V. S., Reynolds, K. A., & Tomich, P. L. (2006). A meta-analytic review of benefit finding and growth. *Journal of Consulting and Clinical Psychology, 74*(5), 797–816. doi:10.1037/0022-006X.74.5.797

Henderson, P. (2012). *Empirical study of the healing nature of artistic expression using mandalas with the positive emotions of love and joy* (Doctoral Dissertation), Texas A&M University, College Station, TX.

Henderson, P., Rosen, S., Sotirova-Kohli, L., & Stephenson, K. (2009). *Expression of positive emotions of love and joy through creating mandalas: A therapeutic intervention.* Paper presented at the First World Congress on Positive Psychology, Philadelphia, PA.

Herth, K. A. (2001). Development and implementation of a Hope Intervention Program. *Oncology Nursing Forum, 28*(6), 1009–1016.

Hicks, J. A., & King, L. A. (2009). Meaning in life as a subjective judgment and a lived experience. *Social and Personality Psychology Compass, 3*(4), 638–653. doi:10.1111/j.1751-9004.2009.00193.x

Hill, A. K. G. (1945). *Art versus illness: A story of art therapy.* London: G. Allen and Unwin.

Hill, C., Thompson, B., & Corbett, M. (1992). The impact of therapist ability to perceive displayed and hidden client reactions on immediate outcome in first sessions of brief therapy. *Psychotherapy Research, 2*(2), 143–155.

Hinz, L. D. (2009). *Expressive therapies continuum: A framework for using art in therapy.* New York: Routledge.

Hinz, L. D. (2011). Embracing excellence: A positive approach to ethical decision making. *Art Therapy: Journal of the American Art Therapy Association, 28*(4), 185–188. doi:10.1080/07421656.2011.622693

Hiscox, A. R., & Calisch, A. C. (1998). *Tapestry of cultural issues in art therapy.* London: Jessica Kingsley.

Hocoy, D. (2005). Art therapy and social action: A transpersonal framework. *Art Therapy: Journal of the American Art Therapy Association, 22*(1), 7–16.

Holmes, T. H., and Rahe, R. (1967). The social readjustment rating scale. *Journal of Psychosomatic Research, 11*(2), 213–218.

Horay, B. J.(2006). Moving towards gray: Art therapy and ambivalence in substance abuse treatment. *Art Therapy: Journal of the American Art Therapy Association, 23*:1, 14–22, doi:10.1080/07421656.2006.10129528

Horney, K. (1951). The individual and therapy. *American Journal of Psychoanalysis, 11*(1), 54–55.

Horovitz, E. G. (2002). *Spiritual art therapy: An alternate path.* 2nd ed. Springfield, IL: Charles C. Thomas Publisher.

Horovitz, E. G. (2014). *The art therapist's primer: A clinical guide to writing assessments, diagnosis and treatment.* Springfield, IL: Charles C. Thomas.

Horwitz, A.V, & Wakefield, J. C. (2007). *The loss of sadness.* New York: Oxford.

Hovick, S. E. (2014). *The effectiveness of an arts based warm-up in facilitating the flow state* (Master of Arts in Art Therapy Thesis), Albertus Magnus College, New Haven, CT.

Howells, V., & Zelnik, T. (2009). Making art: A qualitative study of personal and group transformation in a community arts studio. *Psychiatric Rehabilitation Journal, 32*(3), 215–222. doi:10.2975/32.3.2009.215.222

Huckvale, K., & Learmonth, M. (2009). A case example of art therapy in relation to Dialectical Behaviour Therapy. *International Journal of Art Therapy, 14*(2), 52–63. doi:10.1080/17454830903329196

Huet, V. (2011). Art therapy-based organizational consultancy: A session at Tate Britain. *International Journal of Art Therapy, 16*(1), 3–13.

Hunt, C. (2004). Reading ourselves: Imagining the reader in the writing process. In G. Bolton, S. Howlett, C. Lago, & J. K. Wright (Eds.), *Writing cures: An introductory handbook of writing in counselling and therapy* (pp. 35–44). New York: Routledge.

Huss, E., & Sarid, O. (2014). Visually transforming artwork and guided imagery as a way to reduce work related stress: A quantitative pilot study. *The Arts in Psychotherapy, 41*, 409–412.

Innis, R. E. (2001). Perception, interpretation, and the signs of Art. *Journal of Speculative Philosophy, 15*(1), 20–32.

Isen, A. M. (2004). Positive affect facilitates thinking and problem solving. In A. S. Manstead & N. H. Frijda (Eds.), *Feelings and emotions: The Amsterdam Symposium* (pp. 263–281). Cambridge: Cambridge University Press.

Isis, P. D. (2015). Positive Art Therapy. In D. E. Gussak & M. L. Rosal (Eds.), *The Wiley handbook of art therapy*. Chichester: John Wiley & Sons, Ltd.

Italia, S., Favara-Scacco, C., Di Cataldo, A., & Russo, G. (2008). Evaluation and art therapy treatment of the burnout syndrome in oncology units. *Psycho-Oncology, 17*(7), 676–680. doi:10.1002/pon.1293

Jahoda, M. (1958). *Current concepts of positive mental health*. New York: Basic Books.

James, W. (1890/1950). *The Principles of Psychology*, 2 vols. New York: Dover Publications.

James, W. (1929). *The varieties of religious experience: A study in human nature*. New York: The Modern Library (original edition, 1902, New York and London: Longmans Green and Company).

James, W. (2004/1890). *The principles of psychology*. https://ia600203.us.archive.org/12/items/theprinciplesofp01jameuoft/theprinciplesofp01jameuoft.pdf

Johnson, C. M., & Sullivan-Marx, E. M. (2006). Art therapy: Using the creative process for healing and hope among African American older adults. *Geriatric Nursing, 27*(5), 309–316.

Johnson, K. J., & Fredrickson, B. L. (2005). "We all look the same to me": Positive emotions eliminate the own-race bias in face recognition. *Psychological Science, 16*(11), 875–881. doi:10.1111/j.1467-9280.2005.01631.x

Joseph, C. (2006). Creative alliance: The healing power of art therapy. *Art Therapy: Journal of the American Art Therapy Association, 23*(1), 30–33. doi:10.1080/074216 56.2006.10129531

Jung, C. G. (1959). *The collected works of C. G. Jung*. Volume 9, Part I. *The archetypes and the collective unconscious*. Eds. H. Read, M. Fordham, & G. Adler. Trans. R. F. C. Hull. New York: Pantheon Books.

Jung, C. G. (1965). *Memories, dreams, reflections*. Ed. A. Jaffe. Trans. R. and C. Winston. New York: Random House.

Jung, C. G. (1966/2014). *The spirit of man in art and literature*. London and New York: Routledge.

Jung, C. (1986). *Analytical psychology: Its theory and practice—The Tavistock lectures*. London: Ark Paperbacks.

Jung, C. G. (2009). *The red book: Liber novus.* New York: W.W. Norton & Co.

Jung, C. G. (2014). *The archetypes and the collective unconscious.* London and New York: Routledge.

Jung, C. G. (2015). *Jung on active imagination.* Princeton, NJ: Princeton University Press.

Junge, M. B., Alvarez, J. F., Kellogg, A., & Volker, C. (1993). The art therapist as social activist: Reflections and visions. *Art Therapy: Journal of the American Art Therapy Association, 10*(3), 148–155.

Junge, M. B., & Asawa. P (1994). *A history of art therapy in the United States.* Mundelien, IL: American Art Therapy Association.

Junge, M. B., & Linesch, D. (1993). Our own voices: New paradigms for art therapy research. *The Arts in Psychotherapy, 20*(1), 61–67. doi:10.1016/0197-4556(93)90032-W

Kabat-Zinn, J., (1991). *Full catastrophe living: Using the wisdom of your body and mind to face stress, pain, and illness.* New York: Bantam Doubleday.

Kabat-Zinn, J. (1994). *Wherever you go, there you are: Mindfulness meditation in everyday life.* New York: Hyperion.

Kabat-Zinn, J. (2003). Mindfulness-based interventions in context: Past, present, and future. *Clinical Psychology: Sccience and Practice, 10*(2), 144–156.

Kagin, S. L., & Lusebrink, V. B. (1978). The expressive therapies continuum. *Art Psychotherapy, 5*(4), 171–180.

Kahneman, D., Diener, E., & Schwarz, N. (Eds.). (1999). *Well-being: Foundations of hedonic psychology.* New York: Russell Sage Foundation.

Kaimal, G., Ray, K., & Muniz, J. (2016). Reduction of cortisol levels and participants' responses following art making. *Art Therapy: Journal of the American Art Therapy Association, 33*(2), 74–80.

Kaiser, D. H. (1996). Indications of attachment security in a drawing task. *The Arts in Psychotherapy, 23*(4), 333–340. doi:http://dx.doi.org/10.1016/0197-4556(96)00003-2

Kaiser, D., & Deaver, S. (2013). Establishing a research agenda for art therapy: A Delphi study. *Art Therapy: Journal of the American Art Therapy Association, 30*(3), 114–121.

Kapitan, L. (2010). *Introduction to art therapy research.* New York: Routledge/Taylor & Francis Group.

Kaplan, F. (2000). *Art, science, and art therapy: Repainting the picture.* London: Jessica Kingsley.

Kaplan, F. (2012). Cognitive-behavioral and mind-body approaches. In C. Malchiodi (Ed.), *Handbook of art therapy* (pp. 89–102). New York: Guilford.

Kashdan, T., & Biswas-Diener, R. (2014). *The upside of your dark side: Why being your whole self—not just your "good" self—drives success and fulfillment.* New York: Penguin.

Keen, S. (1974). The golden mean of Roberto Assagioli. *Psychology Today, 8,* 97–107.

Kellogg, J. (1978). *Mandala: Path of beauty.* Baltimore, MD: MARI, Inc.

Kellogg, R. (1967/2007): Rhoda Kellogg child art collection. Digital re-edition by D. Maurer, C. Riboni, K. Wälchli, & B. Gujer. www.early-pictures.ch/kellogg

Keyes, C. L. (2002). The mental health continuum: From languishing to flourishing in life. *Journal of Health and Social Behavior, 43*(2), 207–222.

Keyes, C. L. (2003). *Flourishing.* Wiley Online Library.

Keyes, C. L. (2007). Promoting and protecting mental health as flourishing: a complementary strategy for improving National Mental Health. *American Psychologist, 62,* 95–108.

Kiecolt-Glaser, J. K., McGuire, L., Robles, T. F., & Glaser, R. (2002). Psychoneuroim-munology: Psychological influences on immune function and health. *Journal of Consulting and Clinical Psychology, 70*(3), 537–547. doi:10.1037/0022-006X.70.3.537

Kimport, E. R., & Hartzell, E. (2015). Clay and anxiety reduction: A one-group, pretest/posttest design with patients on a psychiatric unit. *Art Therapy: Journal of the American Art Therapy Association, 32*(4), 184–189. doi: 10.1080/07421656.2015.1092802

King, L. (2001). The health benefits of writing about life goals. *Personality and Social Psychology Bulletin, 27*(7), 798.

Kimport, E. R., & Robbins, S. J. (2012). Efficacy of creative clay work for reducing negative mood: A randomized controlled trial. *Art Therapy: Journal of the American Art Therapy Association, 29*(2), 74–79. doi:10.1080/07421656.2012.680048

King, L. A. (2001). The health benefits of writing about life goals. *Personality and Social Psychology Bulletin, 27*(7), 798–807. doi:10.1177/0146167201277003

King, L. A. (2011). Are we there yet? What happened on the way to the demise of positive psychology. In Sheldon, K. M., Kashdan, T. B., & Steger, M. F. (Eds.), *Designing positive psychology: Taking stock and moving forward* (pp. 439–446). New York: Oxford University Press.

King, L. A. (2012). Meaning: Ubiquitous and effortless. In P. R. Shaver, & M. Mikulincer (Eds.), *Meaning, mortality, and choice: The social psychology of existential concerns.* (pp. 129–144). Washington, DC: American Psychological Association. http://dx.doi.org/10.1037/13748-007

King, L. A., Hicks, J. A., Krull, J. L., & Del Gaiso, A. K. (2006). Positive affect and the experience of meaning in life. *Journal of Personality and Social Psychology, 90*(1), 179–196. doi:10.1037/0022-3514.90.1.179

Kirby, L. D., Morrow, J., Yin, J. (2014). The challenge of challenge. In M. M. Tugade, M. N. Shiota, & L.D. Kirby (Eds.), *Handbook of positive emotions* (pp. 378–395). New York: Guildford Press.

Koch, S. C., Morlinghaus, K., & Fuchs, T. (2007). The joy dance: Specific effects of a single dance intervention on psychiatric patients with depression. *The Arts in Psychotherapy, 34*(4), 340–349.

Kofman, S. (1988). *The childhood of art: An interpretation of Freud's aesthetics.* New York: Columbia University Press.

Koltko-Rivera, M. E. (2004). The psychology of worldviews. *Review of General Psychology, 8*(1), 3–58. doi:10.1037/1089-2680.8.1.3

Kok, B. E., Coffey, K. A., Cohn, M. A., Catalino, L. I., Vacharkulksemsuk, T., Algoe, S. B., ... & Fredrickson, B. L. (2013). How positive emotions build physical health: Perceived positive social connections account for the upward spiral between positive emotions and vagal tone. *Psychological Science, 24*(7), 1123–1132. doi:10.1177/0956797612470827

Kongkasuwan, R., Voraakhom, K., Pisolayabutra, P., Maneechai, P., Boonin, J., & Kuptniratsaikul, V. (2015). Creative art therapy to enhance rehabilitation for stroke patients: A randomized controlled trial. *Clinical Rehabilitation.* doi:10.1177/0269215515607072

Kopytin, A., & Lebedev, A. (2013). Humor, self-attitude, emotions, and cognitions in group art therapy with war veterans. *Art Therapy: Journal of the American Art Therapy Association, 30*(1), 20–29. doi:10.1080/07421656.2013.757758

Kossak, M. (2012). Art-based enquiry: It is what we do! *Journal of Applied Arts and Health, 3*(1), 21–29. doi:10.1386/jaah.3.1.21_1

Kramer, E. (1958). *Art therapy in a children's community.* Springfield, IL: Charles C Thomas.

Kramer, E. (1971). *Art as therapy with children.* New York: Schocken Books.

Kramer, E. (1975). Art and emptiness: New problems in art education and art therapy. In E. Ulman & P. Dachinger (Eds.), *Art therapy in theory and practice,* 1st Ed. (pp. 3–13). New York: Schocken Books.

Kreibig, S. D. (2014). Autonomic nervous system aspects of positive emotions. In M. M. Tugade, M. N. Shiota, and L. D. Kirby (Eds.), *Handbook of positive emotions* (pp. 133–158). New York: Guildford Press.

Kreitler, H., & Kreitler, S. (1972). *Psychology of the arts.* Durham, NC: Duke University Press.

Kübler-Ross, E. (2009). *On death and dying: What the dying have to teach doctors, nurses, clergy and their own families.* New York: Taylor & Francis.

Kuchta, S. (2008). Quantifying the physiological and psychological effects of art making through heart rate variability and mood measurements (Unpublished master's thesis), Albertus Magnus College, New Haven, CT.

Kwiatkowska, H. (1967). Family art therapy. *Family Process, 6,* 37–55. doi:10.111 1/j.1545-5300.1967.00037

Lachman-Chapin, M. (1987). A self-psychology approach to art therapy. In J. A. Rubin (Ed.), *Approaches to art therapy: Theory and technique* (pp. 75–91). New York: Brunner/Mazel.

Lambert, M. J., & Barley, D. E. (2001). Research summary on the therapeutic relationship and psychotherapy outcome. *Psychotherapy: Theory, Research, Practice, Training, 38*(4), 357–361.

Lambert, N. M., Graham, S. M., Fincham, F. D., & Stillman, T. F. (2009). A changed perspective: How gratitude can affect sense of coherence through positive reframing. *Journal of Positive Psychology, 4*(6), 461–470. doi:10.1080/17439760 903157182

Lambert. N. M., Fincham, F. D., Gwinn, A. M. & Ajayi, C. A. (2011). Positive relationship science: A new frontier for positive psychology? In K. Sheldon, T. Kashdan, and M. Steger (Eds.), *Designing the future of positive psychology: Taking stock and moving forward* (pp. 265–279). Oxford: Oxford University Press.

Lambert, J., & Ranger, D. (2009), L'art therapie et la psychologie positive: Ensemble pour le deploiement des forces de vie. *Revue Quebecoise de Psychologie, 30*(30), 57–70.

Landgarten, H. B. (1981). *Clinical art therapy.* New York: Brunner/Mazel.

Langer, S. (1953). *Feeling and form: A theory of art.* New York: Scribner.

Langer, S. (1957). *Philosophy in a new key: A study in the symbolism of reason, rite, and art.* Cambridge, MA: Harvard University Press.

Larsen, R. (2009). The contributions of positive and negative affect to emotional well-being. *Psihologijske teme, 18*(2), 247–266.

Latto, R., (1995). The brain of the beholder. In R. L. Gregory, J. Harris, P. Heard, & D. Rose (Eds.), *The artful eye* (pp. 66–94). Oxford: Oxford University Press.

Lawrence, R. (2008). *Artful inquiry: Reclaiming indigenous knowledge.* Presentation at the Midwest Research-to-Practice Conference in Adult, Continuing, and Community Education, Western Kentucky University, Bowling Green, KY.

Layous, K., Chancellor, J., Lyubomirsky, S., Wang, L., & Doraiswamy, P. M. (2011). Delivering happiness: Translating positive psychology intervention research for treating major and minor depressive disorders. *Journal of Alternative and Complementary Medicine, 17*(8), 1–9.

Lazarus, R. S. (2003). Does the positive psychology movement have legs? *Psychological Inquiry, 14*(2), 93–109.

Leavy, P. (2015). *Method meets art: Arts-based research practice*, 2nd ed. New York: Guilford Press.

Lee, S. Y. (2009). The experience of "flow" in artistic expression: Case studies of immigrant Korean children with adjustment difficulties (Unpublished doctoral dissertation), Teachers College, Columbia University, New York, NY.

Lee, S. Y. (2013). "Flow" in art therapy: Empowering immigrant children with adjustment difficulties. *Art Therapy: Journal of the American Art Therapy Association, 30*(2), 56–63. doi:10.1080/07421656.2013.786978

Lewin K. (1943). Defining the "field at a given time." *Psychological Review, 50,* 292–310. Republished in idem., *Resolving social conflicts and field theory in social science.* Washington, DC: American Psychological Association, 1997.

Lieberman, E. J. (1985). *Acts of will: The life and work of Otto Rank.* New York: Free Press.

Lightsey, O. R. (2006). Resilience, meaning, and well-being. *The Counseling Psychologist, 34*(1), 96–107. doi:10.1177/0011000005282369

Lineham, M. M. (1987). *Dialectical behavior therapy for borderline personality disorder.* New York: Guilford Press.

Linehan, M. M. (1993). *Cognitive behavioral therapy of borderline personality disorder* (Vol. 51). New York: Guilford Press.

Linesch, D. G. (1988). *Adolescent art therapy.* London: Routledge.

Linley, A. P. (2015). Use your strengths to achieve your goals and be happy. http://blog.cappeu.com/2015/01/20/use-your-strengths-to-ach

Linley, A. P., & Dovey, H. (2012). *Technical manual and statistical properties for Realise2.* www.cappeu.com/Portals/3/Files/Realise2_Technical_Manual_V1.3_Dec_2012.pdf

Linley, A. P., & Harrington, S. (2006a). Playing to your strengths. *Psychologist, 19,* 86–89.

Linley, A. P., & Harrington, S. (2006b). Strengths coaching: A potential-guided approach to coaching psychology. *International Coaching Psychology Review, 1*(1), 37–46.

Linley, A. P., Nielsen, K. M., Gillett, R., & Biswas-Diener, R. (2010). Using signature strengths in pursuit of goals: Effects on goal progress, need satisfaction, and well-being, and implications for coaching psychologists. *International Coaching Psychology Review, 5*(1), 6–15.

Linnenbrink-Garcia, L., Rogat, T. K., & Koskey, K.L. (2011). Affect and engagement during small group instruction. *Contemporary Educational Psychology, 36,* 13–24.

Lipton, M. (1996). Demystifying the development of an organizational vision. *Sloan Management Review, 34*(4), 83–92.

Lombardo, T. (2011). Creativity, wisdom, and our evolutionary future. *Journal of Futures Studies, 16*(1), 19–46.

Lowenfeld, V. (1957). *Creative and mental growth,* 3rd. ed. Oxford: Macmillan.

Lundgren, T., Luoma, J. B., Dahl, J., Strosahl, K., & Melin, L. (2012). The bull's-eye values survey: A psychometric evaluation. *Cognitive and Behavioral Practice, 19*(4), 518–526. doi:http://dx.doi.org/10.1016/j.cbpra.2012.01.004

Lusebrink, V. B. (1990). *Imagery and visual expression in therapy.* New York: Plenum Press.

Lusebrink, V. B. (2004). Art therapy and the brain: An attempt to understand the underlying processes of art expression in therapy. *Art Therapy: Journal of the American Art Therapy Association, 21*(3), 125–135. doi:10.1080/07421656.2004.10129496

Lusebrink, V. B. (2010). Assessment and theraputic application of the Expressive Therapies Continuum: Implications for brain stuctures and functions. *Art Therapy: Journal of the American Art Therapy Association, 27*(4), 168–177.

Lykken, D., & Tellegen, A. (1996). Happiness is a stochastic phenomenon. *Psychological Science, 7*, 186–189.

Lyubomirsky, S. (2008). *The how of happiness: A scientific approach to getting the life you want.* New York: Penguin.

Lyubomirsky, S., King, L., & Diener, E. (2005). The benefits of frequent positive affect: Does happiness lead to success? *Psychological Bulletin, 131*(6), 803–855.

Lyubomirsky, S., Sheldon, K., & Schkade, D. (2005). Pursuing happiness: The architecture of sustainable change. *Review of General Psychology, 9*(2), 111–131.

Maclagan, D. (2001). *Psychological aesthetics: Painting, feeling, and making sense.* London: Jessica Kingsley.

Maddux, J. E. (2002). Stopping the "madness." In C. R. Snyder & S. Lopez (Eds.), *Oxford handbook of positive psychology* (pp. 13–25). New York: Oxford University Press.

Maddux, J. E. (2008). Positive psychology and the illness ideology: Toward a positive clinical psychology. *Applied Psychology: An International Review, 57*, 54–70 doi:10.1111/j.1464-0597.2008.00354.x

Maier, S. F., & Seligman, M. E. (1976). Learned helplessness: Theory and evidence. *Journal of Experimental Psychology: General, 105*(1), 3–46. doi:10.1037/0096-3445.105.1.3

Malchiodi, C. A. (2002). *The soul's palette: Drawing on art's transformative powers for health and well-being.* Boston, MA: Shambhala Publications.

Malchiodi, C. A. (2006). *The art therapy sourcebook.* New York: McGraw-Hill.

Malchiodi, C. A. (2011). *Handbook of art therapy,* 2nd ed. New York: Guilford Press.

Malchiodi, C. A., & Loth Rozum, A. (2011). Cognitive-behavioral and mind-body approaches. In C. Malchiodi (Ed.), *Handbook of art therapy* (pp. 89–102). New York: Guilford Press.

Manheim, A. (1998). The relationship between the artistic process and self-actualization. *Art Therapy: Journal of the American Art Therapy Association, 15*(2), 99–106.

Marcia, J. E. (1993). The ego identity status approach to ego identity. In J. E. Marcia, A. S. Waterman, D. R. Matteson, S. L. Archer, & J. L. Orlofsky (Eds.), *Ego identity* (pp. 3–21). New York: Springer.

Maslach, C. (1982). *Burnout: The cost of caring.* Englewood Cliffs, NJ: Prentice-Hall.

Maslow, A. (1943). A theory of human motivation. *Psychological Review, 50*(4), 370–396.

Maslow, A. (1971). *The farther reaches of human nature.* New York: Viking Press.

Masten, A. S., & Coatsworth, J. D. (1998). The development of competence in favorable and unfavorable environments: Lessons from research on successful children. *American Psychologist, 53*(2), 205.

May, R. (1975). *The courage to create.* Oxford: Norton.

McCraty, R., & Childre, D. (2004). The grateful heart: The psychophysiology of appreciation. In R. A. Emmons & M. E. McCullough (Eds.), *The psychology of gratitude* (pp. 230). New York: Oxford University Press.

McCrea, R. R., & Costa, P. T., Jr. (2003). *Personality in adulthood: A five-factor theory perspective.* New York: Guilford Press.

McGregor, I., & Little, B. R. (1998). Personal projects, happiness, and meaning: On doing well and being yourself. *Journal of Personality and Social Psychology, 74*(2), 494.

McKnight, P. E., &. Kashdan, T.B. (2009). Purpose in life as a system that creates and sustains health and well-being: an integrative, testable theory. *Review of General Psychology, 13*(3), 242.

McNamee, C. M. (2005). Bilateral art: Integrating art therapy, family therapy and neuroscience. *Contemporary Family Therapy, 27*(4), 545–557.

McNiff, S. (1974). *Art therapy at Danvers.* Andover, MA: Addison Gallery of American Art (Exhibition brochure, 1972).

McNiff, S. (1992). *Art as medicine: Creating a therapy of the imagination.* Boston, MA: Shambhala.

McNiff, S. (1998). *Art-based research.* London: Jessica Kingsley.

McNiff, S. (2004). *Art heals: How creativity cures the soul.* Boston, MA: Shambhala Publications.

McNiff, S. (2015). *Imagination in action: Secrets for unleashing creative expression.* Boston, MA: Shambhala Publications.

McNiff, S. (2016). Ch'i and artistic expression: An East Asian worldview that fits the creative process everywhere. *Creative Arts Education and Therapy: Frontiers in China—An International Academic Journal for Research and Practice, 2*(2), 12–22.

Miller, E.T., (2012). Benefits of volunteering. *Rehabilitation Nursing, 37*(3), 90.

Miller, W. R., & Rollnick, S. (2002). *Motivational interviewing: Preparing people for change,* 2nd ed. New York: Guilford Press.

Mills, A. (2011). The diagnostic drawing series. In Malchiodi, C. A. (Ed.) *Handbook of art therapy* (pp. 401–409). New York: Guilford Press.

Molnar, A., & de Shazer, S. (1987). Solution-focused therapy: Toward the identification of therapeutic tasks. *Journal of Marital and Family Therapy, 13*(4), 349–358. doi:10.1111/j.1752-0606.1987.tb00716.x

Moneta, G. B. (2004). The flow experience across cultures. *Journal of Happiness Studies, 5*(2), 115–121.

Monti, D., Peterson, C., Kunkel, E., Hauck, W., Pequignot, E., Rhodes, L., & Brainard, G. (2006). A randomized, controlled trial of mindfulness based art therapy (MBAT) for women with cancer. *Psycho-Oncology, 15*(5), 363–373.

Moon, B. L. (2004). *Art and soul: Reflections on an artistic psychology.* Springfield, IL: Charles C. Thomas.

Moon, B. L. (2008). *Introduction to art therapy: Faith in the product.* Springfeld, IL: Charles C. Thomas.

Moon, B. L. (2009). *Existential art therapy: The canvas mirror.* Springfeld, IL: Charles C. Thomas.

Moon, B. L. (2012). *The dynamics of art as therapy with adolescents.* Springfield, IL: Charles C. Thomas Publisher.

Moon, B. L. (2016). Humanism in action. In J. A. Rubin (Ed.), *Approaches to art therapy: Theory and technique* (pp. 203–211). New York: Routledge.

Moon, C. H. (2011). *Materials and media in art therapy: Critical understandings of diverse artistic vocabularies.* New York: Routledge.

Mooney, K. (2000). Focusing on solutions through art: A case study. *Australian and New Zealand Journal of Family Therapy, 21*(1), 34–41.

Moreno, J. (1947). Organization of the social atom. *Sociometry, 10*(3), 287–293. doi:10.2307/2785079

Morrison, L. J. (2013). *Talking back to psychiatry: The psychiatric consumer/survivor/ ex-patient movement.* New York: Routledge.

Moskowitz, J. T. (2010). Coping intereventions and the regulation of positive affect. In S. F. P. E. Nathan (Ed.), *The Oxford handbook of stress, health and coping* (pp. 407–420). Oxford: Oxford University Press.

Mulholland, M. J. (2004). Comics as art therapy. *Art Therapy: Journal of the American Art Therapy Association, 21*(1), 42–43.

Myers, D. G., & Diener, E. (1996). The pursuit of happiness. *Scientific American, 274*(5), 70–72.

Myers, I. B. (1998). *MBTI manual: A guide to the development and use of the Myers-Briggs Type Indicator*. Palo Alto, CA: Consulting Psychologists Press, Incorporated.

Nainis, N., Paice, J. A., Ratner, J., Wirth, J. H., Lai, J., & Shott, S. (2006). Relieving symptoms in cancer: Innovative use of art therapy. *Journal of Pain and Symptom Management, 31*(2), 162–169.

Nakamura, J., & Csíkszentmihályi, M. (2002). The concept of flow. In C. R. Snyder & S. Lopez (Eds.), *Oxford handbook of positive psychology* (pp. 89–105). New York: Oxford University Press.

Naumburg, M. (1958). Art therapy: Its scope and function. In E. F. Hammer (Ed.), *The clinical application of projective drawings* (pp. 511–517). Springfield, IL: Charles C. Thomas.

Naumburg, M. (1966). *Dynamically oriented art therapy: Its principles and practices, illustrated with three case studies*. Orlando, FL: Grune & Stratton.

Neff, K. D. (2003). The development and validation of a scale to measure self-compassion. *Self and Identity, 2*(3), 223–250.

Nickerson, R. S. (1998). Confirmation bias: A ubiquitous phenomenon in many guises. *Review of General Psychology, 2*(2), 175–220. doi:10.1037/1089-2680.2.2.175

Niemiec, R. M. (2013). *Mindfulness and character strengths: A practical guide to flourishing*. USA and Germany: Hogrefe Verlag.

Nobis, W. (2010). *The art of recovery: A reflective and creative path through the Twelve Steps*. Mustang, OK: Tate Publishing.

Nucho, A.O. (2003). *The psychocybernetic model of art therapy*. Springfield, IL: Charles C. Thomas.

Oatley, K., & Djikic, M. (2008). Writing as thinking. *Review of General Psychology, 12*(1), 9–27.

Oishi, S., Diener, E., & Lucas, R. E. (2007). The optimum level of well-being: Can people be too happy? *Perspectives on Psychological Science, 2*(4), 346–360.

Öster, I., Magnusson, E., Thyme, K. E., Lindh, J. & Åström, S. (2007). Art therapy for women with breast cancer: The therapeutic consequences of boundary strengthening. *The Arts in Psychotherapy, 34*(3), 277–288.

Öster, I., Svensk, A. C., Magnusson, E., Thyme, K. E., Sjodin, M., Åström, S. and Lindh, J. (2006). Art therapy improves coping resources: A randomized, controlled study among women with breast cancer. *Palliative and Supportive Care, 4*(1), 57–64.

Otake, K., Shimai, S., Tanaka-Matsumi, J., Otsui, K., & Fredrickson, B. (2006). Happy people become happier through kindness: A counting kindnesses intervention. *Journal of Happiness Studies, 7*, 361–375.

Panksepp, J., & Biven, L. (2012). *The archaeology of mind: Neuroevolutionary origins of human emotions*. New York: Norton.

Park, C. L. (2010). Making sense of the meaning literature: An integrative review of meaning making and its effects on adjustment to stressful life events. *Psychological Bulletin, 136*(2), 257.

Park, C. L. (2011). Meaning and growth within positive psychology: Toward a more complete understanding. In K. M. Sheldon, T. Kashdan, & M. Steger (Eds.), *Designing positive psychology* (pp. 324–334). New York: Oxford University Press.

Park, C. L., & Blumberg, C. J. (2002). Disclosing trauma through writing: Testing the meaning-making hypothesis. *Cognitive Therapy and Research, 26*(5), 597–616. doi:10.1023/a:1020353109229

Park, N., & Peterson, C. (2006). Character strengths and happiness among young children: Content analysis of parental descriptions. *Journal of Happiness Studies, 7*(3), 323–341.

Park, N., & Peterson, C. (2010). Does it matter where we live? The urban psychology of character strengths. *American Psychologist, 65*(6), 535–547. doi:10.1037/a0019621

Pascual-Leone, A., & Greenberg, L. S. (2007). Emotional processing in experiential therapy: Why the only way out is through. *Journal of Consulting and Clinical Psychology, 75*(6), 875.

Pearson, C. (1991). *Awakening the heroes within: Twelve archetypes to help us find ourselves and transform the world.* New York: HarperOne.

Pennebaker, J. W. (1993). Putting stress into words: Health, linguistic, and therapeutic implications. *Behaviour Research and Therapy, 31*(6), 539–548. doi:10.1016/0005-7967(93)90105-4

Perls, F., & Perls, L. (1947). *Ego hunger and aggression: A revision of Freud's theory and method.* Goldsboro, ME: The Gestalt Journal Press.

Perry, B. (2009). Examining child maltreatment through a neurodevelopmental lens: clinical applications of the neurosequential model of therapeutics. *Journal of Loss and Trauma, 14*(4), 240–255.

Peter, C., Geyh, S., Ehde, D., Muller, R., & Jensen, M. (2015). Positive psychology in rehabilitation psychology research and practice. In S. Joseph (Ed.), *Positive psychology in practice: Promoting human flourishing in work, health, education, and everyday life*, 2nd ed. Hoboken, NJ: Wiley.

Peterson, C. (2006). *A primer in positive psychology.* New York: Oxford University Press.

Peterson, C. (2013). Mindfulness-based art therapy. In L. Rappaport (Ed.), *Mindfulness and the arts therapies: Theory and practice* (pp. 64–80). London: Jessica Kingsley.

Peterson, C., & Park, N. (2009). Classifying and measuring strengths of character. In C. R. Snyder & S. J. Lopez (Eds.), *Oxford handbook of positive psychology*, 2nd ed. (pp. 25–33). New York: Oxford University Press.

Peterson, C., Park, N., & Seligman, M. E. (2006). Greater strengths of character and recovery from illness. *Journal of Positive Psychology*, (1), 17–26.

Peterson, C., Park, N., Steen, T. A., & Seligman, M. E. P. (2006). The authentic happiness inventory (Unpublished manuscript), University of Michigan.

Peterson, C., & Seligman, M. E. P. (2004). *Character strengths and virtues: A handbook and classification.* New York: Oxford University Press.

Pham, M. T. (2007). Emotion and rationality: A critical review and interpretation of empirical evidence. *Review of General Psychology, 11*(2), 155.

Physicians' desk reference, 67th ed. (2013). Montvale, NJ: PDR Network

Pinkola Estés, C. (1992). *Women who run with the wolves.* London: Rider.

Pizarro, J. (2004). The efficacy of art and writing therapy: Increasing positive mental health outcomes and participant retention after exposure to traumatic experience. *Art Therapy: Journal of the American Art Therapy Association, 21*(1), 5–12.

Plato (1992). *The Republic.* Rev. C. D. C. Reeve. Trans. G. M. A. Grube. Indianapolis, IN: Hackett.

Pomeroy, L., & Weatherall, A. (2014). Responding to client laughter as therapeutic actions in practice. *Qualitative Research in Psychology, 11*(4), 1–15.

Post, S. G. (2005). Altruism, happiness, and health: It's good to be good. *International Journal of Behavioral Medicine, 12*(2), 66–77.

Potash, J. S. (2005). Rekindling the multicultural history of the American Art Therapy Association, Inc. *Art Therapy: Journal of the American Art Therapy Association, 22*(4), 184–188. doi:10.1080/07421656.2005.10129522

Potash, J. S. (2011). Art therapists as intermediaries for social change. *Journal of Art for Life, 2*(1), 48–58.

Potash, J. S., Mann, S. M., Martinez, J. C., Roach, A. B., & Wallace, N. M. (2016). Spectrum of art therapy practice: Systematic literature review of art therapy, 1983–2014. *Art Therapy: Journal of the American Art Therapy Association, 33*(3), 119–127.

Proctor, C., Tsukayama, E., Wood, A. M., Maltby, J., Eades, J. F., & Linley, P. A. (2011). Strengths gym: The impact of a character strengths-based intervention on the life satisfaction and well-being of adolescents. *Journal of Positive Psychology, 6*(5), 377–388. doi:10.1080/17439760.2011.594079

Puig, A., Lee, S. M., Goodwin, L., & Sherrard, P. A. D. (2006). The efficacy of creative arts therapies to enhance emotional expression, spirituality, and psychological well-being of newly diagnosed Stage I and Stage II breast cancer patients: A preliminary study. *The Arts in Psychotherapy, 33*(3), 218–228.

Radel, D. M. (2015). *The effects of Self-Book© art therapy on emotional distress in female cancer patients: A randomized controlled trial* (Doctoral dissertation), Drexel University, Philadelphia, PA. ProQuest Publication Number 3689731; https://idea. library.drexel.edu/islandora/object/idea%3A6147

Rappaport, L. (2008). *Focusing-oriented art therapy: Accessing the body's wisdom and creative intelligence.* London: Jessica Kingsley.

Rappaport, L. (2013). *Mindfulness and the arts therapies: Theory and practice.* London: Jessica Kingsley.

Rashid, T. (2014). Positive psychotherapy: A strength-based approach. *Journal of Positive Psychology,* 1–16. doi:10.1080/17439760.2014.920411

Rath, T., & Reckmeyer, M. (2009). *How full is your bucket? For kids.* Washington, DC: Gallup Press.

Reis, H. T., & Gable, S. L. (2003). Toward a positive psychology of relationships. In C. L. M. Keyes & J. Haidt (Eds.). *Flourishing: Positive psychology and the life well-lived* (pp. 129–159). Washington, DC: American Psychological Association.

Resnick, S., Warmoth, A., & Serlin, I. A. (2001). The humanistic psychology and positive psychology connection: Implications for psychotherapy. *Journal of Humanistic Psychology, 41*(1), 73–101. doi:10.1177/0022167801411006

Reynolds, F., & Prior, S. (2003). "A lifestyle coat-hanger": A phenomenological study of the meanings of artwork for women coping with chronic illness and disability. *Disability and Rehabilitation, 25*(14), 785–794.

Reynolds, F., & Prior, S. (2006). Creative adventures and flow in art-making: A qualitative study of women living with cancer. *British Journal of Occupational Therapy, 69*(6), no pagination specified.

Rhodes, G., Brake, S., Tan, S., & Taylor, K. (1989). Expertise and configural coding in face recognition. *British Journal of Psychology, 80,* 313–331.

Rhyne, J. (1973). *The gestalt art experience.* Monterey, CA: Brooks/Cole.

Rhyne, J. (2001a). Gestalt art therapy. In J. A. Rubin (Ed.), *Approaches to art therapy: Theory and technique,* 2nd ed. (pp. 134–148). New York: Routledge.

Rhyne, J., (2001b). The gestalt approach to experience, art, and art therapy. *Art Therapy: Journal of the American Art Therapy Association, 40*(1), 109–20.

Ricks, L., Hancock, E., Goodrich, T., & Evans, A. (2014). Laughing for acceptance: A counseling intervention for working with families. *The Family Journal, 22*(4), 397–401. doi:10.1177/1066480714547175

Riddle, J. A., & riddle [*sic*], h. m. (2007). Men and art therapy: A connection through strengths. *Art Therapy: Journal of the American Art Therapy Association, 24*(1), 10–15.

Riley, S. (1999). *Contemporary art therapy with adolescents.* London: Jessica Kingsley.

Riley, S. (2013). *Group process made visible: The use of art in group therapy.* New York: Routledge.

Riley-Hiscox, A. (1997). Interview: Cliff Joseph—Art therapist, pioneer, artist. *Art Therapy: Journal of the American Art Therapy Association, 14*(4), 273–278. doi:10.1 080/07421656.1987.10759297

Rimé, B. (2009). Emotion elicits the social sharing of emotion: Theory and empirical review. *Emotion Review, 1*(1), 60–85.

Roediger, I. H. L. (2004). Presidential column: What happened to behaviorism. www.psychologicalscience.org/index.php/uncategorized/what-happened-to-behaviorism.html

Rogatko, T. (2009). The influence of flow on positive affect in college students. *Journal of Happiness Studies, 10*(2), 133–148.

Rogers, C. R. (1951). *Client-centered therapy: Its current practice, implications, and theory.* Boston, MA: Houghton Mifflin.

Rogers, C. R. (1963). *Actualizing tendency in relation to "Motives" and to consciousness.* Paper presented at the Nebraska Symposium on Motivation.

Rogers, C. R. (1975). Empathic: An unappreciated way of being. *The Counseling Psychologist, 5*(2), 2–10.

Rogers, C. R. (1978). *Carl Rogers on personal power.* New York: Dell.

Rogers, N. (1993). *The creative connection: Expressive arts as healing.* Palo Alto, CA: Science & Behavior Books.

Rosal, M. (2016). Cognitive-behavioral art therapy. In J. A. Rubin (Ed.), *Approaches to art therapy: Theory and technique,* Vol. 3 (pp. 210–225). New York: Routledge.

Rose, S., Elkis-Abuhoff, D., Goldblatt, R., & Miller, E. (2012). Hope against the rain: Investigating the psychometric overlap between an objective and projective measure of hope in a medical student sample. *The Arts in Psychotherapy, 39*(4), 272–278. doi:http://dx.doi.org/10.1016/j.aip.2012.04.003

Rubak, S., Sandbæk, A., Lauritzen, T., & Christensen, B. (2005). Motivational interviewing: a systematic review and meta-analysis. *British Journal of General Practice, 55*(513), 305–312.

Rubin, J. A. (1978). *Child art therapy: Understanding and helping children grow through art.* New York: Van Nostrand Reinhold.

Rubin, J. A. (1982). Art therapy: What it is and what it is not. *Art Therapy: Journal of the American Art Therapy Association, 21*(2), 57–58.

Rubin, J. A. (1999). *Art therapy: An introduction.* Philadelphia, PA: Brunner-Routledge.

Rubin, J. A. (2011). *The art of art therapy: What every art therapist needs to know.* New York: Routledge.

Rubin, J. A. (2016). *Approaches to art therapy,* 3rd ed. New York: Routledge.

Ruvolo, A. P. (1998). Marital well-being and general happiness of newlywed couples: Relationships across time. *Journal of Social and Personal Relationships, 15*(4), 470–489.

Ryan, M. B. (2008). The transpersonal William James. *Journal of Transpersonal Psychology, 40*(1), 20–40.

Ryan, R. M. & Deci, E. L. (2000). Self-determination theory and the facilitation of intrinsic motivation, social development, and well-being. *American Psychologist, 55*(1), 68–78. doi.org/10.1037/0003-066X.55.1.68

Ryan, R. M., & Deci, E. L. (2001). On happiness and human potentials: A review of research on hedonic and eudaimonic well-being. *Annual Review of Psychology, 52*(1), 141–166.

Ryan, R. M. & Frederick C. M. (1997). On energy, personality, and health: Subjective vitality as a dynamic reflection of well-being. *Journal of Personality, 65*(3), 529–565.

Ryff, C. D. (1989). Happiness is everything, or is it? Explorations on the meaning of psychological well-being. *Journal of Personality and Social Psychology, 57*(6), 1069.

Ryff, C. D. (2014). Psychological wellbeing revisited: Advances in the science and practices of eudaimonia. *Psychotherapy and Psychosomatics, 83*, 10–28. doi:10.1159/000353263

Ryff, C. D., & Keyes, C. L. M. (1995). The structure of psychological well-being revisited. *Journal of Personality and Social Psychology, 69*(4), 719.

Saleebey, D. (1996). The strengths perspective in social work practice: Extensions and cautions. *Social Work, 41*(3), 296–305.

Salovey, P., Rothman, A. J., Detweiler, J. B., & Steward, W. T. (2000). Emotional states and physical health. *American Psychologist, 55*(1), 110–121. doi:10.1037/0003-066X.55.1.110

Salzano, A. T., Lindemann, E., & Trotsky, L. N. (2013). The effectiveness of a collaborative art-making task on reducing stress in hospice caregivers. *The Arts In Psychotherapy, 40*(1), 45–52. doi:10.1016/j.aip.2012.09.008

Sandmire, D. A., Rankin, N. E., Gorham, S. R., Eggleston, D. T., French, C. A., Lodge, E. E., . . . & Grimm, D. R. (2015). Psychological and autonomic effects of art making in college-aged students. *Anxiety, Stress, and Coping,* 1–9. doi:10.1080/10615806.2015.1076798

Schaverien, J., (1999). *The revealing image: Analytical art psychotherapy in theory and practice.* London: Jessica Kingsley.

Scheier, M. F. & Carver, C. S. (1993). On the power of positive thinking: The benefits of being optimistic. *Current Directions in Psychological Science, 2*(1), 26–38.

Scheinberg, P. (2012). *Exploring hope and quality of life: A proposal for a group art therapy hope intervention for individuals diagnosed with lupus* (Master's Thesis), Eastern Virginia Medical School, Norfolk, VA.

Scherer, K. R. (2005). What are emotions? And how can they be measured? *Social Science Information, 44*(4), 695–729. doi:10.1177/0539018405058216

Schreibman, R., & Chilton, G. (2012). Small waterfalls in art therapy supervision: A poetic appreciative inquiry. *Art Therapy: Journal of the American Art Therapy Association, 29*(4), 188–191. doi:10.1080/07421656.2012.730924

Schwartz, C., Meisenhelder, J. B., Ma, Y., & Reed, G. (2003). Altruistic social interest behaviors are associated with better mental health. *Psychosomatic Medicine, 65*(5), 778–785.

Schwartz, S. H. (2012). An overview of the Schwartz theory of basic values. *Online Readings in Psychology and Culture, 2*(1). http://dx.doi.org/10.9707/230

Sears, S., Stanton, A., & Danoff-Burg, S. (2003). The Yellow Brick Road and the Emerald City: Benefit finding, positive reappraisal coping, and posttraumatic growth in women with early-stage breast cancer. *Health Psychology*, *22*(5), 487–497.

Seery, M. D. (2011). Resilience: A silver lining to experiencing adverse life events? *Current Directions in Psychological Science*, *20*(6), 390–394.

Seligman, M. E. P. (1998). Building human strength: Psychology's forgotten mission. *APA Monitor*, *29*(1).

Seligman, M. E. P. (1999). The president's address. *American Psychologist*, *54*, 559–562.

Seligman, M. E. P. (2002a). *Authentic happiness: Using the new positive psychology to realize your potential for lasting fulfillment.* New York: Free Press.

Seligman, M. E. P. (2002b). Positive psychology, positive prevention, and positive therapy. In C. R. Synder & S. Lopez (Eds.), *Oxford handbook of positive psychology* (pp. 3–12). New York: Oxford University Press.

Seligman, M. E. P. (2006/2011). *Learned optimism: How to change your mind and your life.* New York: Vintage.

Seligman, M. E. P. (2011). *Flourish: A visionary new understanding of happiness and well-being.* New York: Free Press.

Seligman, M. E. P. (2014). Chris Peterson's unfinished masterwork: The real mental illnesses. *Journal of Positive Psychology*, *10*(1), 3–6.

Seligman, M. E. P., & Csíkszentmihályi, M. (2000). Positive psychology: an introduction. *American Psychologist*, *55*(1), 5.

Seligman, M. E., Parks, A. C., & Steen, T. (2004). A balanced psychology and a full life. *Philosophical Transactions—Royal Society of London Series B: Biological Sciences*, *359*, 1379–1382.

Seligman, M. E. P., Rashid, T., & Parks, A. (2006). Positive psychotherapy. *American Psychologist*, *61*(8), 774–788.

Seligman, M. E. P., Steen, T. A., Park, N., & Peterson, C. (2005). Positive psychology progress: Empirical validation of interventions. *American Psychologist*, *60*(5), 410–421. www.psykologtidsskriftet.no/pdf/2005/874-884.pdf

Selye, H. (1955). Stress and disease. *The Laryngoscope*, *65*(7), 500–514.

Shapiro, F., & Laliotis, D. (2010). EMDR and the adaptive information processing model: Integrative treatment and case conceptualization. *Clinical Social Work Journal*, *39*(2), 191–200.

Shapiro, J. P., McCue, K., Heyman, E. N., Dey, T., & Haller, H. S. (2010). A naturalistic evaluation of psychosocial interventions for cancer patients in a community setting. *Journal of Psychosocial Oncology*, *28*(1), 23–42. doi:10.1080/07347330903438891

Sharot, T., Riccardi, A. M., Raio, C. M., & Phelps, E. A. (2007). Neural mechanisms mediating optimism bias. *Nature*, *450*(7166), 102–105. www.nature.com/nature/journal/v450/n7166/suppinfo/nature06280_S1.html

Sharpe, J. P., Martin, N. R., & Roth, K. A. (2011). Optimism and the Big Five factors of personality: Beyond neuroticism and extraversion. *Personality and Individual Differences*, *51*(8), 946–951.

Shearer, C. B. (1996). Multiple intelligences developmental assessment scales (MIDAS). United States of America: Author.

Sheldon, K. M., & Elliot, A. J. (1999). Goal striving, need-satisfaction, and longitudinal well-being: The self-concordance model. *Journal of Personality and Social Psychology*, *76*, 482–497.

Sheldon, K. M., Frederickson, B., Rathunde, K., Csíkszentmihályi, M., & Haidt, J. (2000). *Positive psychology manifesto.* www. positivepsychology.org/akumalmanifesto.htm.

Sheldon, K. M., Kashdan, T. B., & Steger, M. F. (Eds.). (2011). *Designing positive psychology: Taking stock and moving forward.* New York: Oxford University Press.

Sheldon, K. M., & King, L. (2001). Why positive psychology is necessary. *American Psychologist, 56*(3), 216.

Sheldon, K. M., & Lyubomirsky, S. (2006). How to increase and sustain positive emotion: The effects of expressing gratitude and visualizing best possible selves. *Journal of Positive Psychology, 1*(2), 73–82.

Silver, R. (2002). *Three art assessments: The Silver drawing test of cognition and emotion, draw a story, screening for depression, and stimulus drawing techniques.* New York: Psychology Press.

Silver, R. A. (2001). *Art as language: Access to thoughts and feelings through stimulus drawings.* New York: Psychology Press.

Silverstone, L. (1997). *Art therapy, the person-centred way: Art and the development of the person,* 2nd ed. London: Jessica Kingsley.

Simonton, D. K. (1990). Creativity in the later years: Optimistic prospects for achievement. *The Gerontologist, 30*(5), 626–631. doi:10.1093/geront/30.5.626

Sin, N. L., & Lyubomirsky, S. (2009). Enhancing well being and alleviating depressive symptoms with positive psychology interventions: A practice friendly meta analysis. *Journal of Clinical Psychology, 65*(5), 467–487.

Smith, E. J. (2006). The strength-based counseling model. *The Counseling Psychologist, 34*(1), 13–79.

Smith, T. W., Glazer, K., Ruiz, J. M., & Gallo, L. C. (2004). Hostility, anger, aggressiveness, and coronary heart disease: An interpersonal perspective on personality, emotion, and health. *Journal of Personality, 72*(6), 1217–1270. doi:10.1111/j.1467-64 94.2004.00296.x

Smith-Jones, E. (2014). *Strengths-based therapy: Connecting theory practice and skills.* Los Angeles, CA: Sage.

Smolarski, K., Leone, K., & Robbins, S. J. (2015). Reducing negative mood through drawing: Comparing venting, positive expression, and tracing. *Art Therapy: Journal of the American Art Therapy Association, 32*(4), 197–201. doi:10.1080/07421656.20 15.1092697

Snyder, C. (Ed.) (2000). *Handbook of hope: Theory, measures and applications.* San Diego, CA: Academic Press.

Snyder, C., & Lopez, S. (2002). *Oxford handbook of positive psychology.* New York: Oxford University Press.

Snyder, C., Ritschel, L. A., Rand, K. L., & Berg, C. J. (2006). Balancing psychological assessments: Including strengths and hope in client reports. *Journal of Clinical Psychology, 62*(1), 33–46.

Sonne, J. L. & Jochai, D. (2014), The "vicissitudes of love" between therapist and patient: A review of the research on romantic and sexual feelings, thoughts, and behaviors in psychotherapy. *Journal of Clinical Psychology, 70:* 182–195. doi:10.1002/jclp.22069

Spaniol, S. (1998). Towards an ethnographic approach to art therapy research: People with psychiatric disability as collaborators. *Art Therapy: Journal of the American Art Therapy Association, 15*(1), 29–37.

Spaniol, S. (2003). Art therapy with adults with severe mental illness. In C.A. Malchiodi (Ed.), *Handbook of art therapy* (pp. 268–281). New York: Guilford Press.

Stamm, B. H. (1997). Work-related secondary traumatic stress. *PTSD Research Quarterly, 8*(2), 1–6.

Stamm, B. H. (2002). Measuring compassion satisfaction as well as fatigue: Developmental history of the compassion satisfaction and fatigue test. In C. R. Figley (Ed.), *Treating compassion fatigue* (pp. 107–119). New York: Brunner-Routledge.

Stamm, B. H. (2010). The ProQOL Manual, 2nd ed. Pocatello, ID: ProQOL.org.

Steele, W., Malchiodi, C, & Kuban, C. (2008). Drawing as intervention with child witnesses to violence. In C. Maichiodi (Ed.), *Creative Interventions with Traumatized Children* (pp. 133–166). New York: Guilford Press.

Steger, M. F., Frazier, P., Oishi, S., & Kaler, M. (2006). The Meaning In Life Questionnaire: Assessing the presence of and search for meaning in life. *Journal of Counseling Psychology, 53*(1), 80–93. doi:10.1037/0022-0167.53.1.80

Steger, M. F., & Kashdan, T. B. (2006). Stability and specificity of meaning in life and life satisfaction over one year. *Journal of Happiness Studies, 8*(2), 161–179. doi:10.1007/s10902-006-9011-8

Steger, M. F., Sheline, K., Merriman, L., & Kashdan, T. B. (2013a). Acceptance, commitment, and meaning: Using the synergy between ACT and meaning in life research to help. In T. B. Kashdan & J. Ciarrochi (Eds.), *Cultivating well-being: Treatment innovations in positive psychology, acceptance and commitment therapy, and beyond.* Oakland, CA: New Harbinger.

Steger, M. F., Sheline, K., Merriman, L., & Kashdan, T. B. (2013b). Using the science of meaning to invigorate values-congruent, purpose-driven action. In T. B. Kashdan & J. Ciarrochi (Eds.), *Mindfulness, acceptance, and positive psychology: The seven foundations of well-being* (pp. 240–266). Oakland, CA: Context Press.

Stone, D. (2008). Wounded healing: Exploring the circle of compassion in the helping relationship. *The Humanistic Psychologist, 36*(1), 45–51. doi:10.1080/0887326070 1415587

Striker, S & Kimmel, E. (1984). *The anti-coloring book.* New York: Holt.

Stuckey, H. L., & Nobel, J. (2010). The connection between art, healing, and public health: A review of current literature. *American Journal of Public Health, 100*(2), 254.

Sullivan, H. S. (1953). *The interpersonal theory of psychiatry.* New York: Routledge.

Suls, J. Martin, R, & Wheeler, L. (2002). Social comparison: Why, with whom, and with what effect? *Current Directions in Psychological Science, 11*(5): 159–163. doi:10.1111/1467-8721.00191

Svensk, A., Öster, I., Thyme, K., Magnusson, E., Sjödin, M., Eisemann, M., . . . & Lindh, J. (2009). Art therapy improves experienced quality of life among women undergoing treatment for breast cancer: A randomized controlled study. *European Journal of Cancer Care, 18*(1), 69–77.

Swan-Foster, N. (2016). Jungian art therapy. In J. A. Rubin (Ed.), *Approaches to Art Therapy: Theory and Technique*, 3rd ed. (pp. 167–193). New York: Routledge.

Sweeney,T. (2001/2002). Merging art therapy and applied ecopsychology for enhanced therapeutic benefit. www.ecopsychology.org/journal/gatherings6/html/Overview/overview_art_therapy.html

Talwar, S. (2007). Accessing traumatic memory through art making: An art therapy trauma protocol (ATTP). *The Arts in Psychotherapy, 34*(1), 22–35.

Talwar, S. (2010). An intersectional framework for race, class, gender, and sexuality in art therapy. *Art Therapy: Journal of the American Art Therapy Association, 27*(1), 11–17.

Talwar, S., Moon, C., Timm-Bottos, J., & Kapitan, L. (2015). *Decolonizing art therapy: Social justice and new paradigms of care.* Paper presented at the 46th Annual Conference of the American Art Therapy Association, Minneapolis, MN.

Tamir, M. (2009). What do people want to feel and why? Pleasure and utility in emotion regulation. *Current Directions in Psychological Science, 18,* 101–105.

Taylor, S. E. (2011). Social support: A review. In H. S. Friedman (Ed.), *The handbook of health psychology* (pp. 189–214). New York: Oxford University Press.

Tedeschi, R. G., & Calhoun, L. G. (1996). The posttraumatic growth inventory: Measuring the positive legacy of trauma. *Journal of Traumatic Stress, 9*(3), 455-471.

Tedeschi, R. G., & Calhoun, L. G. (2004). Posttraumatic growth: Conceptual foundations and empirical evidence. *Psychological Inquiry, 15*(1), 1–18. doi:10.1207/s15327965pli1501_01

Tennen, H., & Affleck, G. (1999). Finding benefits in adversity. In C. R. Snyder (Ed.), *Coping: The psychology of what works* (pp. 279–304). New York: Oxford University Press.

Terr, L. (2008). *Unchained memories: True stories of traumatic memories lost and found.* New York: Basic Books.

Thomson, J. A. K. (1953). *The ethics of Aristotle: The Nicomachean ethics.* London: Penguin Books.

Thyme, K. E., Sundin, E. C., Wiberg, B., Öster, I., Åström, S., & Lindh, J. (2009). Individual brief art therapy can be helpful for women with breast cancer: a randomized controlled clinical study. *Palliative and Supportive Care, 7*(1), 87.

Tomasulo, D. J., & Pawelski, J. O. (2012). Happily ever after: The use of stories to promote positive interventions. *Psychology, 3*(12A), 1189–1195.

Tracy, J. L., Weidman, A. C., Cheng, J. T., & Martens, J. P. (2014). Pride: The fundamental emotion of success, power and status. In M. M. Tugade, M. N. Shiota, & L.D. Kirby (Eds.), *Handbook of positive emotions* (pp. 294–310). New York: Guildford Press.

Trauger-Querry, B., & Haghighi, K. R. (1999). Balancing the focus: Art and music therapy for pain control and symptom management in hospice care. *Hospice Journal, 14*(1), 25–38. doi:http://dx.doi.org/10.1300/J011v14n01_03

Tripp, T. (2007). A short term therapy approach to processing trauma: Art therapy and bilateral stimulation, *Art Therapy: Journal of the American Art Therapy Association, 24*(4), 176–183. doi:10.1080/07421656.2007.10129476

Trout, D. (2009). *Journal spilling: Mixed-media techniques for free expression.* Cincinnati, OH: North Light Books.

Tsang, J. A. (2006). Gratitude and prosocial behaviour: An experimental test of gratitude. *Cognition and Emotion, 20*(1), 138–148.

Turner, J. H. (2000). *On the origins of human emotions: A sociological inquiry into the evolution of human affect.* Palo Alto, CA: Stanford University Press.

Turner, Y. & Clark-Schock, K. (1990). Dynamic corporate training for women: A creative arts therapies approach. *The Arts in Psychotherapy, 17,* 217–222.

Ullen, F., de Manzano, O., Theorell, T., & Harmat, L. (2010). The physiology of effortless attention: Correlates of state flow and flow proneness. In B. Bruya (Ed.), *Effortless attention: A new perspective in the cognitive science of attention and action.* Cambridge, MA: MIT Press.

Ulman, E. (1986). Variations on a Freudian theme: Three art therapy theorists. *American Journal of Art Therapy: Journal of the American Art Therapy Association, 24*(4), 125–134.

Ulman, E. (2001). Art therapy: Problems of definition. *Art Therapy: Journal of the American Art Therapy Association, 40*(1), 16.

Ulman, E., & Dachinger, P. (1996). *Art therapy in theory and practice.* Chicago, IL: Magnolia Street Publishers.

Vaish, A., Grossmann, T., & Woodward, A. (2008). Not all emotions are created equal: The negativity bias in social-emotional development. *Psychological Bulletin, 134*(3), 383–403. doi:10.1037/0033-2909.134.3.383

Vallerand, R. J. (2008). On the psychology of passion: In search of what makes people's lives most worth living. *Canadian Psychology/Psychologie Canadienne, 49*(1), 1–13.

Vella-Broderick, D. (2009, June). *Interventions for enhancing wellbeing: The role of person-activity fit.* Workshop presented at the First World Congress on Positive Psychology, Philadephia, PA.

Vick, R. M. (2003). A brief history of art therapy. In C. A. Malchiodi (Ed.), *Handbook of art therapy* (pp. 5–15). New York: Guilford Press.

Victorson, D., Kentor, M., Maletich, C., Lawton, R. C., Kaufman, V. H., Borrero, M., . . . & Berkowitz, C. (2015). Mindfulness meditation to promote wellness and manage chronic disease: A systematic review and meta-analysis of mindfulness-based randomized controlled trials relevant to lifestyle medicine. *American Journal of Lifestyle Medicine, 9*(3), 185–211. doi:10.1177/1559827614537789

Visser, A. and Op'T Hoog, M. (2008). Education of creative art therapy to cancer patients: Evaluation and effects. *Journal of Cancer Education, 23*(2): 80–84. doi:10. 1080/08858190701821204

Voytilla, A. (2006). *Flow states during art making* (MA thesis), The School of the Art Institute of Chicago, Chicago, IL.

Wadeson, H. (1980/2010). *Art psychotherapy.* New York: Wiley.

Wadeson, H. (2002). Confronting polarization in art therapy. *Art Therapy: Journal of the American Art Therapy Association, 19*(2), 77–84.

Walker, C. J. (2010). Experiencing flow: Is doing it together better than doing it alone? *Journal of Positive Psychology, 5*(1), 3–11.

Wallas, G. (1926). *The art of thought.* London: Jonathan Cape.

Walter, J. L., & Peller, J. E. (1992). *Becoming solution-focused in brief therapy.* New York: Psychology Press/Routledge.

Watson, D. (2000). *Mood and temperament.* New York: Guilford Press.

Weiner, H. B., & Sacks, J. M. (1969). Warm-up and sum-up. *Group Psychotherapy, 22*(1–2), 85–102.

Whelton, W. J. (2004). Emotional processes in psychotherapy: Evidence across therapeutic modalities. *Clinical Psychology and Psychotherapy, 11*(1), 58–71.

White, M. & Epston, D. (1990). *Narrative means to therapeutic ends.* New York: Norton.

Whitney, D., Trosten-Bloom, A., & Rader, K. (2010). Leading positive performance: A conversation about appreciative leadership. *Performance Improvement, 49*(3), 5–10. doi:10.1002/pfi.20131

Wilkinson, R. A., & Chilton, G. (2013). Positive art therapy: Linking positive psychology to art therapy theory, practice, and research. *Art Therapy: Journal of the American Art Therapy Association, 30*(1), 4–11. doi:10.1080/07421656.2013.757513

Wilson, T. D., & Gilbert, D. T. (2003). Affective forecasting. In M. P. Zanna (Ed.), *Advances in experimental social psychology*, vol. 35 (pp. 345–411). San Diego, CA: Academic Press.

Wilson, T. D., & Gilbert, D. T. (2005). Affective forecasting: Knowing what to want. *Current Directions in Psychological Science, 14*(3), 131–134. doi:10.1111/j.0963-7214.2005.00355.x

Winkel, M., & Junge, M. (2012). *Graphic facilitation and art therapy imagery and metaphor in organizational development.* Springfield, IL: Charles C. Thomas.

Winnicott, D. (1971). *Playing and reality.* London: Tavistock/Routledge.

Wix, L. (2000). Looking for what's lost: The artistic roots of art therapy—Mary Huntoon. *Art Therapy: Journal of the American Art Therapy Association, 17*(3), 168–176. doi: 10.1080/07421656.2000.10129699

Wolin, S. J., & Wolin, S. (1993). *The resilient self: How survivors of troubled families rise above adversity.* New York: Villard.

Wong, P. T. (2011). Positive psychology 2.0: Towards a balanced interactive model of the good life. *Canadian Psychology, 52*(2), 69–81.

Wood, A. M., Froh, J. J., & Geraghty, A. W. A. (2010). Gratitude and well-being: A review and theoretical integration. *Clinical Psychology Review, 30*(7), 890–905.

Wood, A. M., Linley, P. A., Maltby, J., Kashdan, T. B., & Hurling, R. (2011). Using personal and psychological strengths leads to increases in well-being over time: A longitudinal study and the development of the strengths use questionnaire. *Personality and Individual Differences, 50*(1), 15–19.

Wood, A. M., & Tarrier, N. (2010). Positive clinical psychology: A new vision and strategy for integrated research and practice. *Clinical Psychology Review, 30*(7), 819–829. doi:http://dx.doi.org/10.1016/j.cpr.2010.06.003

Wood, J. V., Taylor, S. E., & Lichtman, R. R. (1985). Social comparison in adjustment to breast cancer. *Journal of Personality and Social Psychology, 49* (50), 1169–1183. doi:10.1037/0022-3514.49.5.1169

Wood, M. J., Molassiotis, A. and Payne, S. (2011), What research evidence is there for the use of art therapy in the management of symptoms in adults with cancer? A systematic review. *Psycho-Oncology, 20,* 135–145. doi:10.1002/pon.1722

World Health Organization, 2014. Mental Health a State of Wellbeing. www.who.int/features/factfiles/mental_health/en/

Xu, J., & Roberts, R. E. (2010). The power of positive emotions: It's a matter of life or death—Subjective well-being and longevity over 28 years in a general population. *Health Psychology, 29*(1), 9.

Yalom, I. D. (1995). *The theory and practice of group psychotherapy.* New York: Basic Books.

Young-Eisendrath, P. (2003). Response to Lazarus. *Psychological Inquiry, 14* (2), 170–172.

Zadra, J. R., & Clore, G. L. (2011). Emotion and perception: The role of affective information. *Wiley Interdisciplinary Reviews: Cognitive Science, 2*(6), 676–685. doi:10.1002/wcs.147

Zinker, J. (1977). *Creative process in gestalt therapy.* New York: Brunner/Mazel.

Index

270

Printed and bound by CPI Group (UK) Ltd, Croydon, CR0 4YY

22/10/2024

01777613-0004